Living Well with Dementia: The Importance of the Person and the Environment for Wellbeing

DR SHIBLEY RAHMAN

Queen's Scholar, BA (1st Class Honours), MA, MB, BChir, PhD (all Cambridge); MRCP(UK); Graduate Diploma in Law and LLB(Hons) (BPP Law School); LLM (with Commendation) (College of Law of England and Wales); MBA (BPP Business School); BPP Postgraduate Diploma in Legal Practice; FRSA

Forewords by
PROFESSOR JOHN R HODGES, SALLY-ANN MARCIANO AND PROFESSOR FACUNDO MANES

Radcliffe Publishing
London • New York

Radcliffe Publishing Ltd
St Mark's House
Shepherdess Walk
London N1 7LH
United Kingdom

www.radcliffehealth.com

British Library Cataloguing in Publication Data

A catalogue record for this book is available from the British Library.

ISBN-13: 978 190891 197 1

The paper used for the text pages of this book is FSC® certified. FSC (The Forest Stewardship Council®) is an international network to promote responsible management of the world's forests.

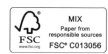

Typeset by Darkriver Design, Auckland, New Zealand
Printed and bound by TJI Digital, Padstow, Cornwall, UK

Contents

Foreword by Professor John R Hodges

It was a great honour to be asked by Shibley to write a foreword to his amazing book. I have known Shibley for over a decade, since he undertook his PhD in Cambridge in conjunction with his medical studies, and we have kept in contact since. When he told me about the book I knew that he would make a good job of it, but I had no idea of the scope and depth of scholarship until I read the draft. It is a truly unique and multifaceted contribution.

The topic of 'Wellbeing' has moved from the fringes of psychology to be central to the health agenda. This alone makes the book important but it is well known that we are entering into a potentially epidemiologically tricky phase of dementia with our ageing population, which makes the topic of wellbeing in dementia particularly poignant and relevant. Another trend is the need to consider the person suffering from dementia in the context of his or her family and society, rather than from the viewpoint of a medical model, which emphasises the disease and its treatment. Shibley has summarised the complex literature on quality of life and carer burden in dementia through wellness spectacles.

Parallel developments in the medical world have been the improvements in the early diagnosis of dementia and characterisation of subtypes, which again Shibley has dealt with expertly. Decision-making and capacity in dementia are vitally important and clinically relevant to the thrust of this book. Shibley's unique qualifications in medicine and law make him well placed to draw together these disparate strands. A look at Shibley's qualifications might lead the reader erroneously to expect the writing to be dry and academic. Nothing could be further from the truth. The whole book is infused with passion and the desire to make a difference to those living with dementia.

As well as providing a lucid overview of diverse academic topics, the book is a fantastic resource and user guide, covering topics such as communication and living well with dementia, home and ward design, assisted technology, and built environments. Shibley should be congratulated for this unique synthesis of ideas and practice. I am sure that the book will find a wide audience. I shall certainly be recommending it to professions but particularly to families living with these horrendous diseases.

Professor John R Hodges
Professor of Cognitive Neurology for Neuroscience
University of New South Wales, Sydney
Emeritus Professor of Behavioural Neurology
University of Cambridge
October 2013

Foreword by Sally-Ann Marciano

I feel a tremendous honour that I have been asked to write a foreword to Shibley's outstanding book. I am not an academic but I am a nurse, whose wonderful father died of Alzheimer's in September 2012. Nothing during my training or nursing career could have prepared me for the challenge that came with supporting my mother in my father's journey with dementia. I have never met Shibley in person, which makes being asked to write this even more special. What we do have in common, however, is real passion for raising the profile of dementia and a hope that we can – one day – improve care for all those living with dementia.

Many people with dementia will live for many years after their diagnosis, and it should be everyone's ambition in health and social care to ensure that those living with dementia do so as well as possible for all of the remaining years of their life. Diagnosis is just the start of the journey, and, with that, should come full care and support to allow those with dementia to live where they wish, and with their closest present every step of the way.

Sadly, my father's experience revealed a system where no one appeared to take direct responsibility for his care or support. He was, rather, classified as a 'social care problem', and as a result, he had to fund his own care. Even when he was dying, his care was classified as 'basic' so that he did not even qualify for funded healthcare. Our only visit was once a year from the memory nurse, and, as his condition declined, my once intelligent, articulate father, who did not even know my name towards the end, needed total care.

Dementia of the Alzheimer type destroyed his brain so badly that my father was unable to feed himself, mobilise or verbalise his needs. He became totally dependent on my mother 24/7. As the condition advanced, my father became increasingly frail, with recurrent chest infections due to aspiration from swallowing difficulties. Each time the GP would be called out, antibiotics prescribed, and so the cycle would begin again. As a nurse, I wanted to see proactive management of my father's condition. The system locally, however, was quite unable to provide this service. I feel that dementia of the Alzheimer type is a terminal condition, and, as such, should be treated like other similar conditions in care models. What we instead experienced was a 'reactive' system of care where the default option was admission to hospital into an environment where my father would quickly decline.

Dementia awareness and training among staff must be better; many staff within health and social care will come into contact with people living with dementia as part of their everyday work. That is why I am so excited about Shibley's book. It is written in a language that is easy to read, and the book will appeal to a wide readership. He has tackled many of the big topics 'head on', and put the people living with dementia and their families at the centre of his writing. You can tell this book is written by someone who 'understands' dementia; someone who has seen its joy but who has also felt the pain.

My father was cared for at home right up until he died, mostly through the sheer determination of my mother to ensure she fulfilled his wishes. Not everyone is so fortunate, and for these individuals we really need to be their champion and advocate. Everyone should be allowed to live well with dementia for however long that may be, and, with this book, we can go some way to making this a reality for all.

Sally-Ann Marciano
Project Specialist, Skills Utilisation Project
Skills for Health
October 2013

Foreword by Professor Facundo Manes

A timely diagnosis of dementia can be a gateway to appropriate care for that particular person. While historically an emphasis has been given to medication, there is no doubt that understanding the person and his or her environment is central to dementia care. Shibley's book will be of massive help to dementia researchers worldwide in my view, as well as to actual patients and their carers, and is a great example of the practical application of research. For patients with dementia, the assistance of caregivers can be necessary for many activities of daily living, such as medication management, financial matters, dressing, planning, and communication with family and friends. The majority of caregivers provide high levels of care, yet at the same time they are burdened by the loss of their loved ones. Interventions developed to offer support for caregivers to dementia patients living at home include counselling, training and education programmes, homecare/healthcare teams, respite care and information technology–based support. There is evidence to support the view that caregivers of patients with dementia especially benefit from these initiatives.

I am currently the Co-Chair of Aphasia/Cognitive Disorders Research Group of the World Federation of Neurology. In this group, we also have a specialist interest in world dementia research. 'Wellbeing' is notoriously difficult to define. Indeed, the World Health Organization (WHO, 2011) indirectly defines wellbeing through its definition of mental health:

> Mental health is defined as a state of well-being in which every individual realizes his or her own potential, can cope with the normal stresses of life, can work productively and fruitfully, and is able to make a contribution to her or his community.

Such a definition necessarily emphasises the potential contribution of a person to society. Some people who participate in research are voluntarily contributing to society. Irrespective of the importance that they assign to their own wellbeing, it is the duty and responsibility of researchers to protect participants' wellbeing and even to contribute towards it if possible. Participating in research can and should be a positive experience.

I feel that there is much 'positive energy' in dementia research around the world. Dementia research is very much a global effort, and many laboratories work in partnership both nationally and internationally, where expertise can be pooled and more progress can be made through collaborative efforts.

In England, the support and funding of world-class health research in the best possible facilities by the National Institute for Health Research, the Medical Research Council, the Economic and Social Research Council and the Research Charities is vital to the development of new and better treatments, diagnostics and care. Likewise, the 'World Brain Alliance' is working towards making the brain, its health, and its disorders the subject of a future United Nations General Assembly meeting. As part of this effort, a 'World Brain Summit' is being planned for 2014, Europe's 'Brain Year', to create a platform involving professional organisations, industry, patient groups and the public, in an effort to set a World Brain Agenda.

It is certainly appropriate to think these are exciting times, at last, for living well with dementia.

Professor Facundo Manes
Director, Institute of Neurosciences
Professor of Neurology and Cognitive Neuroscience
Favaloro University, Buenos Aires
Co-Chair, Aphasia/Cognitive Disorders Research Group
World Federation of Neurology
October 2013

REFERENCE

World Health Organization (WHO) (2011) *Mental Health: A State of Wellbeing.* Geneva: WHO, available at: www.who.int/features/factfiles/mental_health/en/

Acknowledgements

I have written this book as a tribute to the work you never seem to hear about, concerning 'living well with dementia'. I have been particularly mindful of the smaller charities who do outstanding work for this important societal issue, researchers who have been quietly getting on with seminal work here in England, and the 'unsung' individuals.

I think it was very clever of Radcliffe Publishing to realise the value of this topic of wellbeing in dementia as relevant, significant and important. There have been so many recent developments in the interdisciplinary strands of this field that an attitude for lifelong learning is an attribute necessary for embracing it. I hope that I have captured some of the excitement in this new emerging area.

I would like to say a special 'thank you' to Professor John Hodges, Sally-Ann Marciano and Professor Facundo Manes for writing the forewords to my book.

I would also like to thank Professors Felicia Huppert, Peter Lansley, Roger Orpwood, Marcus Ormerod, Andrew Sixsmith and Catherine Ward Thompson for sending to me personally recent papers from their laboratories.

My late father, before, sadly, he passed away in 2010, reckoned it was much better than to seek to 'add life to years', at a time when in fact his own wellbeing was not good. This is something that I have never forgotten. He was a very wise man.

I continue to be impressed by the wonderful commitment and enthusiasm of #dementiachallengers and people interested in innovation whom I meet on Twitter virtually daily. These include Shirley Ayres, Helen Bevan, Beth Britton, Dr Martin Brunet, Professor Alistair Burns (the National Clinical Lead for Dementia in England), Anne Cooper, Dr John Cosgrove, Simona Florio, Dr Peter Gordon, Darren Gormley, Stephen Hale, Professor Tricia Hart, Anna Hepburn, Tony Jameson-Allen ('Sporting memories'), Helen Jones, Sue Learner, Lucy Jane Masters, Dr Edana Minghella, Marian Naidoo, Rachel Niblock, Kim Pennock, Gill Phillips, Sarah Reed, Dr Karim Saad, Andrea Sutcliffe, Dr Jonathon Tomlinson, Suzy Webster and Thomas Whitelaw ('Tommy on Tour'). Of course, there are very many more. Charmaine Hardy is also a valued member of our community, with awe-inspiring pictures of the fruits of gardening (often quite literally)!

In general, I have acknowledged people in the main text, and cited the sources of extracts clearly wherever possible. I should particularly like to thank the following for being very kind in providing for me relevant copyright permissions: Beth Britton (specialist blogger on dementia issues), BMJ Publishing Group Limited (for extracts from original articles in the *British Medical Journal* and the *Journal of Medical Ethics*), Dr Martin Brunet (for extracts of articles written in the *British Medical Journal* and *Journal of Dementia Care*), Department of Health (for extracts under open license of crown copyright publications from their Government department and for extracts from the 'NHS Choices' website), Guardian News and Media Limited (for short extracts from the *Guardian* newspaper/website), Hawker Publications Limited (for an extract from *Journal of Dementia Care*), Sue Learner (for an extract from one of her articles in www.carehome.co.uk), Local Government Association, National Council for Palliative Care, Nuffield Council on Bioethics, Gill Phillips (for 'Whose Shoes' material, on behalf of Nutshell Communications Limited), and the World Health Organization (and Alzheimer's Disease International, for extracts from *Dementia: a public health priority*).

I am also especially grateful to Simona Florio and her management team, and individuals pictured themselves and their relatives, at the 'Healthy Living Club' (in Stockwell, London) for kind permission for photographs provided in Figures 7.1 and 10.1 of this book.

Finally, I sincerely hope very much I have done justice to all of these remarkable influences to my thesis.

This book is dedicated to Professor Felicia Huppert, professor of psychology and the Founding Director of the Wellbeing Institute at the University of Cambridge.

Professor Huppert's research has had a profound impact on the literature of wellbeing and positive ageing, and her varied career includes leading the consortium that has developed national indicators of wellbeing for Europe.

CHAPTER 1

Introduction

OPENING REMARKS

Living well with dementia is fundamentally about what an individual can do, rather than what he or she cannot do. For example, on an evening in March 2013, filmmakers and scientists came together at an event hosted by the University of Bristol to increase the public understanding of dementia. A series of short films about dementia, curated by local filmmaker James Murray-White, preceded a discussion with researchers from the University of Bristol and other institutions supported by 'BRACE', a local charity that funds research into Alzheimer's disease and other forms of dementia (BRACE, 2013).

At the start of this book, I begin a long journey into 'living well with dementia', but this is a journey that will only begin in English public health policy really where this book finishes. The main actors of the play are now well known. Wellbeing is more than the absence of illbeing, just as health is more than the absence of disease (Huppert, 2014, citing WHO, 1947). Huppert – only this year, 2013 – remarks, *'Yet it is remarkable how resistant large sectors of the academic, practitioner, and policy communities are to recognising the importance of positive wellbeing or of positive health'.*

This has been an incredibly challenging book to write, but also an incredibly exciting one. It is a massively complex issue, but an extremely significant one for society. Dementia in the UK is a huge issue, but so is wellbeing; any attempt to write a book on both of these issues is bound to be an ambitious task. I have been fortunate in that I have written this book completely unfunded, with no income in the form of sponsorship even. This means that I can write freely, without any conflicts of interest at all. This book does not give any medical or legal advice, and you are encouraged anyway to read this book in conjunction with other sources of useful information. You are, in particular, advised to be guided by professional lawyers and physicians for aspects of advice that require their expertise (such as capacity-related issues, pain or hydration), but I hope this book will provide an interesting and thought-provoking introduction to the ever-enlarging field of 'living well with dementia'.

THE SCALE OF THE 'CHALLENGE'

According to the Department of Health's *Improving Care for People with Dementia* (2013a), there are around 800 000 people with dementia in the UK, and the disease 'costs' the economy £23 billion a year. By 2040, the number of people affected is expected to double – and the costs are likely to treble. There is no doubt, therefore, about the scale of the societal issue, and it needs the finest minds in showing leadership on how to enable individuals with dementia to live better, and indeed to live well. **The Prime Minister's Dementia Challenge** ('Challenge') (Department of Health, 2012) sets out a renewed ambition 'to go further and faster' on substantial progress in previous policy, building on the work of the National Dementia Strategy, so that people with dementia, their carers and families essentially get the services and support that they need. This Challenge wished to address in particular certain issues, such as the observation that the number of people with dementia is increasing, that currently the diagnosis rates are thought to be relatively *low*, and that there is sadly a lack of awareness and skills needed to support people with dementia and their carers. While it is possibly difficult to find a 'miracle cure' for dementia, it is a reasonable aspiration for individuals with dementia (and their immediates) to have as best a quality of life as possible, and it is not necessarily the case that subtle but significant improvements in quality of life will *'cost the earth'*.

It is intended that this book should be *not* just of interest in the UK, as the problems in healthcare are relevant to all jurisdictions. This story will be of interest to patients, families, friends, geriatricians, psychiatrists, nurses, students, social workers, economists, lawyers, managers, leaders, journalists, public health professionals, GPs, commissioners, politicians and many more. Thinking about how society should respond inevitably does pose some jurisdiction-specific issues; for example, this book refers to legislation in the UK such as the **Equality Act** 2010 or the **Mental Capacity Act** 2005, or regulations in health and safety relevant to building design in the UK. However, a consideration of the global issues in public health leads one quickly to appreciate the complexity of the economic case for improving wellbeing in individuals in dementia and their immediates, and that there are many people who are genuinely interested.

RESPONDING TO THE 'CHALLENGE'

While indeed there has been a lead through the Prime Minister's Dementia Challenge (Department of Health, 2012), previous administrations in England have latterly decided to prioritise dementia as a public health priority (e.g. the

National Dementia Strategy, *Living Well with Dementia*, 2009). The **'ecosystem'** of interested parties is large, and it is striking that there are so many passionate '#dementiachallengers' on Twitter daily, for example, who are always a source of contemporary information, enthusiasm and innovation. There are currently huge advances being made in research and policy, and it is only possible through dementia communities 'working together' to keep abreast of them all. For that reason, this book has necessarily had to include electronic references, and I have tried to maintain links as correct and up to date at the time of publication. However, please feel free to look for any related information anywhere, and please do not use this book as an authoritative source of information to rely on necessarily. This book is intended simply as an introduction to a vibrant field, and certainly please be guided by healthcare professionals regarding individual care. The text of this book provides general principles, which I hope you might find interesting.

THE NICE QUALITY STANDARD ON 'SUPPORTING PEOPLE TO LIVE WELL WITH DEMENTIA'

The original clinical guidance by the National Institute for Health and Clinical Excellence (NICE) for dementia (**CG42**) was published as far back as 2006, and yet the importance of wellbeing in dementia is clearly seen even then. This in part has been driven by a relative lack of strong neuropharmacological interventions in early dementia of the Alzheimer type, perhaps. As recently as April 2013, NICE published its **Quality Standard 30** on **'supporting people to live well with dementia'**. This quality standard was intended to cover the care and support of people with dementia. It applies to all social care settings and services working with and caring for people with dementia.

NICE quality standards are supposed to describe high-priority areas for quality improvement in a defined care or service area. Each standard consists of a prioritised set of specific, concise and measurable statements. NICE quality standards draw on existing guidance, which provide an underpinning, comprehensive set of recommendations, and are designed to support the measurement of improvement.

The areas covered in this **'quality standard'** include:

- **Statement 1**, Chapter 12. People worried about possible dementia in themselves or someone they know can discuss their concerns, and the options of seeking a diagnosis, with someone with knowledge and expertise.
- **Statement 2**, Chapter 10. People with dementia, with the involvement of their carers, have choice and control in decisions affecting their care and support.
- **Statement 3**, Chapter 10. People with dementia participate, with the involvement of their carers, in a review of their needs and preferences when their circumstances change.

- **Statement 4**, Chapter 7. People with dementia are enabled, with the involvement of their carers, to take part in leisure activities during their day based on individual interest and choice.
- **Statement 5**, Chapter 6. People with dementia are enabled, with the involvement of their carers, to maintain and develop relationships.
- **Statement 6**, Chapter 6. People with dementia are enabled, with the involvement of their carers, to access services that help maintain their physical and mental health and wellbeing.
- **Statement 7**, Chapter 14. People with dementia live in housing that meets their specific needs.
- **Statement 8**, Chapter 13. People with dementia have opportunities, with the involvement of their carers, to participate in and influence the design, planning, evaluation and delivery of services.
- **Statement 9**, Chapter 11. People with dementia are enabled, with the involvement of their carers, to access independent advocacy services.
- **Statement 10**, Chapter 11. People with dementia are enabled, with the involvement of their carers, to maintain and develop their involvement in and contribution to their community.

OVERVIEW

The aim of this book was not to provide a prescriptive text for this quality standard, but to make occasional reference to it where appropriate. I am hoping especially that the book will be interesting to what I have called 'immediates' – by which I mean people who are close to an individual with a diagnosis of dementia, which might include a friend or relative. It is, therefore, extremely hard to find all this information 'in one place', and it is hoped that this book will help to provide a much-needed overview and to build bridges between different 'silos' of thinking.

The approach of the **national dementia strategy** *Living Well with Dementia* (Department of Health, 2009) devotes the whole of its chapter 5 to the issue of living well with dementia. In the preceding chapter in this strategy, chapter 4 on early diagnosis, the approach described is obviously inclusive:

From our consultation, and based on a successful DH pilot and the DH cost-effectiveness case, it appears that new specialist services need to be commissioned to deliver good-quality early diagnosis and intervention. Such services would need to provide a simple single focus for referrals from primary care, and would work locally to stimulate understanding of dementia and referrals to the service. They would provide an inclusive service, working for people of all ages and from all ethnic backgrounds.

A 'timely diagnosis' is only of benefit, it is felt, if there is a 'useful' intervention in dementia or appropriate support can be given in keeping with the wishes of the patient. The diagnosis has to be correct, and appropriate to the patient at that particular time. This is described in the strategy's **chapter 4** as having three essential components: (1) making the diagnosis well, (2) breaking the news of the diagnosis well to the individual with dementia and his or her immediates, and (3) providing directly appropriate treatment, information, care and support for such individuals. The present book is part of a drive to dispel the notion that *'nothing can be done'* in the context of management of dementia, even if current pharmacological therapies might have limited efficacy. This book is an overview of the field, describing what 'wellbeing' actually means, and why it is important in the context of national policy.

This book quickly establishes the importance of the 'person' in discussing dementia care, including independence, leisure and other activities, and, in the final stages, end-of-life care, which is an unavoidable discussion. No individual with dementia should be abandoned in relation to his or her environment, and, indeed, there is much evidence to support the idea that the environment can be optimised to improve the wellbeing of an individual with dementia and the people who are closest to him or her. Considerations include home and ward design, the use of assistive technologies and telecare, and the 'built environment'. A constructive interaction of an individual with his or her environment is clearly vital, and this includes understanding communication issues, how to champion the rights of an individual living well with dementia through independent advocacy, and the way in which 'dementia-friendly communities' can be supported.

CHAPTER HEADINGS

1. Introduction
2. What is 'living well'?
3. Measuring living well with dementia
4. Socio-economic arguments for promoting living well with dementia
5. A public health perspective on living well with dementia, and the debate over screening
6. The relevance of the person for living well with dementia
7. Leisure activities and living well with dementia
8. Maintaining wellbeing in end-of-life care for living well with dementia
9. Living well with specific types of dementia: a cognitive neurology perspective
10. General activities that encourage wellbeing
11. Decision-making, capacity and advocacy in living well with dementia
12. Communication and living well with dementia
13. Home and ward design to promote living well with dementia
14. Assistive technology and living well with dementia

CHAPTER SYNOPSES

It is possible to read each chapter in this book independently, and, indeed, each chapter is independently referenced. However, I feel the book makes much more sense if read from beginning to end – not at one go, obviously!

Chapter 2 is an introduction to the whole book. It introduces the concept of what is like to 'live well with dementia'. Investigating wellbeing has broadened the scope of previously overly narrow approaches to healthcare in measuring outcomes. This chapter also introduces the idea that it is grossly unfair to consider 'dementia' as a unitary diagnosis, as in fact the term is a *portmanteau* of hundreds of different conditions at least. There has been an incorrect growing trend that 'dementia' and 'memory problems' are entirely synonymous, and this has added unnecessary noise to the debate. Dementia care is currently undertaken in a number of different settings, and assisted living may be of increasing relevance in a drive to encourage individuals to live well independently with dementia.

Chapter 3 presents the formidable challenges of how 'living well' might be measured in general. There are issues about how quality of life measures change as a dementia progresses, what the relationship might be between wellbeing and physical health, and how wellbeing in dementia could be measured accurately at all.

Chapter 4 looks at the current socio-economic arguments for promoting a wellbeing approach in dementia. There are a number of converging cases for considering wellbeing, such as the economic case, the ethical case and a case based on social equality. While resources are always limited, serious considerations have to be made as to which interventions are truly cost-effective, including, of course, the assistive technologies and ambient-living innovations.

Chapter 5 presents the background for dementia as a public health issue in the UK. There is also a very active debate as to whether one should 'screen' for dementia, although the general consensus at present is that screening for dementia as a whole would be inadvisable. A core aim of the national dementia strategy *Living Well with Dementia* (Department of Health, 2009) is therefore to ensure that effective services for early diagnosis and intervention are available for all on a nationwide basis. It is argued, in this strategy, that, '*the evidence available also points strongly to the value of early diagnosis and intervention to improve quality of life and to delay or prevent unnecessary admissions into care homes.*'

Chapter 6 considers how and why being a 'person' has become so central to living well with dementia in academic and practitioner circles. In a way, the approach of 'person-centred care' is a historic one, but it has been a consistent strand of English health policy, developing into contemporaneous views of integrated and whole person care. This chapter also introduces 'personhood', and the approach of 'dementia care approach'.

Chapter 7 addresses the specific rôle of leisure activities for an individual with dementia. Leisure activities are generally considered for many to be beneficial for the mental and physical wellbeing of individuals with dementia, and there are specific problems to be addressed, such as the reported levels of relative inactivity in care homes.

Chapter 8 details how wellbeing is relevant also to end of life in dementia. This chapter considers the importance of support for carers, for the wellbeing of individuals with dementia and their carers. This chapter considers where optimal care could be given for individuals with dementia, the contribution of medication, and how it is vital to address specific issues in advanced dementia that have a direct impact on wellbeing (such as pain control). This is of course an extremely complicated professional area, with deeply rooted ethical issues, and this chapter only at best skims the surface of this huge sub-discipline from a general perspective.

Chapter 9 further elaborates the idea that it is impossible to consider dementia as a unitary diagnosis, and that specific forms of dementia can present their own formidable demands and issues. This chapter considers in detail how and why memory problems can be a presenting feature of dementia of the Alzheimer type, and the implications for interventions in wayfinding that could rationally improve wellbeing in such patients. The chapter also includes recent elegant work about the distributed neuronal networks that are hypothesised to be important in behavioural variant frontotemporal dementia, and proposes an initial view of how this 'social context network model' fundamentally affects our notion of wellbeing in such individuals.

Chapter 10 introduces 'general activities that encourage wellbeing'. Certain memories, once revived, can be particularly potent in the dementia of the Alzheimer type, and, while the 'jury is possibly out' on the experimental robustness of reminiscence therapy, the chapter discusses the possible benefits of the CIRCA project on the wellbeing of individuals with dementia. Other activities are also considered; how they may help wellbeing, such as dancing, exercise and music.

Chapter 11 takes up an important theme in living well with dementia – that is, empowering the invididual to make decisions, the law relating to capacity, and how independent advocacy services have a beneficial rôle to play. Independent dementia advocacy is a critical area of a statement in **NICE QS30**, and this chapter reviews types of advocacy (and its relevance to wellbeing and person-centred care), the current mental capacity legislation, and the crucial importance of diversity and equality in policy.

Chapter 12 explains why good communication is so crucial in the setting of individuals living well with dementia, and this is not simply restricted to healthcare professionals. This appears to be in terms of not only providing information about the condition locally but also face-to-face communication with people living well with dementia. This chapter looks in detail at both verbal and non-verbal methods of communication, with a view to raising awareness of their impact on living well with dementia.

Chapter 13 analyses the importance of home and ward design for improving wellbeing in dementia. 'Therapeutic design' is a central philosophy of good design, and this chapter has as its focus a number of different settings. This is a philosophy that has been warmly embraced by a number of different stakeholders, ranging from the King's Fund to the Royal Institute of British Architects, the professional body for architects in this jurisdiction. General principles for the improvement of wellbeing through careful design of certain parts of the house (such as balconies, bathrooms, bedrooms, living rooms and dining rooms) are described, and this chapter considers some basic neuroscience of sensory considerations at play (e.g. in lighting and vision, and sound and hearing.)

Chapter 14 is the *first* of two chapters on 'assistive technologies' in dementia, providing an overview of this important area for living well with dementia. This chapter explains what 'assistive technology' is, what its potential limitations are, the INDEPENDENT project, the importance of 'telehealth' (and important ethical considerations), and the design of 'smart homes'.

Chapter 15 is the *second* of two chapters on 'assistive technologies' in dementia, looking specifically at an approach called 'ambient assisted living' (AAL). The rationale behind the use of AAL in improving wellbeing is explained, as well as the general issue of how to encourage adoption of innovations in an older population. Detailed examples of specific AAL projects in improving wellbeing are described, including SOPRANO, COACH and NOCTURNAL.

Chapter 16 introduces the general emphasis on the 'built environment' setting, and how inclusivity still drives this area of work in living well with dementia. Ageing presents its own challenges, including opportunities and threats, but this chapter focuses on the remarkable initiatives that have recently taken place in improving the outside environment for individuals with dementia. The chapter details the I'DGO project, and highlights the especial importance of inclusive design for furthering wellbeing in dementia outside environments. The chapter concludes with an evolving theme in the research that the quality of wellbeing of an individual with dementia is a highly personal affair. It is very much dependent on that person's unique interaction with his or her environment.

Chapter 17 considers how an individual with dementia lives as part of the rest of a community and society, and policy initiatives that have sought to address this. The discussion is unexpectedly problematic about a need to define what a 'community' might be, but the chapter includes domestic and international approaches to the 'dementia-friendly community', including the RSA's 'Connected Communities' and the World Health Organization's 'age-friendly communities' initiatives.

As a central policy plank that is thought to be critical for developing wellbeing in individuals with dementia and their immediates, this chapter considers why dementia-friendly communities are worth encouraging at all, why there is a societal need to involve individuals with dementia in their communities, what aspects individuals with dementia wish from such communities (including the 'Four Cornerstones' model), and the benefits of 'resilient communities'.

Chapter 18 completes my thesis. It concludes with a review of some of the themes that emerge in this book, but puts especial focus on the language of the debate regarding 'prompt diagnosis' or 'timely diagnosis' and tries to put current policy on living well with dementia into a realistic and achievable perspective.

FURTHER INFORMATION

You are advised to look at specialty websites that are devoted to all the dementias (such as medical charities), which often have useful information fact sheets and booklets.

Also, the Department of Health and their 'Dementia Challenge' website is an impressive source of information (2013b). You are also advised to consult the National Health Service (NHS) website (www.evidence.nhs.uk), which has access to a number of useful contemporaneous clinical evidence sources. Online medical journals are also an excellent source of peer-reviewed research, such as the *BMJ*, the *Lancet*, and the *New England Journal of Medicine*. You are also strongly recommended to become familiar with the output of the King's Fund, the Royal College of Physicians and the Royal College of Psychiatrists, which have all produced interesting contributions in this field.

In the references, I have decided to include some **electronic references**, but only where I feel this would really help, given the problems that these links may become dead 'in due course'. All links are to citations that were accessible on the internet at the time of submission of the manuscript, on 1 August 2013. I apologise if you are unable to find links as updated, although it might be worth using a search engine to discover whether links have been relocated. They are, by and large, important documents that are unlikely to be taken 'off' the internet.

LOOKING TO THE FUTURE

There are, of course, no '*right answers*' to many issues, and a wise person is a person who knows where to find relevant information. However, the sense of optimism and goodwill is a genuine one in UK health policy, regarding dementia. While there will often be difficult debates regarding dementia – such as 'How willing should a GP be to make a diagnosis of dementia when a patient has only gone to see his GP because of a sore throat?' or 'Should we look to research a drug that can immunise people against dementia?' – the fact there are so many bright people in the UK working in areas relating to dementia is a real credit to English health policy, as it faces formidable challenges of its own.

Developments in neuroscience and cognitive neurology have helped to shape this policy, but also there are formidable converging strands of thinking in social care, bioengineering, general medicine, economics, social and cognitive psychology and innovation management, to name but a few. The impact of the English law – for example, in equality and mental capacity – cannot be underestimated either, and helps to see some of the policy elements as enforceable rights rather than well-meant aspirations. Understanding how elements of this jigsaw all produce a coherent picture of living well in dementia is certainly challenging, but undeniably rewarding.

Dr Shibley Rahman
Queen's Scholar, BA (1st Class Honours),
MA, MB, BChir, PhD (all Cambridge); MRCP(UK);
Graduate Diploma in Law and LLB(Hons) (BPP Law School);
LLM (with commendation) (College of Law of England
and Wales); MBA (BPP Business School); BPP Postgraduate
Diploma in Legal Practice; FRSA
October 2013

REFERENCES

BRACE (2013) *An Evening of Short Films about Dementia*, available at: www.alzheimers-brace.org/events/evening-short-films-about-dementia

Department of Health (2009) *Living Well with Dementia: A National Dementia Strategy; Putting people first.* London: The Stationery Office, available at: www.gov.uk/government/uploads/system/uploads/attachment_data/file/168220/dh_094051.pdf

Department of Health (2012) *The Prime Minister's 'Dementia Challenge': Delivering Major Improvements in Dementia Care and Research by 2015.* London: The Stationery Office, available at: www.gov.uk/government/policies/improving-care-for-people-with-dementia

Department of Health (2013a) *Improving Care for People with Dementia.* London: The Stationery Office, available at: www.gov.uk/government/policies/improving-care-for-people-with-dementia

Department of Health (2013b) *The Dementia Challenge.* London: The Stationery Office, available at: dementiachallenge.dh.gov.uk

Huppert, F. (2014) The state of well-being science: concepts, measures, interventions and policies. In: Huppert, F.A., and Cooper, C.L. (eds) *Interventions and Policies to Enhance Wellbeing*, vol. 6. Oxford: Wiley-Blackwell. pp. 1–49.

National Institute for Health and Clinical Excellence (NICE) and Social Care Institute for

Excellence (2006) *CG42: Dementia.* A NICE–SCIE Guideline on supporting people with dementia and their carers in health and social care, available at: www.nice.org.uk/CG42

National Institute for Health and Care Excellence (NICE) (2013) *Supporting People to Live Well with Dementia (QS30)*, available at: http://guidance.nice.org.uk/QS30

UK Government. *Mental Capacity Act* 2005, available at: www.legislation.gov.uk/ukpga/2005/9/contents

UK Government. *Equality Act 2010*, available at: www.legislation.gov.uk/ukpga/2010/15/contents

World Health Organization (WHO) (1947) *The Constitution of the World Health Organization.* Geneva: WHO.

CHAPTER 2

What is 'living well'?

The most elder-rich period of human history is upon us. How we regard and make use of this windfall of elders will define the world in which we live.

> W H Thomas, *What are Old People For?*
> *How Elders Will Save the World*

Before contemplating approaches to **'living well with dementia'**, and how you could even measure it, we need to have an understanding of what **'wellbeing'** might be, and why it is currently considered important in public health policy circles and beyond.

DEFINITION OF WELLBEING

There has been a shift in thinking to appreciate that 'happiness', 'wellbeing' and 'contentment' may be valid outcomes for measuring how healthy an individual or society is (e.g. report by Mark Easton on the BBC website from 2006).

The first thing, in analysing this issue critically, to think about is: what does it *actually mean to live well – in other words, wellbeing?*

Historically, Jahoda (1958) is usually regarded as the first person to have promoted the idea of positive mental health, which she defined in terms of six elements of positive functioning: (1) 'attitudes of an individual towards his own self', (2) 'self-actualisation', (3) 'integration', (4) 'autonomy', (5) 'perception of reality' and (6) 'environmental mastery'.

Huppert, Baylis and Keverne (2004), for their Royal Society meeting in 2004, further proposed a definition of **'wellbeing'** as follows:

For the purposes of the Discussion Meeting, we defined wellbeing in broad terms as 'a positive and sustainable state that allows individuals, groups or nations to thrive and flourish'.

This means that at the level of an individual, wellbeing refers to psychological, physical and social states that are distinctively positive. Positive psychological states are exemplified by emotions such as happiness and contentment, attitudes such as generosity and empathy, and mental processes such as cognitive capabilities, interest and motivation. Positive physical states are characterized [*sic*] by vitality and physical capabilities, while positive social states include satisfying social bonds and loving relationships. Our definition of wellbeing also encompasses human resilience – the ability to survive and thrive in the face of the setbacks inherent in the process of living.

Wellbeing can be used to describe an objective state as well as a subjective experience. **Objective** wellbeing refers to wellbeing at the societal level; the objective facts of people's lives, in contrast to **subjective** wellbeing, which concerns how people actually experience their lives.

WELLBEING AS A GOAL

Wellbeing has become an important goal in itself, both here and in the United States among many other jurisdictions.

Wellbeing is truly a concept that crosses over a number of different subject disciplines, and for many there are common attractions in using it as a national policy goal. Quoted by Juliet Michaelson (2012) of the New Economics Foundation's Centre for Well-being, the head of the central bank of the United States, Federal Reserve chair Ben Bernanke, offered:

'The ultimate purpose of economics, of course, is to understand and promote the enhancement of wellbeing. Economic measurement accordingly must encompass measures of wellbeing and its determinants.'

There are currently at least **four** good key reasons at least for a focus on wellbeing:

1. *Wellbeing indicators directly capture information about human lives.* **There is now substantial evidence showing that we may be able robustly to measure how people 'feel' about their lives, using indicators that converge with a whole range of other types of data. This is explored further in Chapter 3. These have also been shown to predict future behaviour.**
2. *Measuring wellbeing broadens the scope of an overly narrow politics.* It is widely argued that politicians have become so used to their success or failure being judged according to the headline measure of economic growth that their scope of action (the gross domestic product) has become rather

narrow. This may indeed have contributed to apathy and disenfranchisement with the contemporaneous 'political process'.

3. *People support wellbeing as a goal for governments as well as themselves.* There has long been evidence that people think wellbeing is an important goal for governments to pursue. For example, a BBC poll of 1996 found that 81% of people in the UK supported the idea that government's prime objective should be the 'greatest happiness' rather than the 'greatest wealth'.

4. *Measuring wellbeing is a fundamentally democratic approach.* Directly measuring how people feel about their lives avoids the need for others making decisions about what is important to them: this is the much respected *'no decision about me without me'* approach. In principle, then, this brings people's voices into the heart of policy.

According to Norton, Matthews and Brayne (2013), population ageing over the first half of this century is likely to lead to dramatic increases in the prevalence of dementia. This will affect all regions of the world, but also (it is said) particularly developing regions. Dementia projections have been used extensively to support policy. It is therefore important these projections are as accurate as possible. By the middle of this century, around 1 in 5 of the estimated 9 billion world population are expected to be aged over 60 years, compared with around 1 in 10 in the year 2000 (United Nations, 2004).

Furthermore, according to Luengo-Fernandez, Leal and Gray (2011), dementia was estimated to cost the European Union €189 billion in 2007. Sixty-eight per cent of total costs were due to informal care, 26% to social care, 5% to healthcare and 1% to 'productivity losses'. Therefore, dementia has posed a significant economic burden to European health and social care systems, and society overall, and it is extremely likely that it will continue to do so. The EURODEM consortium found that among European studies, using similar methodologies and diagnostic criteria, there were only trivial differences in the age-specific prevalence of dementia (twelve studies) and **dementia of the Alzheimer type (DAT)** (six centres), concluding that ecological comparisons were unlikely to be informative about aetiology (Rocca *et al.*, 1991).

WHAT IS DEMENTIA?

One of the biggest misconceptions is that 'dementia' is a unitary condition.

'Dementia' is a term that covers a number of different conditions, different causes and different presentations. Therefore, it can have an extremely variable timecourse.

Some forms are reversible, while others are not. A dementia can be part of a wider general illness, or it might not be. Telling the difference between these types, in making a diagnosis of dementia at all, is clearly going to be important and should be done in competent hands. One cannot underestimate the tragedy of advising someone that they have dementia, when he or she does not, as that person's life will be thrown upside down. Likewise, knowing a correct diagnosis of dementia can allow individuals and their nearest to make realistic plans for the future.

Indeed, some people estimate that there are hundreds of different types of dementia. Descriptions of all these types of dementias are contained in specialist textbooks on dementia, and are clearly outside of the scope of this particular text.

While in other illnesses there may be simple association between health-related quality of life and an easily measurable clinical variable, in dementia this is not so (Banerjee *et al.*, 2008). Dementia is one of the most common and serious conditions, not exclusively confined to later life. Most cases are sporadic, but a few run in families. It can cause ultimately an irreversible decline in global intellectual and physical functioning, and it has a significant personal, social, health and economic impact on people with dementia, their family carers, and health and social services. This has been a pervasive concept in all national documents about dementia policy.

Overall, the term 'dementia' describes a set of symptoms that include loss of memory, mood changes, and problems with communication and reasoning. Dementia is progressive, which means the symptoms will gradually get worse. How fast dementia progresses will depend on the individual person, and what type of dementia he or she has. Each person is unique, and each person will experience dementia in his or her own way. It is often the case that the person's family and friends are more concerned about the symptoms than the person may be him- or herself, and this will particularly be the case if an individual with dementia lacks insight. There is considerable heterogeneity within diagnostic groups as well as between diagnostic groups in the course of illness and abnormalities in behaviour, insight, judgement and symptoms such as psychosis, anxiety and depression. Given this complexity, there has been discussion about how best to measure the impact of dementia on individuals and the effects of interventions.

Broadly speaking, symptoms of dementia may include the following:

- **Loss of memory** – this particularly affects short-term memory; for example, forgetting what happened earlier in the day, not being able to recall conversations, being repetitive or forgetting the way home from the shops. Long-term memory is usually still quite good. Often it is said that an individual with Alzheimer's disease will remember very clearly what happened 30 or 40 years ago, but will have genuine trouble in remembering what he or she had for breakfast.
- **Mood changes** – people with dementia may be withdrawn, sad, frightened or angry about what is happening to them.
- **Communication problems** – including problems finding the right words for things (e.g. describing the function of an item instead of naming it).

Communication issues are in fact discussed in greater detail in **Chapter 12** of this book.

- **Personality and behavioural change** – this can be quite slow and subtle, and very often not noticed by the patient him- or herself, but noticed by an immediate such as family member. This can be a prominent feature of some particular types of dementia, such as the behavioural variant of frontotemporal dementia.

In the later stages of dementia, the person affected will have problems carrying out everyday tasks and will become increasingly dependent on other people.

There are several *common* diseases and conditions that result in dementia. These include:

- *Dementia of the Alzheimer type.* This is most common cause of dementia among the older age groups. During the course of the disease the chemistry and structure of the brain change, leading to the death of brain cells. Problems of short-term memory are usually the first noticeable sign, reflecting pathology initially in the hippocampal formation, in the temporal lobe, by the ear. Spatial navigation can be a particular problem, and this is described in detail in **Chapter 9**.
- *Post-stroke (vascular) dementia.* If the oxygen supply to the brain fails due to vascular disease, or blood vessels burst into the brain, brain cells are likely to suffer some form of damage, causing the symptoms of vascular dementia. These symptoms can occur either suddenly, following a stroke, or over time through a series of small strokes. Such strokes can happen anywhere in the brain, and an experienced neurologist may be able to tell where the stroke has occurred from the presenting features, even before he or she has access to a high-quality brain scan.
- *Dementia with Lewy bodies.* This form of dementia gets its name from tiny abnormal structures that develop inside nerve cells. Their presence in the brain leads to the degeneration of brain tissue. Symptoms can include disorientation and hallucinations, as well as problems with planning, reasoning and problem-solving. Memory may be affected to a lesser degree. This form of dementia shares some characteristics with Parkinson's disease. As patients with the dementia with Lewy bodies can react very badly to some medications, it is clearly essential for a medical doctor to be able to diagnose the condition accurately. The relevance of this accurate diagnosis, in relation to home and ward design, is described in **Chapter 13**.
- *Frontotemporal dementia.* In frontotemporal dementia, damage is usually focused in the front part of the brain. At first, personality and behaviour changes are the most obvious signs. The clinical syndromes of frontotemporal lobar degeneration include behavioural variant frontotemporal dementia (bvFTD) and semantic and non-fluent variants of primary progressive aphasia. A concern here is that individuals with bvFTD may have

a profound change in personality and behaviour, noticed by partners, relatives or friends, unknown to the patient him- or herself, with the general absence of impairment in general conventional IQ domains. Patients with bvFTD might have specific cognitive deficits, however, in decision-making behaviour. This problem of effective social interactions is described in detail in **Chapter 9**.

There is a suggestion from a French study using one of the well-known measurement instruments (Thomas *et al.*, 2006) that people with Lewy body dementia may have lower 'health-related quality of life' scores than people with DAT or mixed dementia. This might possibly reflect the impact of the hallucinations and other symptoms that are part of Lewy body dementia but are not necessarily found in DAT.

There are **many other rarer causes** that may lead to dementia, including progressive supranuclear palsy, metabolic conditions (such as Wilson's disease or neuroferritinopathy) Korsakoff's syndrome, Binswanger's disease, HIV/AIDS and Creutzfeldt–Jakob disease. Some people with multiple sclerosis, motor neurone disease, Parkinson's disease and Huntington's disease may also develop dementia as a result of the natural course of their diseases.

In the alternative, some individuals may have noticed problems with their memory, but a medical doctor may feel that the symptoms are not severe enough to warrant a diagnosis of DAT or another type of dementia, particularly if a person is still managing well. When this occurs, some doctors will use the term 'mild cognitive impairment' (MCI). Recent research has shown that individuals with MCI have an increased risk of developing dementia. The conversion rate from MCI to dementia of the Alzheimer type is 10%–20% each year, so a diagnosis of MCI does not always mean that the person will go on to develop dementia.

THE IMPORTANCE OF THE ENVIRONMENT FOR WELLBEING

It can be too tempting to see 'dementia' as a disease, and not to get to know the person behind a label. The notion of *'what is a person?'* is first introduced in **Chapter 6**, and continues to be a major influence in English health policy on dementia. There has been much discussion of the contributing factors to an individual's wellbeing. It is clear the environment, while not the only factor, is a prominent consideration.

A relatively recent report from the **MRC Institute for Environment and Health** summarised the situation thus, as per Green (2000).

The socio-economic model of health (adopted by the Independent Enquiry into Inequalities in Health) focuses on the main determinants of health and wellbeing as layers of influence.

These layers include fixed constitutional factors (e.g. age), lifestyle behaviours (e.g. smoking habit) and social and community influences (e.g. family, local community). Broader aspects such as living and working conditions and access to services are, in turn, bounded by the overall economic, cultural and environmental conditions of a society as a whole. Importantly, the model emphasises the interaction between these layers of influence. For example, individual life-styles are embedded in social networks and in living and working conditions, which, in turn, are related to the wider socio-economic environment.

THE IMPACT OF WELLBEING IN DEMENTIA: UK HEALTH POLICY

Dementia is now a central part of English health policy.

In the *Report of the National Audit of Dementia Care in General Hospitals* (Royal College of Psychiatrists, 2011), it is cited that an appropriate 'ward action plan' might be to 'celebrate good practice – reinforcing how the positives impact on patients' wellbeing'. Indeed, Professor Alistair Burns, the National Clinical Lead for Dementia (at the time of writing) and Professor Philippe Robert (2009), wrote that, *'The benefits of early diagnosis and intervention are highlighted – for economic reasons and for individual wellbeing.'*

However, the impression unfortunately has evolved that there is too little joined-up working between health and social care services for people with dementia, a situation echoed by Professor Carol Brayne, Director of the Cambridge Institute of Public Health on the University of Cambridge website in 2012:

What patients and families tell us is that there are problems with fragmentation of care for dementia, with not enough information about what's available and what pattern of services works best.

Larson and Langa (2008) helpfully reviewed new findings from a paper that had just been published in the *Lancet* (Llibre Rodriguez *et al.* (2008), for the '10/66 Dementia Research Group'). They wrote:

The rising tide of late-life dementia is both a triumph of public health and an opportunity. Increased worldwide prevalence reflects gains in life expectancy, perhaps made more evident in present knowledge-based societies. Cognitive skills are probably more essential for survival and sustain wellbeing better in cities, where people are increasingly concentrated. Because the rates rise considerably in late old age, delaying the onset of functional impairment would represent true prevention or at least compression of morbidity.

We are now, arguably, living in a 'technological explosion', and this is bound to have an impact upon how individuals with dementia and their families are included in the development of UK policy. For example, in Scotland, the Dementia Managed Knowledge Network ('Dementia MKN') is a growing virtual network of people interested in improving the care, support and quality of life of people with dementia. Within the network, there are a number of 'Communities of Practice' focusing on dementia. The Dementia MKN thus provides an opportunity for health and social services staff to share knowledge and experience, and support one another in the shared goal to promote excellence in dementia support and care. On a positive note, this technological explosion might pave the way for more effective social inclusion.

In the UK, the remarkable **'dementia-friendly communities'** initiatives focus on improving the inclusion and wellbeing of people with dementia. This is part of a wider, successful global initiative. In such communities, people will be aware of and understand more about dementia; people with dementia and people who know them the closest will be encouraged to seek help and support; and people with dementia will not only feel included in their community but also perceive themselves as more independent, and have more choice and control over their lives.

It is envisaged that a 'dementia-friendly community' is one that shows a high level of public awareness and understanding so that people with dementia and their carers are supported by their community. Many villages, towns and cities in England are already taking steps towards becoming, or have an ambition to become, 'dementia friendly'. However, it is acknowledged that realising dementia-friendly communities will take a number of years. Through the programme, an aim is to give public recognition and support to villages, towns, cities and national organisations taking steps towards being more inclusive of people with dementia. These communities are considered in detail in **Chapter 17**.

THE 'PRIME MINISTER'S DEMENTIA CHALLENGE'

According to Professor Sube Banerjee (2010), *'Strategy and policy evolves and, as the evidence base has grown, so the last decade has seen a growing acknowledgement and understanding of the challenge posed by dementia and the need for service improvement.'*

Banerjee cites *Forget Me Not: Mental Health Services for Older People* (Audit Commission, 2000), as a starting point. Key findings of that included:

- only a half of GPs believed it important to look actively for signs of dementia and to make an early diagnosis
- less than half of GPs felt that they had received sufficient training in how to diagnose dementia
- a lack of clear information, counselling, advocacy and support for people with dementia and their family carers

- an insufficient supply of specialist home care
- poor-quality assessment and treatment, with little joint health and social care planning and working.

All of these are, of course, extremely important points.

Following the launch of *Living Well with Dementia: A National Dementia Strategy* (Department of Health, 2009) in England and the development of similar plans elsewhere in the UK, there has been an increasing focus on the needs of people with dementia. Clearly, this is significant, as other chronic illnesses and diseases will also need resources with a finite source of funding for the NHS.

BOX 2.1 Key features of the Prime Minister's Dementia Challenge (Department of Health, 2012)

Driving improvements in health and care
- Increased diagnosis rates through regular checks for over-65s
- Financial rewards for hospitals offering quality dementia care
- An Innovation Challenge Prize of £1m
- A Dementia Care and Support Compact signed by leading care home and home care providers
- Promoting local information on dementia services

Creating dementia-friendly communities that understand how to help
- Dementia-friendly communities across the country
- Support from leading businesses for the Prime Minister's Challenge
- Awareness-raising campaign
- A major event, bringing together UK leaders from industry, academia and the public sector

Better research
- More than doubling overall funding for dementia research to over £66m by 2015
- Major investment in brain scanning
- £13m funding for social science research on dementia (the National Institute for Health Research (NIHR) and the Economic and Social Research Council)
- £36m funding over 5 years for a new NIHR dementia translational research collaboration to pull discoveries into real benefits for patients; four new NIHR biomedical research units in dementia and biomedical research centres that include dementia-themed research will share their considerable resources and world-leading expertise to improve treatment and care
- Participation in high-quality research

The key features of the Prime Minister's Dementia Challenge ('Challenge') are shown in Box 2.1.

The Challenge was launched in March 2012 by UK prime minister David Cameron to tackle one of the most important issues we face as the population ages. The Challenge is undoubtedly an ambitious programme of work designed to make a real difference to the lives of people with dementia and their families and carers.

The Dementia Challenge in particular wished to approach the following issues:

- the number of people with dementia is *increasing*
- the diagnosis rates are *low*
- there is a *lack of awareness and skills* needed to support people with dementia and their carers.

The Challenge on dementia therefore set out a renewed ambition to pursue dementia policy, building on progress made through the National Dementia Strategy, so that people with dementia, their carers and families get the services and support they need.

Likewise, wellbeing has become firmly footed in the NHS nursing strategy. A critical policy priority has been to prioritise both health and wellbeing, reflected in the **Care Bill** 2013 and **Health and Social Care Act** 2012, helping people to stay independent. It is also advised that nurses should contribute to dementia-friendly communities that understand how to help, and help to lead, deliver and evaluate care nearer home.

A QUESTION OF LANGUAGE: 'PROMPT', 'EARLY' OR 'TIMELY'?

According to the Dementia Challenge, prompt diagnosis is a genuine policy problem.

Currently only 42% of people with dementia in England have a formal diagnosis. The diagnosis rate varies – from 27% in the worst-performing areas to 59% in the best. Too often, diagnosis comes too late – during a crisis or beyond the point where people can plan for the future and make informed choices about how they would like to be cared for. This is not good enough.

Surveys show us that people with dementia would like early diagnosis., and we know that with early intervention, and access to the right services and support, people with dementia can continue to live well for many years.

The people most at risk of developing dementia (the over-75s) see their GP at least once, if not several times, a year. Around 97% of people aged over 75 go to their GP surgery at least once a year, and around 87% at least once every six months.

It is likely that there is going to be greater scrutiny of what type of dementia diagnosis exactly is being provided in primary care, such as 'prompt', 'early' or 'timely', and beyond in the NHS. This debate, to be discussed further in **Chapter 5** and in **Chapter 18**, needs to be handled extremely responsibly by senior policymakers, as any economic perverse incentives for early diagnosis, especially from non-clinicians, might have the disastrous unintended consequence of driving up rates of misdiagnosis too. It is vital that this discussion is open, transparent and strongly footed in accurate evidence. Any underactive thyroid, misdiagnosed as DAT, would, of course, be a disaster for all concerned. This is a hugely important topic, with a realisation currently in public health circles that the media (and entities with a potential commercial stake in the progression of English dementia policy) have a responsible part to play in avoiding a culture of **'moral panic'**.

THE OPTIMISATION OF THE ENVIRONMENT

Traditional analysis of the environment has looked at the impact of common factors in the environment, such as air quality or water quality, on general health and wellbeing. However, there has been a growing appreciation in the literature that the local environment of an individual with dementia may be particularly relevant to his or her wellbeing.

For example, Day, Carreon and Stump (2000) in the *Gerontologist* journal reviewed the empirical research on design and dementia, including research concerning facility planning (relocation, respite and day care, special care units, group size), research on environmental attributes (non-institutional character, sensory stimulation, lighting, safety), studies concerning building organisation (orientation, outdoor space), and research on specific rooms and activity spaces (bathrooms, toilet rooms, dining rooms, kitchens and resident rooms). The authors indeed concluded, *'For greatest impact, design professionals and researchers must continue to educate administrators and families on the potential role of environmental design for improving quality of life in a comprehensive way. These recommendations, if implemented, will ensure continued progress in the study and design of therapeutic environments for people with dementia.'*

WARD ENVIRONMENTS

With people aged 65 and over making up the largest number of households in the future, the importance of ensuring that all types of housing provide a flexible, adaptable living environment to meet people's changing needs throughout the life-course is apparent. Future-proofing of all housing would give people more housing choice and less likelihood of having to face disruptive adaptations or unwanted moves when circumstances change. For housing to be both inclusive and dementia friendly, they also need to address sensory and other neurocognitive challenges. In terms of making neighbourhoods more dementia friendly, much can be done at the design level. Indeed, the design of the environment can make a big difference to the level of independence and ability to use and find their way around the neighbourhood of people with dementia.

Importantly, in 'Streets for Life' (Mitchell and Burton, 2006), the authors identified six principles of **'dementia-friendly environments'**: (1) familiarity, (2) legibility, (3) distinctiveness, (4) accessibility, (5) safety and (6) comfort. This is not too dissimilar to the formulation of such environments by Kerr (1997), who states that for people with learning disabilities and dementia, it is important to think about the environment in terms of the environment being calm and stress-free, predictable and easy to understand, familiar, suitably stimulating and safe.

The tragedy of poor design is well known to many (e.g. Cohen-Mansfielda *et al.*, 2010). Nursing home residents with dementia most often spend their time without any activity and with minimum stimulation, which can magnify the apathy, boredom, depression, loneliness and behaviour problems that often accompany the progression of dementia. Interventions that involve objects or tasks with meaning specific to the person with dementia will be more likely to engage that person.

According to the Royal College of Physicians of London (RCP, 2012), the demand on clinical services is increasing to the point where acute care cannot arguably keep pace. This is according to the *Hospitals on the Edge? The Time for Action* report. This quite hard-hitting report highlights that there are a third fewer general and acute beds now than there were 25 years ago (Imison, Poteliakhoff, and Thompson, 2012), yet the last decade alone has seen a 37% increase in emergency admissions. This is coupled with a change in patients' needs. Nearly two-thirds (65%) of people admitted to hospital are over 65 years old (Cornwell *et al.*, 2012), and an increasing number are frail or have a diagnosis of dementia. However, all too often hospital buildings, services and staff are not equipped to deal with those with multiple, complex needs including dementia.

Hospital stays in particular are recognised to have detrimental effects on some people with dementia. Yet the evidence from the King's Fund **'Enhancing the Healing Environment' programme** is that relatively straightforward and inexpensive changes to the design and fabric of the care environment can have a considerable impact on the wellbeing of people with dementia, as well as improving staff morale and reducing overall costs. However, the *Report of the National Audit of Dementia Care in General Hospitals* (Royal College of Psychiatrists, 2011) suggested that most hospitals had yet to implement such changes. These design principles are offered as practical resource to help healthcare organisations develop dementia-friendly healthcare environments.

ASSISTIVE TECHNOLOGY

Assistive technology (AT) can be defined as

> an umbrella term for any device or system that allows an individual to perform a task they would otherwise be unable to do or increases the ease and safety with which the task can be performed (Cowan and Turner-Smith, 1999).

An alternative definition, which emphasises the rôle of AT in maximising the independence of older people, is:

> *AT is any product or service designed to enable independence for disabled and older people* (The King's Fund, 2001 – *see* website references).

The technologies embraced by these definitions include devices that might form part of 'telecare' and 'telehealth' service packages (that is, assistance devices linked to response teams via a person's telephone, such as community alarm services, detectors or monitors of fire, gas or falls). The definitions also embrace a range of technologies from low-level to high-tech devices, however. These may also include more general technologies (such as access to the internet) that might have a rôle in promoting the independence and wellbeing of older people.

Such technologies clearly require more analysis, and they raise important ethical issues about empowering patients at the risk of potentially making them more 'socially excluded', definitely an 'unintended consequence'. ATs, including ambient assisted living, are discussed in **Chapters 14 and 15**, in particular in relation to what might constitute a 'successful innovation' for an individual with dementia.

WHERE TO NEXT?

The next chapter considers that, if you think observing wellbeing is a worthwhile activity, how should wellbeing be measured?

WEBSITES

- 'Dementia MKN website' can be accessed on the Scottish NHS site: www. knowledge.scot.nhs.uk/dementia.aspx
- 'Enhancing the Healing Environment', an initiative from the King's Fund: www.enhancingthehealingenvironment.org.uk

REFERENCES

Audit Commission (2000) *Forget Me Not: Mental Health Services for Older People.* Abingdon, Oxon; Audit Commission Publications, available at: archive.audit-commission.gov.uk/auditcommission/nationalstudies/health/mentalhealth/pages/forgetmenot.aspx.html

Banerjee, S. (2009) *The Use of Antipsychotic Medication for People with Dementia: Time for Action; A report for the Minister of State for Care Services.* London; Department of Health.

Banerjee, S. (2010) Living well with dementia: development of the National Dementia Strategy for England. *Int J Geriatr Psychiatry,* **25**(9), pp. 917–22.

Banerjee, S., Samsi, K., Petrie, C.D., *et al.* (2008) What do we know about quality of life in dementia? A review of the emerging evidence on the predictive and explanatory value of disease specific measures of health related quality of life in people with dementia. *Int J Geriatr Psychiatry,* **24**(1), pp. 15–24.

Brayne, C. (2012) 'Rooted in evidence: a public health perspective to dementia', available at: www.cam.ac.uk/research/news/rooted-in-evidence-a-public-health-response-to-dementia.

Brayne, C., Bayer, A., Boustani, M., *et al.* (2013). Rapid response to 'There is no evidence base for proposed dementia screening' (27 February 2013): 'A rallying call for an evidence based approach to dementia and related policy development', available at: www.bmj.com/content/345/bmj.e8588/rr/633370

Burns, A., and Robert, P. (2009) The National Dementia Strategy in England: a 'smorgasbord' of evidence, economics, and obligation, *BMJ,* **338**: b931.

Cohen-Mansfielda, J., Theina, K., Dakheel-Alia, M., *et al.* (2010) The underlying meaning of stimuli: Impact on engagement of persons with dementia, *Psychiatry Res,* **177**(1–2), pp. 216–22.

Cornwell, J., Sonola, L., Levenson, R., *et al.* (2012) *Continuity of Care for Older Hospital Patients: A Call for Action.* London: King's Fund, available at: www.kingsfund.org.uk/publications/continuity-care-older-hospital-patients

Cowan, D., and Turner–Smith, A. (1999) The role of assistive technology in alternative models of care for older people. In: Tinker, A., *et al.* (eds.) *Alternative Models of Care for Older People: Royal Commission on Long Term Care Research Volume 2.* London: The Stationery Office. pp. 325–46.

Day, K., Carreon, D., and Stump, C. (2010) The therapeutic design of environments for people wih dementia: a review of the empirical research, *Gerontologist,* **40**(4), pp. 397–416.

Department of Health (2009) *Living Well with Dementia: A National Dementia Strategy.* London: The Stationery Office, available at: www.gov.uk/government/publications/living-well-with-dementia-a-national-dementia-strategy

Department of Health (2012) *The Prime Minister's 'Dementia Challenge': Delivering Major Improvements in Dementia Care and Research by 2015.* London: Department of Health, available at: http://media.dh.gov.uk/network/353/files/2012/11/The-Prime-Ministers-Challenge-on-Dementia-Delivering-major-improvements-in-dementia-care-and-research-by-2015-A-report-of-progress.pdf

Easton, M. (2006) *Britain's Happiness in Decline,* BBC website, 2 May 2006, available at: http://news.bbc.co.uk/1/hi/programmes/happiness_formula/4771908.stm

Green, E. on behalf of the MRC Institute for Environment and Health (2000) *Health and Wellbeing: Does our Environment Matter? A report of an open seminar organised by the MRC*

Institute for Environment and Health and held at the NSPCC National Training Centre, Leicester, on 28 November 2000, available at: www.cranfield.ac.uk/health/researchareas/ environmenthealth/ieh/ieh%20publications/handwreport.pdf

Jahoda, M. (1958) *Current Concepts of Positive Mental Health*. New York, NY: Basic Books.

Hodges, J.R. (2010) Dementia. In: London. In: Warrell, D.A., Cox, T.M., and Firth, J.D. (eds) *Oxford Textbook of Medicine*. Fifth edition. Oxford: Oxford University Press. Chapter 24.2.2.

Huppert, F.A., Baylis, N., and Keverne, B. (2004) Introduction: why do we need a science of well-being? *Philos Trans R Soc Lond B Biol Sci*, **359**(1449), pp. 1331–2.

Imison, C., Poteliakhoff, E., and Thompson, J. (2012) *Older People and Emergency Bed Use: Exploring Variation*. London: King's Fund, available at: www.kingsfund.org.uk/sites/ files/kf/field/field_publication_file/older-people-and-emergency-bed-use-aug-2012.pdf

Kerr, D. (1997) *Down's Syndrome and Dementia: Practitioner's Guide*. Birmingham: Venture Press.

King's Fund (2001) A description of a consultation meeting on assistive technology cited in: www.fastuk.org/about/definitionofat.php

Larson, E.B., and Langa, K.M. (2008) The rising tide of dementia worldwide, *Lancet*, **372**(9637), pp. 430–2.

Llibre Rodriguez, J.J., Ferri, C.P., Acosta, D., *et al.* (2008) Prevalence of dementia in Latin America, India, and China: a population-based cross-sectional survey, *Lancet*, **372**(9637), pp. 464–74.

Luengo-Fernandez, R., Leal, J., and Gray, A.M. (2011) Cost of dementia in the pre-enlargement countries of the European Union, *J Alzheimers Dis*, **27**(1), pp. 187–96.

Michaelson, J. (2012) *The Importance of Measuring Well-being*, New Economics Foundation, 7 August, available at: www.neweconomics.org/blog/entry/the-importance-of-measuring-well-being

Mitchell, L., and Burton, E. (2006) Neighbourhoods for Life: designing dementia-friendly outdoor environments. *Qual Ageing Older Adults*, **7**(1), 26–33.

Norton, S., Matthews, F.E., and Brayne, C. (2013) A commentary on studies presenting projections of the future prevalence of dementia, *BMC Public Health*, 13, p. 1.

Rahman, S., and Sahakian, B.J. (2001) Dementia, chapter 12 (pp. 127–42) *in*: Sirtori, C., Reidenberg, M., Kuhlmann, J., *et al.* (eds) *Clinical Pharmacology*, London: McGraw Hill Publishers.

Rahman, S., Sahakian, B.J., and Gregory, C.A. (2001) Therapeutic strategies in early onset dementia. In: Hodges, J.R. (ed.) *Early Onset Dementia*, Oxford: Oxford University Press. pp. 422–44.

Rahman, S., Swainson, R., and Sahakian, B.J. (2001) Dementia of the Alzheimer type. In: Owen, A.M. (ed.) *Cognitive Deficits in Brain Disorders*, London: Martin-Dunitz. pp. 139–68.

Rocca, W.A., Hofman, A., Brayne, C., *et al.* (1991) Frequency and distribution of Alzheimer's disease in Europe: a collaborative study of 1980–1990 prevalence findings. The EURODEM-Prevalence Research Group. *Ann Neurol*, **30**(3): pp. 381–90.

Royal College of Physicians of London (RCP) (2012) *Hospitals on the Edge? The Time for Action* (quoted in RCP, *Acute Hospital Care Could Be on the Brink of Collapse, warns RCP*, Press Release, London: RCP; 13 September, available at: www.rcplondon.ac.uk/ press-releases/acute-hospital-care-could-be-brink-collapse-warns-rcp).

Royal College of Psychiatrists (2011) *Report of the National Audit of Dementia Care in General Hospitals*, London: Healthcare Quality Improvement Partnership.

Thomas, P., Lalloué, F., Preux, P.M., *et al.* (2006) Dementia patients' caregivers quality of life: the PIXEL study, *Int J Geriatr Psychiatry*, **21**(1), pp. 50–6.

Thomas, W.H. (2004) *What are Old People For? How Elders Will Save the World.* Acton, MA: VanderWyk & Burnham.

UK Government. (2012) *Health and Social Care Act 2012*, available at: www.legislation.gov.uk/ukpga/2012/7/contents/enacted

United Nations (2004) *World Population to 2300*, available at: www.un.org/esa/population/publications/longrange2/WorldPop2300final.pdf

CHAPTER 3

Measuring living well with dementia

In 2011, the most senior civil servant in the UK government, Gus O'Donnell, said in a speech about well-being 'If you treasure it, measure it'. If we accept well-being as a fundamental human goal, and recognise that GDP [gross domestic product] and other indicators beloved of governments are just the means to that goal, we need to measure well-being – and we need to measure it well. This requires the use of subjective indicators to establish how people experience their lives and this in turn requires us to measure how people feel, and how well they perceive themselves to be functioning. So how good are our measures of well-being and what do they tell us about the causes of well-being and how to improve it?

F.A. Huppert, 'Interventions and policies to enhance wellbeing'

Starting from the premise that it would be useful to consider wellbeing at all as a policy outcome, or something to strive for at least, it would seem a natural development to think about how this is measured. Such endeavours have necessarily been challenging, as, to measure wellbeing, one must presumably have a strong mental construct of what wellbeing is. Strikingly, Huppert (2014) observes, 'the plethora of different approaches to identifying the key components of well-being, and the huge number and variety of available scales, can cause confusion for investigators who wish to establish whether their intervention has increased well-being.'

WHY IS WELLBEING IMPORTANT FOR PUBLIC HEALTH?

Over the past 10 years, experts in the field of dementia have increasingly turned their attention to consideration of patient '**quality of life**' (QoL). The importance of measuring QoL outcomes in clinical trials and for the clinical management of dementia was debated and discussed among leaders in dementia research and treatment, the pharmaceutical industry and government agencies (Small *et al.*, 1997; Whitehouse *et al.*, 1997).

Any sensible definition of 'wellbeing' integrates mental health (mind) and physical health (body), resulting in more holistic approaches to disease prevention and health promotion. That the two are in some way linked, particularly in notions such as distress, is likely to be an important area of research in future. Wellbeing is a valid population outcome measure beyond morbidity, mortality and economic status, and it tells us how people perceive their life is going from their own perspective. Wellbeing is an outcome that is meaningful to the public. Advances in cognitive and social psychology, neuroscience, and measurement theory suggest that wellbeing can be measured with some degree of accuracy.

Results from cross-sectional, longitudinal and experimental studies find that wellbeing is associated with a number of aspects (e.g. Diener and Seligman, 2004; Lyubomirsky, King and Diener, 2005):

- self-perceived health
- longevity
- healthy behaviours
- mental and physical illness
- social connectedness
- productivity
- factors in the physical and social environment.

Wellbeing can provide a common metric that can help policymakers shape and compare the effects of different policies (e.g. loss of green space might affect wellbeing more so than commercial development of an area) (Frey and Stutzer, 2002; Diener *et al.*, 2009). Wellbeing is associated with numerous health-, job-, family-, and economically related benefits (Lyubomirsky, King and Diener, 2005). For example, higher levels of wellbeing are thought to be associated with decreased risk of disease, illness and injury; better immune functioning; speedier recovery; and increased longevity. Individuals with high levels of wellbeing are often thought to be more productive at work, and are more likely to contribute to their communities. The link between mental and physical wellbeing might explain why the physical health of individuals with dementia may be dependent on their mental wellbeing, as determined by a new environment. Clearly, this will be an interesting area to explore, in future.

Previous research meanwhile lends some support to the view that the negative affect component of wellbeing can be strongly associated with neuroticism and that positive affect component has a similar association with extraversion. This research also supports the view that positive emotions – central components of wellbeing – are not merely the opposite of negative emotions but, rather, are independent dimensions of mental health that can and should be fostered (Bradburn, 1969; Barry and Jenkins, 2007). Positive emotions can be the *consequence* of certain cognitive or behavioural processes, as well as their cause. Although a substantial proportion of the variance in wellbeing can be attributed to inherited or heritable factors, environmental factors play an equally if not more important rôle. Taken together, these findings suggest that positive emotions lead to positive cognitions, positive behaviours and increased cognitive capability, and that positive cognitions, behaviours and capabilities in turn fuel positive emotions (Fredrickson and Joiner, 2002).

HOW IS WELLBEING DEFINED?

Reviewed in Friedli (2009) on behalf of WHO Europe, although definitions vary, **positive mental health** is generally seen as including the following:

- emotion (affect or feeling)
- cognition (perception, thinking, reasoning)
- social functioning (relations with others and society)
- coherence (sense of meaning and purpose in life).

There is admittedly, however, no consensus around a single definition of wellbeing, but there is general agreement that at minimum, wellbeing includes the presence of positive emotions and moods (e.g. contentment, happiness), the absence of negative emotions (e.g. depression, anxiety), satisfaction with life, fulfilment and positive functioning. In simple terms, wellbeing can be described as judging life positively and feeling good. For public health purposes, physical wellbeing (e.g. feeling very healthy and full of energy) is also viewed as critical to overall wellbeing.

Researchers from convergent different disciplines have examined different aspects of wellbeing that include the following:

- physical wellbeing
- economic wellbeing
- social wellbeing
- development and activity
- emotional wellbeing
- psychological wellbeing
- life satisfaction
- domain-specific satisfaction
- engaging activities and work.

WELLBEING AS A PUBLIC HEALTH POLICY GOAL

Economics, even if unfairly called the 'dismal science', has its unique perspective on the importance of wellbeing and 'happiness' to economic society (Rahman, 2011). Traditional economics has focused on the 'rational' agent in decision-making, but policy has increasingly seen wellbeing as a subjective measure that is not necessarily rational and certainly difficult to measure. Metcalfe and Mischel (1999), in a famous paper by Jonathan Haidt (2001), describe how the human brain might be organised into 'hot' and 'cold' processing sytems:

> Metcalfe and Mischel (1999) proposed a dual process model of willpower in which two separate but interacting systems govern human behavior in the face of temptation. The 'hot' system is specialized [sic] for quick emotional processing, and it makes heavy use of amygdala-based memory. The 'cool' system is specialized [sic] for complex spatiotemporal and episodic representation and thought. It relies on hippocampal memory and frontal lobe planning and inhibition areas. It can block the impulses of the hot system, but it develops later in life, making childhood and adolescence seem like a long struggle to overcome impulsiveness and gain self-control.

Professor Felicia Huppert (2009) at the distinguished Wellbeing Institute of the University of Cambridge has been seminal in this field. She has described that the recent flowering of research on mental wellbeing has come about for a number of reasons, chief among them being:

- the recognition that, since wellbeing is more than the absence of illbeing, it needs to be studied in its own right
- the need to distinguish between these approaches to improving psychological wellbeing: (a) treating disorder when it is present; (b) preventing disorder from occurring; and (c) enhancing wellbeing (i.e. increasing flourishing)
- evidence that many of the drivers of wellbeing are not the same as the drivers of illbeing
- the strong possibility that, by increasing flourishing in the population, we might do more to reduce common mental and behavioural problems than by focusing exclusively on the treatment and prevention of disorder.

A growing consensus has thus emerged within the research community regarding the robustness of such global measures for accurately reflecting individuals' feelings about their own lives. However, there remains a lack of agreement concerning precisely how the emotional aspects of wellbeing relate to the overall definition and measurement of subjective wellbeing.

The relationship between these aspects of subjective wellbeing is best summarised by the following diagram, adapted from Hird's (2003) review.

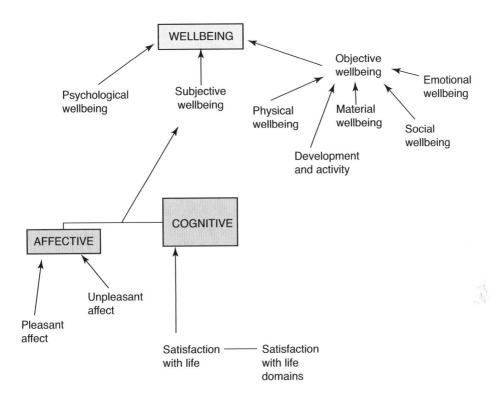

FIGURE 3.1 The relationship between different aspects of subjective wellbeing (adapted from McAllister, 2005, and based on Hird, 2003)

Figure 3.1 demonstrates how psychological definitions of subjective wellbeing occupy a grey area, with some viewing psychological wellbeing as synonymous with subjective wellbeing, and others seeing it as distinct. While sensing value in models that measure wellbeing in terms of the balance between positive and negative feelings, and affect, Hird (2003) concludes that in practice the distinctions drawn between 'happiness', 'affect' and 'life satisfaction' may not be so important.

Economists and sociologists also use data related to individuals' *perception* of their circumstances, such as self-rated physical healthiness or whether individuals think that they have a lot of money or live in a safe neighbourhood. These somewhat disparate approaches to subjective wellbeing reflect the breadth of definitions given to it, and the large number of potential influences upon it.

IMPLEMENTING WELLBEING DOMAINS IN NATIONAL AND INTERNATIONAL POLICY

The **Stroud/ADI Dementia Quality Framework** is one very good example of a mechanism that tries to structure assessment of the quality-of-life effects at a population level (Banerjee *et al.*, 2010). Information available can be mapped onto the framework. With its international approach, the Stroud/ADI Dementia Quality Framework even has validity across cultures within and between countries. It is intended as a useful aid for the assessment of services and policies for people with dementia and their family carers. The five themes, interestingly, included a 'supra-national' and 'transcedent'. This offers a systematic way to judge the efficacy of a service and policy, and can be used by the individuals in the service themselves, clients and inspectors.

The 'inner' ring refers to individual factors of the 'domains' of quality of care, health, communication, environment and personhood; the outer ring refers to societal factors of service funding, public attitudes and policy (*see* **Figure 3.2**).

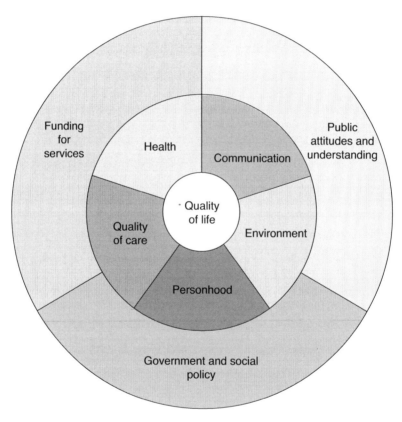

FIGURE 3.2 The Stroud/ADI Dementia Quality Framework: a cross-national population-level framework for assessing the quality-of-life effects of services and policies for people with dementia and their family carers (Banerjee *et al.*, 2010)

MEASURING 'HEALTH-RELATED QUALITY OF LIFE'

Although measures of cognitive, functional and behavioural outcomes are widely used to evaluate interventions for dementia, **the challenge of measuring**

broader outcomes such as health-related quality of life (HRQoL) has only recently begun to be addressed.

This presents challenges about how to assess the subjective perceptions and experiences of the person with dementia in a reliable and valid way.

What happens to 'quality of life' as dementia progresses?

Measuring quality of life in dementia is challenging, not least because of potentially poor recall, time perception and communication on the part of the person with dementia. Furthermore, subjective evaluation of QoL by people with dementia may be influenced by their cognitive limitations and may reflect reduced insight; however, they represent the best way of understanding the experience of life with dementia (Albrecht and Devleiger, 1999). Medical models of QoL have traditionally assumed that the more symptoms present, and the more advanced the disease, the poorer the QoL.

However, an apparent paradox is that people with chronically limiting conditions often report a high QoL. Woods (1999) suggests that there is an implicit assumption in many studies that increased independent function must be associated with a better QoL. He concludes that if wellbeing is to be increased through efforts to improve independent functioning, then there needs to be a better understanding of how the person with dementia cognitively processes these changes. Therefore, an understanding of people's perceptions, behaviours and experiences is needed if the concept of subjective QoL is to be adequately described.

Individuals with dementia may have a range of cognitive and behavioural symptoms that can interfere with their ability to answer QoL questions. Communication, attention, memory and judgement are necessary skills to answer survey questions (e.g. Tourangeau, Rips and Rasinski, 2000) and these are all cognitive areas that may be impaired in people with dementia. Similarly, altered psychological states such as depression, may have an impact on QoL assessment, particularly when this involves reports about subjective wellbeing.

Katschnig, Freeman and Sartorius (1997) highlight the rôle of momentary affective states, reality distortion and poor cognition in the distortion of responses to questions about functioning in social rôles, and about material and social living conditions. People vary widely in their typical emotional style – that is, whether they tend to feel generally positive or generally negative. It might be that the key to understanding individual differences in emotional style is the extraordinarily protracted period of human brain development, which is sensitive to environmental influences. Unlike the other major organs of the body, our brain undergoes most of its development postnatally, and is exquisitely designed to respond to the environmental conditions in which a child happens to grow up. This is entirely relevant to our discourse about living well with dementia, as my thesis will articulate.

A further challenge for the direct assessment of QoL in people with dementia is the apparent lack of insight demonstrated by many individuals. For example, patients with mild behavioural variant frontotemporal dementia can have complete lack of insight (Rahman *et al.*, 1999). This deficit can relate to awareness of specific memory or cognitive deficits, awareness of global memory or cognitive deficits, awareness of the impact of memory problems or dementia, or awareness of dementia as a whole (Ansell and Bucks, 2006). Insight varies across domains such as self-care, memory, health status and language abilities (Green *et al.*, 1993).

However, Brod and colleagues (Brod *et al.*, 1999b) suggest that 'awareness of feelings may be preserved, even in instances where awareness of cognitive deficits is impaired'; awareness of cognitive symptoms has traditionally been a very important strand in the cognitive neurology literature (e.g. Agnew and Morris, 1998). Brod and colleagues (1999b) cite evidence (e.g. Seltzer and colleagues (Seltzer *et al.*, 1995) that reports good correlations between patient and proxy measures, such as mood, energy, health and sense of self, alongside poor agreement on measures of memory and functional ability. There is growing evidence to suggest that people with dementia can respond accurately to questions about QoL (Brod *et al.*, 1999b). Although investigations of cognitively impaired individuals show that proxies consistently rate QoL lower for the patient than they would rate themselves (Logsdon *et al.*, 1999), this lack of agreement is not entirely attributable to the level of patient cognitive impairment (Teri and Wagner, 1991). It currently appears likely that mild to moderately cognitively impaired individuals can articulate feelings, concerns and preferences, and provide evaluations of their health and QoL.

Trigg, Jones and Skevington (2007) conducted a study to examine the reliability of the item pool of a new measure of self-reported QoL, the Bath Assessment of Subjective Quality of Life in Dementia. They found that participants were able to complete items relating to feelings and evaluations of a range of QoL domains. The consistency of responses over a 2-week period suggests that self-reported QoL assessments are feasible and appropriate for people with mild to moderate dementia.

Cross-sectional studies

Cross-sectional studies have generally not compared HRQoL in clinical groups with either age-matched normative data or a general population control group.

There are currently few longitudinal or cohort studies of HRQoL in dementia. González-Salvador and colleagues (González-Salvador *et al.*, 2000) found that assisted-living residents with dementia reported consistently better HRQoL than those living in skilled nursing facilities, although the former group also had higher Mini-Mental State Examination scores (mean 9.5, as compared to 2.6). One of the few available longitudinal studies of psychosocial outcomes in dementia (Albert *et al.*, 2001) provides a baseline profile of people with dementia in terms of activity, confinement to home and affect. Longitudinal data collected at 6-monthly intervals for 4 or more years suggested that when severity of dementia increased over follow-up, subjects were more likely to experience poor QoL (indicated by reduced activity, reduced positive affect and increased confinement).

Comparisons with normative populations

The lack of data comparing HRQoL in people with dementia with age-matched normative data or controls ultimately means that it is often difficult to draw conclusions about whether the impact on HRQoL is due to dementia or reflects a more general age-related pattern. It is important to document these disease effects because a treatment could not, in general, be expected to improve HRQoL unless it was known that the disease itself has a negative impact on HRQoL. Furthermore, it is essential to know the magnitude of the disease effect. Treatment effects are likely to be smaller than disease effects, so knowledge of the magnitude of the disease effect can inform estimation of the expected treatment effect, thus enabling more accurate power calculations for evaluation studies and clinical trials.

IMPACT ON CARERS

The impact on carers depends on the characteristics of the carer as well as the person with dementia.

Levin and colleagues (Levin, Sinclair and Gorbach, 1989) have usefully defined **four** main sources of stress and burden:

1. *practical*: need for help with personal care and housework;
2. *behavioural*: including active problems (e.g. aggression, wandering, night disturbance, incontinence) and passive problems (e.g. apathy, decreased social interaction), which may be particularly difficult to deal with;
3. *interpersonal*: difficulty in communication and change in the nature of the relationship with the person with dementia;
4. *social*: restrictions on the carer leaving the home, socialising or going to work.

Logiudice and colleagues (Logiudice *et al.*, 1998) found that the psychosocial health of carers of people with dementia was impaired, although in a different way to chronically ill patients, with social interaction and recreation most affected. It has also been suggested that carers who are co-resident with the person with dementia, socially isolated, and/or who have previously had a poor relationship, are at increased risk of distress (Brodaty and Hadzi-Pavlovic, 1990).

As Cuijpers (2005) reviewed, it has been well-established that caregivers of dementia patients suffer disproportionately from severe stress, associated with the necessity to cope with behavioural problems of the elderly person, inability to communicate, and feelings of intense loneliness and loss, comparable to losing a loved one. On account of these serious disruptions in their lives, it is hardly surprising that caregivers of dementia patients often suffer from health problems (Vitaliano, Zhang and Scanlan, 2003), and especially from mental health problems, such as depressive symptomatology and anxiety. In the past few decades, dozens of studies have shown that levels of depressive symptomatology are seriously increased in caregivers of dementia patients (e.g. Schulz *et al.*, 1995).

As the dementia illness progresses, people with dementia appear to require more help with self-care and other aspects of daily functioning. The burden of care usually falls on close family members, typically co-resident spouses or daughters, with most of the caring carried out by one relative (Schneider *et al.*, 1992), and with the tasks rarely equally shared. Caring for people with dementia can be extremely stressful; carers have been found to have poorer physical and mental health than age-matched controls (Livingston, Manela and Katona, 1996).

WELBEING AND PHYSICAL HEALTH

A key question is *whether there are any significant differences in outcomes for people who have good mental health, compared with those with average or poor mental health* (among people who do not have a diagnosable mental disorder).

Some evidence shows that compared with those who are flourishing, moderately mentally healthy and languishing adults have significant psychosocial impairment and poorer physical health, lower productivity and more limitations in daily living (Keyes 2005). Keyes found that cardiovascular disease was lowest in adults who were the most mentally healthy, and higher among adults with major depressive episodes, minor depression and moderate mental health. This is consistent with review level evidence that coronary heart disease risk is directly related to the severity of depression: a 1–2× increase in coronary heart disease for minor depression and 3–5× increase for major depression (Bunker *et al.*, 2003). In other words, intermediate levels of mental health are different from mental illness, as well as from 'flourishing'.

GENERAL MODELS OF HEALTH-RELATED QUALITY OF LIFE

The World Health Organization (WHO) (WHO, 1947; WHO, 1948) definition recognises health as a multidimensional concept that includes physical, mental and social wellbeing.

Autonomy has more recently been added as a fourth component (WHO, 1984). Autonomy is generally a very important principle to apply correctly in considering individuals living well with dementia, and will be discussed again in **Chapters 11** and **14** of this book.

More recently, the WHO has defined positive mental health as '*a state of wellbeing in which the individual realizes* [sic] *his or her own abilities, can cope with the normal stresses of life, can work productively and fruitfully, and is able to make a contribution to his or her community*' (WHO, 2001). Most general models of HRQoL indeed now reflect the importance of physical, psychological and social functioning, often including the ability to perform usual rôles within each of these domains. In addition, several models (Patrick and Bergner, 1990; Patrick and Erikson, 1993; Ware, 1987; Wilson and Cleary, 1995) include general health perceptions as a domain of HRQoL. Some models also include another potentially important component – '**opportunity for health**' (Patrick and Bergner, 1990; Patrick and Erickson, 1993) or '**health potential**' (Bergner, 1985) – that is, the ability to withstand stress and the extent to which an individual has physiological reserves. The construct HRQoL is therefore sometimes described as having elements of '**positive health**', which includes the ability to fulfil potential, in addition to the absence of illness and the ability to function adequately. These positive aspects of health and HRQoL are difficult to measure, and are rarely included in instruments to measure HRQoL.

Well-established generic measures of HRQoL and health status, such as the Short Form 36 (Ware, Kosinski and Keller 1994), Health Utilities Index (Furlong *et al.*, 2001), EQ-5D (EuroQoL group, 1990) and WHOQoL (WHOQoL group, 1996), may also all include additional domains such as pain, general health perceptions, energy, independence, environment and spirituality. Most conceptual work on HRQoL has latterly aimed to provide a description of the construct, but few studies have explored the relationship between different domains of HRQoL or between HRQoL and other relevant constructs (Bergner, 1985).

DEMENTIA-SPECIFIC MODELS OF HEALTH-RELATED QUALITY OF LIFE

Other neurodegenerative conditions can present with a much more consistent pattern of cognitive and affective symptoms, compared to the dementias. For example, idiopathic Parkinson's disease presents with a classic diagnostic triad of tremor, bradykinesia and rigidity. Rahman and colleagues (Rahman *et al.*, 2008) found that anxiety and depression can predict quality of life in Parkinson's disease.

As explored previously in my thesis, dementia is a complex heterogeneous entity, not least because 'dementia' is a portmanteau term for different conditions with different aetiology; progression is non-linear, and can be very unpredictable. In this way, it is a similar to the problems posed by 'cancer' as a term.

Conceptual work to identify the specific domains of HRQoL that are relevant to people with dementia is still relatively underdeveloped. There is an emerging body of literature that suggests that people with dementia have a meaningful experience of HRQoL and are able to report this subjective experience (Cohen and Eisdorfer, 1986; Ronch, 1996; Cotrell and Shultz 1993). Most studies of HRQoL in dementia are descriptive; few have compared findings with general models or explored the relationship among different aspects of HRQoL or between HRQoL and other relevant variables.

More recent perspectives, especially the work of Tom Kitwood (1997), have re-evaluated the concept of QoL of people with dementia and developed care concepts that have been framed by social–psychological theories and models. This alternative perspective argues that many people with dementia can experience a reasonable QoL, despite their condition, and focuses on the 'personhood' in terms of a sense of personal worth, agency, confidence and social reciprocity. While the dementing illness can undermine aspects of personhood, some or many other aspects may remain intact. The rôle of care is to facilitate the maintenance of personhood (a coherent self), through providing care and support that encourages and supports the person in their everyday lives.

Kitwood's '**Dementia Care Mapping**' (DCM) (Kitwood and Bredin, 1992) approach suggests that there are four sentient states relevant to quality of life in dementia:
1. sense of personal
2. growth sense of agency
3. social confidence
4. hope.

Parse (1996) describes four emerging dimensions of quality of life based on interviews with people with dementia:
1. calm/turbulence
2. freedom/restriction
3. certainty/uncertainty
4. togetherness/aloneness.

Brod and colleagues (Brod, Stewart and Sands, 1999a) conducted three focus groups: one with five co-resident carers of people with dementia, one with six service providers, and one with six people in the early stages of dementia who were regular participants in a support group. They then proposed a conceptual framework that includes:
- **aesthetics** (including enjoying/appreciating beauty, nature and surroundings)
- **positive affect** (including humour, feeling happy, content and hopeful)
- **absence of negative affect** (including worry, frustration, depression, anxiety, sadness, loneliness, fear, irritability, nervousness, embarrassment and anger)
- **self-esteem** (including feeling accomplished, confident or satisfied with self, able to make own decisions)
- **feelings of belonging** ('feeling loveable, liked and useful').

These models conceptualise HRQoL in terms of subjective components. The Brod model (Brod, Stewart and Sands, 1999a), which builds on the generic conceptual models of Lawton (Lawton, 1983; Coen *et al.*, 1993; Novella *et al.*, 2001) and the approach of Wilson and Cleary (1995), proposes a conceptual model of the relationship between domains of HRQoL and other areas of impact in dementia. Further work is needed to test the hypothesised relationships between these aspects of health.

An alternative narrative (Lawton, 1994) has developed to suggest that quality of life in dementia includes both subjective and physical/social-normative components. The subjective component includes perceived quality of self (psychological wellbeing) and the environment (the person's own evaluation of housing, income, leisure activities). The physical/social-normative component includes behavioural competence (activities of daily living, cognitive performance and social behaviour) and the quality of the external environment (observer ratings of the living environment or amount of private space or homeliness). Lawton argues that because people with dementia who are beyond the early stages of the condition are not able reliably to report verbally on their subjective experience, the external or observable components are often the only aspect of quality of life that can be assessed. Other authors have suggested that this reliance on external observations does not allow for the individual nature of values, needs and ability to adapt (Brod, Stewart and Sands, 1999a).

A further important aspect of the re-evaluation of dementia is an emphasis on 'ecological' perspectives of QoL. From this perspective (Torrington, 2006), a person's activities and wellbeing are seen to be influenced by a number of factors, such as attributes of the person (functional ability, cognitive ability, psychological factors, etc.) and attributes of the context (formal support network, social network, physical environment and cultural context). Everyday activities can be seen to be either facilitated or constrained by these personal and contextual factors. How a person derives meaning from their everyday activities is central to their wellbeing. Positive wellbeing (e.g. happiness, life satisfaction) derives from being involved in activities and situations that are personally meaningful and valued, whereas negative life experiences derive from being unable to be involved in these.

Figure 3.3 shows the ecological model that was developed to help to conceptualise this. It developed as a result of the discussion of the INDEPENDENT project as a framework for guiding the user research and technology development. It provides a structure for carrying out user research in order to develop a sound understanding of QoL among people with dementia, using this knowledge to develop an agenda for the development of technology and design solutions, and an iterative development of technologies with users and carers. This framework is discussed further in **Chapter 14**.

Lawton's idea of '**person–environment fit**' (Lawton and Nahemow, 1973) also appears to have clear parallels. This suggests that increasing frailty in old

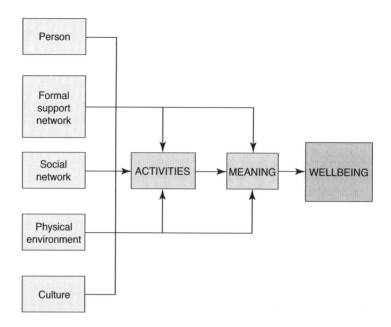

FIGURE 3.3 Ecological model of wellbeing and dementia (Torrington, 2006) – this has been an important aspect in the re-evaluation of dementia is an emphasis on 'ecological' perspectives of quality of life

age leads to a reduction in the ability to perform activities of daily living, and that people with reduced personal capacities are more vulnerable to environmental demands compared with people whose capacities remain intact. In this context, environmental factors become very important in terms of their everyday tasks of living and QoL. Lawton (1991) extended his model by introducing subjective wellbeing and described QoL in terms of four overlapping sub-domains: (1) behavioural competence – the capacity to deal with the demands of everyday life; (2) objective environment – physical and social context within which a person lives; (3) perceived QoL or the subjective evaluation of their function and circumstances; and (4) psychological wellbeing – wellbeing, happiness, and so on.

DISEASE-SPECIFIC MEASURES

Because disease-specific measures are designed to be relevant to a particular condition, they are generally more sensitive in detecting change following an intervention. The disadvantage of disease-specific instruments is that they do not allow comparisons across different conditions. Ideally, the evaluation of HRQoL should include both generic and disease-specific instruments, although the additional respondent burden imposed by administering an extra questionnaire may make this unfeasible.

Major advances have been made in evaluating disease-specific, patient-based health outcomes such as HRQoL. Several disease-specific instruments are available for use in a wide range of conditions (Bowling, 1997; Bowling, 2001; McDowell and Newell, 1996; Wilkin, Hallam and Doggett, 1992). In dementia, however, the development of patient-based measures of HRQoL has been slower and more limited. This lag is likely to be due to the methodological challenges in measuring patient-reported outcomes such as HRQoL in dementia.

Activity and affect indicators of quality of life

Albert and colleagues (Albert *et al.*, 1996) created a measure of QoL that incorporates assessment of patients' activity and affect. These domains were measured because they are observable, quantifiable, behavioural, and they were hypothesised to be indicators of subjective, internal states of patients. A strength of this measure is that it is appropriate for use with a broad range of patients, from mild to severe stages of dementia severity. Furthermore, the measures can be used in both institutional and home-care settings. A potential drawback of this inventory, however, is that it provides a fairly narrow measurement of QoL that is confined to two dimensions, activity and affect.

The **Cornell-Brown Scale for Quality of Life in Dementia** (CBS) (Ready *et al.*, 2002) provides a global assessment of QoL. The scale was developed based on the conceptualisation that high QOL is indicated by the presence of positive affect, physical and psychological satisfactions, self-esteem and the relative absence of negative affect and experiences. Initial psychometric evidence has been obtained from patients in the mild to moderate stages of dementia severity, who are still living at home.

Dementia Care Mapping

DCM (Beavis, Simpson and Graham, 2002) is a structured, observational assessment of dementia patient experiences that was introduced in 1992. DCM was developed for use in residential care settings with dementia patients who are unable to provide valid and reliable reports about their experiences. Thus, it is most appropriate for use with moderate to severely impaired patients. Patient wellbeing and activities are coded with an emphasis on behaviours that are hypothesised to be related to QoL. Well versus illbeing of patients is rated on a 6-point ordinal scale and ratings are based on signs from patients and on the behaviour of staff towards the patient. There are 24 activity rating categories, and indicators of social withdrawal also can be coded.

DEM-QoL

Smith and colleagues (Smith *et al.*, 2005) have described an elegant 28-item **DEMQoL** and the 31-item DEMQoL-Proxy provide a method for evaluating HRQoL in dementia. The (relatively) new measures show comparable psychometric properties to the best available dementia-specific measures, provide both self- and proxy-report versions for people with dementia and their carers, are appropriate for use in mild or moderate dementia, and are considered suitable for use in the UK. DEMQoL-Proxy also shows promise in severe dementia. As DEMQoL and DEMQoL-Proxy give different but complementary perspectives on quality of life in dementia, the use of both measures together is recommended. (In severe dementia, only DEMQoL-Proxy should be used.)

Dementia Quality of Life Instrument

The **Dementia Quality of Life Instrument (DQoL)** (Brod *et al.*, 1999b) was developed through an iterative conceptual and statistical process that included a literature review and consultation with expert panels comprising dementia patients, caregivers, and professional care providers. It is a 29-item scale, plus one global item ('Overall, how would you rate your quality of life?') that measures 5 domains of QoL: Positive Affect (6 items), Negative Affect (11 items), Feelings of Belonging (3 items), Self-esteem (4 items) and Sense of Aesthetics (5 items). The DQoL yields scores on five subscales but subscale scores are not summed to reach an overall or global measure of QoL.

The scale is remarkable, as it has been developed for administering to patients. Item-stems were made as simple as possible and a 5-point visual scale is used to present multiple-choice response options to patients. All points on the response scale are associated with verbal descriptors. Screening questions ensure that patients understand questionnaire instructions and the response format for the scale. Because it relies solely on patient input, the DQoL is appropriate for use with patients in the mild to moderate stages of dementia.

Quality of Life–Alzheimer's Disease

Items for the **Quality of Life–Alzheimer's Disease (QoL-AD)** (Logsdon *et al.*, 1999) were selected to reflect domains of QoL in older adults based on a literature review of QoL in geriatric populations. Face validity and comprehensiveness was ensured by having patients with dementia of Alzheimer type, caregivers, non-demented older adults, and dementia experts review potential items. The final scale is composed of 13 items that measure the domains of physical condition, mood, memory, funcational abilities, interpersonal relationships, ability to participate in meaningful activities, financial situation, and global assessments of self as a whole and QoL as a whole. Response options are 4-point multiple-choice options (1 = poor, 4 = excellent). Scale scores range from 13 to 52, with higher scores indicating greater QoL. Strengths of this scale are its brevity and that it relies on reports from patients, caregivers or both.

A drawback is that it relies on a conceptualisation of QoL that may be regarded by some investigators as somewhat broad because it includes items about memory and functional abilities.

Alzheimer's Disease–Related Quality of Life

The **Alzheimer's Disease–Related Quality of Life (ADRQL)** (Rabins *et al.*, 1999) was developed to assess domains that caregivers of Alzheimer's disease patients and Alzheimer's disease experts identified as important for health-related QoL in dementia. Focus groups and expert panels guided scale development. The scale measures both positive and negative behaviours across five domains: (1) social interaction, (2) awareness of self, (3) feelings and mood, (4) enjoyment of activities, and (5) response to surroundings. The majority of items measure observable behaviours and actions, although some rely on assessment of subjective and internal states. Caregiver respondents are used for the ADRQL. Scores are calculated using a preference-based weighting approach, where weights for QoL indicators differ according to the importance of the domain.

Quality of Life Assessment Schedule

A strength of the **Quality of Life Assessment Schedule (QoLAS)** (Selai *et al.*, 2001) is that it is the only dementia QoL instrument that is tailored to individual patients and employs both qualitative and quantitative measurement approaches. Patients are interviewed and asked to identify what is important for their QoL and two issues from each of the following domains are identified: physical, psychological, social/family, usual activities, and cognitive functioning. Patients then rate how much of a problem he or she is currently experiencing with regard to each of the 10 issues on a 6-point scale (0 = no problem; 5 = it could not be worse). Scores range from 0 to 50, with higher scores reflecting poorer QoL. A drawback of the QoLAS is that psychometric properties have been evaluated in a small sample of patients, to date.

WHAT FACTORS GENERALLY AFFECT WELLBEING AND HEALTH-RELATED QUALITY OF LIFE?

There is no sole determinant of individual wellbeing, but in general, wellbeing is dependent upon good health, positive social relationships, and availability and access to basic resources (e.g. shelter, income).

Numerous studies have examined the associations between determinants of individual and national levels of wellbeing. Many of these studies have used different measures of wellbeing (e.g. life satisfaction, positive affect, psychological wellbeing), and different methodologies resulting in occasional inconsistent findings related to wellbeing and its predictors. In general, life satisfaction is dependent more closely on the availability of basic needs being met (e.g. food, shelter, income) as well as access to modern conveniences (e.g. electricity). Pleasant emotions are more closely associated with having supportive relationships.

Some general findings on associations between wellbeing and its associations with other factors are as follows.

- *Genes and personality.* At the individual level, genetic factors, personality, and demographic factors are related to wellbeing. Some personality factors that are strongly associated with wellbeing include optimism, extroversion and self-esteem. Genetic factors and personality factors are closely related, and can interact in influencing individual wellbeing. While genetic factors and personality factors are important determinants of wellbeing, they are beyond the realm of public policy goals.

- *Age and gender.* Depending on which types of measures are used (e.g. life satisfaction *versus* positive affect), age and gender also have been shown to be related to wellbeing. In general, men and women have similar levels of wellbeing, but this pattern changes with age, and has changed over time. According to Huppert (2009), the association between age and mental wellbeing is also complex. Large surveys using single-item measures of wellbeing (e.g. overall rating of life satisfaction) usually find a U-shaped relationship with age: younger and older people tend to have higher wellbeing scores than the middle aged, although there may be a decline in wellbeing among the very old. Middle-aged adults also have the highest prevalence of common mental disorders.

- *Income and work.* The relationship between income and wellbeing is complex. Depending on which types of measures are used and which comparisons are made, income correlates only modestly with wellbeing. In general, associations between income and wellbeing (usually measured in terms of life satisfaction) are stronger for those at lower economic levels, but studies also have found effects for those at higher income levels. Major socio-economic factors tend to have comparable effects on mental wellbeing and mental illbeing. In general, there is a social gradient whereby higher levels of income and socio-economic status are associated with higher levels of wellbeing and lower rates of disorder (e.g. Dolan, Peasgood and White, 2008; Ryff and Singer, 1998), although this effect diminishes at progressively higher levels of income.

- *Relationships.* Having supportive relationships is one of the strongest predictors of wellbeing, having a notably positive effect.

WHAT CAN BE DONE TO IMPROVE WELLBEING IN DEMENTIA?

A focus of this book is improving wellbeing through the environment for individuals with dementia, and those closest to them. However, this is not to give especial attention to factors involving the personhood of individuals with dementia.

According to the International School for Communities, Rights and Inclusion, addressing mental wellbeing can simultaneously achieve three objectives, and

TABLE 3.1 Objectives and targets

Objective	Target
Assist the general population to improve mental wellbeing, with concomitant improvements in mental and physical health, reductions in human service usage and wider social gains – a universal population-based approach	Improved population mental wellbeing
Improve the wellbeing, and associated gains, of those at risk of developing mental health problems and prevent such problems occurring through targeted interventions	Reduction in the number of people of all ages developing mental health problems and associated with this reducing the levels of suicide and self-harm
Improve wellbeing and assist those who have mental health problems and through recovery to achieve more fulfilled lives	Reduced numbers experiencing mental distress, recovery and inclusion of people with mental illness

'Making sense of mental wellbeing, mental health and mental illness' in 'Commissioning wellbeing' (p. 8) from the International School for Communities, Rights and Inclusion at University of Central Lancashire (the National Mental Health Development Unit (NMHDU)). This document is available at: www.nmhdu.org.uk/silo/files/commissioning-wellbeing-for-all.pdf

enable stronger communities and help local economies. **Three main proposed objectives** are shown in **Table 3.1**.

Woods (2011) suggests helpfully a number of different potential strategies in dementia care.

Improve mood

As low mood is the major predictor of poor QoL, this would appear to be a prime target of intervention, both pharmacologically and non-pharmacologically. People in the early stages of dementia are able to engage in cognitive behaviour therapy, with some adaptations, with some benefits reported in preliminary studies.

Maintain health

Physical health limitations lead to constraints on activities, and may be associated with discomfort and pain. Part of supporting someone with dementia is to ensure they are as free from pain as possible (and this is a focus of discussion in Chapter 8 on end-of-life issues, particularly). Different pain assessment tools can be helpful in identifying whether the person with dementia is communicating that they are experiencing pain. Physical health limitations, taken together, may also be a significant contributor to low mood. It is therefore appropriate to ensure that the person's physical health needs are carefully and sympathetically evaluated and appropriate actions taken.

Staff attitudes

Staff with hopeful attitudes recognise that people with dementia can respond and that there can be small but significant achievements.

Reduce use of antipsychotic medication

More effective ways of responding to behaviour that challenges will be needed in the long term to reduce reliance on pharmacological approaches with their associated adverse side effects.

Enhance relationship with carer

There is scope for more development of approaches that may help to maintain and improve the relationship between the person with dementia and the carer.

Encourage family involvement

In the care home context, supporting relatives with continued involvement is important.

Improving cognitive function?

Given the clear and consistent finding that cognitive function is not related to self-reported QoL in people with dementia, it appears unlikely that approaches that focus on cognitive function will have an effect on QoL. However, there is now a growing body of evidence that approaches such as cognitive stimulation and cognitive rehabilitation may indeed result in improved QoL.

Creative approaches

There is currently great interest in the involvement of people with dementia in creative artistic activities, which may well have the potential to influence QoL. Typical projects involve visits to art galleries, in some cases with subsequent work with an artist to produce art work inspired by the visit, that can then form the basis of a future exhibition. Involvement in choirs, through the *Singing for the Brain* project, for example, or in other music-based activities, is increasingly popular.

This theme is resumed in **Chapter 10**.

CONCLUSION

This chapter has established various different methods for measuring 'living well' in dementia, and one can see immediately that this is a very complicated area of ongoing research. The next chapter (**Chapter 4**), meanwhile, is an introduction to some of the socio-economic arguments in considering living with dementia.

REFERENCES

Agnew, S.K., and Morris, R.G. (1998) The heterogeneity of anosognosia for memory impairment in Alzheimer's disease: a review of the literature and a proposed model. Alzheimer's disease: a review of the literature and a proposed model, *Aging Ment Health*, 2(1), pp. 7–19.

Albert, S.M., del Castillo-Castanada, C., Sano, M., *et al.* (1996) Quality of life in patients with Alzheimer's disease as reported by patient proxies, *J Am Geriatr Soc*, 44(11), pp. 1342–7.

Albert, S.M., Jabobs, D.M., Sano, M., *et al.* (2001) Longitudinal study of quality of life in people with advanced Alzheimer's disease, *Am J Geriatr Psychiatry*, 9(2), pp. 160–8.

Albrecht, G.L., and Devleiger, P.J. (1999) The disability paradox: high quality of life against all the odds, *Soc Sci Med*, 48(8), pp. 977–88.

Ansell, E.L., and Bucks, R.S. (2006) Memory anosognosia in Alzheimer's disease: a test of Agnew and Morris (1998), *Neuropsychologia*, 44(7), pp. 1095–102.

Banerjee, S., Willis, R., Graham, N., *et al.* (2010) The Stroud/ADI dementia quality framework: a cross-national population-level framework for assessing the quality of life impacts of services and policies for people with dementia and their family carers, *Int J Geriatr Psychiatry*, 25(3), pp. 249–57.

Barry, M.M., and Jenkins, R. (2007) *Implementing Mental Health Promotion*. Oxford: Churchill Livingstone, Elsevier.

Beavis, D., Simpson, S, and Graham, I. (2002) A literature review of Dementia Care Mapping: methodological considerations and efficacy, *J Psychiatr Ment Health Nurs*, 9(6), pp. 725–73.

Bergner M. (1985) Measurement of health status, *Med Care*, 23(5), pp. 696–704.

Bowling, A. (1997) *Measuring Health: A Review of Quality of Life Measurement Scales*. Milton Keynes: Open University Press.

Bowling, A. (2001) *Measuring Disease*. Milton Keynes: Open University Press.

Bradburn, N.M. (1969) *The Structure of Psychological Wellbeing*. Chicago, IL: Aldine.

Brod, M., Stewart, A.L., and Sands, L. (1999a) Conceptualisation of quality of life in dementia, *J Ment Health Aging*, 5, pp. 7–19.

Brod, M., Stewart, A.L., Sands, L., *et al.* (1999b) Conceptualisation and measurement of quality of life in dementia: the dementia quality of life instrument (DQoL), *Gerontologist*, 39(1), pp. 25–35.

Brodaty, H., and Hadzi-Pavlovic, D. (1990) Psychosocial effects on carers of living with persons with dementia, *Aust NZ J Psychiatry*, 24(3), pp. 351–61.

Bunker S.J., Colquhoun D.M., Esler M.D., *et al.* (2003) 'Stress' and coronary heart disease: psychosocial risk factors. *Med J Aust*, 178(6), pp. 272–6.

Coen, R., O'Mahony, D., O'Boyle, C.A., *et al.* (1993) Measuring the quality of life of dementia patients using the Schedule for the Evaluation of Individualised Quality of Life, *Irish J Psychol*, 14: 154–63.

Cohen, D., and Eisdorfer, C. (1986) *The Loss of Self*. New York, NY: W.W. Norton.

Cotrell, V., and Shultz, R. (1993) The perspective of the patient with Alzheimer's disease: a neglected dimension of dementia research, *Gerontologist*, 33(2), pp. 205–11.

Cuijpers, P. (2005) Depressive disorders in caregivers of dementia patients: a systematic review, *Aging Ment Health*, 9(4), pp. 325–30.

Diener, E., and Seligman, M.E. (2004) Beyond money: toward an economy of wellbeing, *Psychol Sci Public Interest*, **5**(1), pp. 1–31.

Diener, E., Lucas, R., Schimmack, U., and Helliwell, J. (2009) *Wellbeing for Public Policy.* New York, NY: Oxford University Press.

Dolan, P., Peasgood, T., and White, M. (2008) Do we really know what makes us happy? A review of the economic literature on the factors associated with subjective wellbeing, *J Econ Psychol*, **29**, pp. 94–122.

EuroQol Group (1990) A new facility for the measurement of health-related quality of life, *Health Policy*, **16**(3), pp. 199–208.

Fredrickson B.L., and Joiner T. (2002) Positive emotions trigger upward spirals toward emotional well-being, *Psychol Sci*, **13**(2), pp. 172–5.

Fredrickson, B.L., Mancuso, R.A., Branigan, C., *et al.* (2000) The undoing effect of positive emotions, *Motiv Emot*, **24**(4), pp. 237–58.

Frey, B.S., and Stutzer, A. (2002) *Happiness and Economics.* Princeton, NJ: Princeton University Press.

Friedli, L., on behalf of the World Health Organization: Europe; National Institute for Mental Health in England, Child Poverty Action Group, Faculty of Public Health and Mental Health Foundation (2009) *Mental Health, Resilience and Inequalities*, available at: www.euro.who.int/__data/assets/pdf_file/0012/100821/E92227.pdf

Furlong, W.J., Feeny, D.H., Torrance, G.W., *et al.* (2001) The Health Utilities Index (HUI) system for assessing health-related quality of life in clinical studies, *Ann Med*, **33**(5), pp. 375–84.

González-Salvador, T., Lyketsos, C.G., Baker, A., *et al.* (2000) Quality of life in dementia patients in long-term care, *Int J Geriatr Psychiatry*, **15**(2), pp. 181–9.

Green, J., Goldstein, F.C., Sirockman, B.E., *et al.* (1993) Variable awareness of deficits in Alzheimer's disease, *Neuropsychiatry Neuropsychol Behav Neurol*, **6**, pp. 159–65.

Haidt, J. (2001) The emotional dog and its rational tail: a social intuitionist approach to moral judgment, *Psychol Rev*, **108**(4), pp. 814–34.

Hird, S. (2003) *What is Wellbeing? A Brief Review of Current Literature and Concepts.* Glasgow: NHS Health Scotland.

Huppert, F.A. (2009) Psychological wellbeing: evidence regarding its causes and consequences, *Appl Psychol Health Well Being*, 2009, **1**(2), pp. 137–64.

Huppert, F. (2014) The state of well-being science: concepts, measures, interventions and policies. In: Huppert, F.A., and Cooper, C.L. (eds) *Interventions and Policies to Enhance Well-being*, vol. 6. Oxford: Wiley-Blackwell. pp. 1–49.

International School for Communities, Rights and Inclusion, and University of Central Lancashire (2010) *Commissioning Mental Wellbeing: A Leadership Brief for Boards and Senior Managers; The role of wellbeing and mental health promotion in achieving whole system improvement.* Preston, Lancashire: University of Central Lancashire, available at: www.nmhdu.org.uk/silo/files/commissioning-for-wellbeing-and-population-mental-health.pdf

Katschnig, H., Freeman, H., Sartorius, N. (1997) *Quality of Life in Mental Disorders*, Chichester: John Wiley.

Keyes, C.L.M. (2005) Mental illness and/or mental health? Investigating axioms of the complete state model of health, *J Consult Clin Psychol*, **73**(3), pp. 539–48.

Kitwood, T. (1997) *Dementia Reconsidered: The Person Comes First.* Buckingham: Open University Press.

Kitwood T., and Bredin, K. (1992) Towards a theory of dementia care: personhood and well-being, *Ageing Soc*, **12**, pp. 269–87.

Lawton, M. P. (1983) Environment and other determinants of well-being in older people, *Gerontologist*, **23**, pp. 349–57.

Lawton, M. P. (1991) A multidimensional view of quality of life. In: Birren, J. E., Lubben, J. E., Rowe, J. C., *et al.* (eds.) *The Concept and Measurement of Quality of Life in the Frail Elderly*. New York: Academic Press. pp. 3–27.

Lawton, M.P. (1994) Quality of life in Alzheimer disease. *Alzheimer Dis Assoc Disord*, **8**(Suppl. 3), pp. 138–50.

Lawton, M.P., and Nahemow, L. (1973) Ecology and the aging process. In: Eisdorfer, C., Lawton, M.P., (eds.) *The psychology of adult development and aging*. Washington, DC: American Psychological Association. pp. 619–74.

Levin E, Sinclair I, and Gorbach P. (1989) Families, services and confusion in old age. Aldershot: Avebury.

Livingston, G., Manela, M., and Katona, C. (1996) Depression and other psychiatric morbidity in carers of elderly people living at home, *BMJ*, **312**(7024), pp. 153–6.

Logiudice, D., Kerse, N., Brown, K., *et al.* (1998) The psychosocial health status of carers of persons with dementia: a comparison with the chronically ill, *Qual Life Res*, **7**(4), pp. 345–51.

Logsdon, R., Gibbons, L.E., McCurry, S.M., *et al.* (1999) Quality of life in Alzheimer's disease: patient and caregiver reports, *J Ment Health Aging*, **5**, pp. 21–31.

Lyubomirsky, S., King, L., and Diener, E. (2005) The benefits of frequent positive affect: does happiness lead to success? *Psychol Bull*, **131**(6), pp. 803–55.

McAllister, F. (2005) *Wellbeing Concepts and Challenges*, discussion paper for the Sustainable Development Research Network, available at: www.sd-research.org.uk/research-and-resources/wellbeing-concepts-and-challenges-discussion-paper

McDowell, I., and Newell, C. (1996) *Measuring Health: A Review of Quality of Life Measurement Scales*. Oxford: Oxford University Press.

Metcalf, J., and Mischel, W. (1999) A hot/cool-system analysis of delay of gratification: dynamics of willpower, *Psychol Rev*, **106**(1), 3–19.

Novella, J.L., Ankri, J., Morrone, I., *et al.* (2001) Evaluation of the quality of life in dementia with a generic quality of life questionnaire: the Duke Health Profile, *Dement Geriatr Cogn Disord*, **12**(2), pp. 158–66.

Parse, R.R. (1996) Quality of life for persons living with Alzheimer's disease: the human becoming perspective, *Nurs Sci Q*, **9**(3), pp. 126–33.

Patrick, D.L., and Bergner, M. (1990) Measurement of health status in the 1990s, *Ann Rev Public Health*, **11**, pp. 165–83.

Patrick, D.L., and Erickson, P. (eds) (1993) Concepts of health-related quality of life. In: Patrick, D.L., and Erickson, P., *Health Status and Health Policy: Quality of Life in Health Care Evaluation and Resource Allocation*. Oxford: Oxford University Press. pp. 76–112.

Rabins, P.V., Kasper J,D., Kleinman, L., *et al.* (1999) Concepts and methods in the development of the ADRQL: an instrument for assessing health-related quality of life in persons with Alzheimer's disease, *J Ment Health Aging*, **5**, pp. 33–48.

Rahman, S. (2011) Shibley Rahman on Carol Graham: the pursuit of happiness; toward an economy of well-being, *World Economics*, **12**(3), pp. 213–18.

Rahman, S., Griffin, H.J., Quinn, N.P., *et al.* (2008) Quality of life in Parkinson's disease: the relative importance of the symptoms, *Mov Disord*, **23**(10), pp. 1428–34.

Rahman, S., Sahakian, B.J., Hodges, J.R., *et al.* (1999) Specific cognitive deficits in mild frontal variant frontotemporal dementia, *Brain*, **122**(8), pp. 1469–93.

Ready, R.E., Ott, B.R., Grace, J., *et al.* (2002) The Cornell-Brown Scale for Quality of Life in Dementia, *Alzheimer Dis Assoc Disord*, **16**(2), pp. 109–15.

Ronch, J.L. (1996) Assessment of quality of life: preservation of the self, *Int Psychogeriatr*, **8**, pp. 267–75.

Ryff, C.D., and Singer, B. (1998). Middle age and wellbeing. In: Friedman, H.S. (ed.) *Encyclopedia of Mental Health*, 1st Edition, New York, NY: Academic Press, pp. 707–19.

Schneider, J., Kavanagh, S., Knapp, M., *et al.* (1992) Elderly people with advanced cognitive impairment in England: resource use and costs, *Ageing Soc*, **13**, pp. 27–50.

Schneider, L.S, Streim, J.E., Sunderland, T., *et al.* (1997) Diagnosis and treatment of Alzheimer disease and related disorders. Consensus statement of the American Association for Geriatric Psychiatry, the Alzheimer's Association, and the American Geriatrics Society, *JAMA*, **278**(16): 1363–71.

Schulz R., O'Brien A.T., Bookwala J., *et al.* (1995) Psychiatric and physical morbidity effects of dementia caregiving: prevalence, correlates, and causes, *Gerontologist*, **35**(6), pp. 771–91.

Selai, C.E., Trimble, M.R., Rossor, M.N., *et al.* (2001) Assessing quality of life in dementia: preliminary psychometric testing of the Quality of Life Assessment Schedule, *Neuropsychol Rehabil*, **11**, 219–43.

Seltzer, B., Vasterling, J.J., Hale, M.A., *et al.* (1995) Unawareness of memory defect in Alzheimer's disease: relation to mood and other disease variables, *Neuropsychiatry, Neurophysiol Behav Neurol*, **8**, pp. 176–81.

Small, G.W., Rabins, P.V., Barry, P.P., *et al.* (1997) Diagnosis and treatment of Alzheimer disease and related disorders. Consensus statement of the American Association for Geriatric Psychiatry, the Alzheimer's Association, and the American Geriatrics Society, *JAMA*, **278**(16), pp. 1363–71.

Smith, S.C., Lamping, D.L., Banerjee, S., *et al.* (2005) Measurement of health-related quality of life for people with dementia: development of a new instrument (DEMQOL) and an evaluation of current methodology, *Health Technol Assess*, **9**(10), pp. 1–93, iii-iv.

Teri, L., and Wagner, A. (1991) Assessment of depression in patients with Alzheimer's disease: Concordance among informants, *Psychol Aging*, **6**, pp. 280–5.

Torrington, J. (2006) What has architecture got to do with dementia care? Explorations of the relationship between quality of life and building design in two EQUAL projects, *Qual Ageing*, **7**(1), pp. 34–49. Quoted in Vaarama, M., Pieper, R., and Sixsmith, A. (eds) *Care-Related Quality of Life in Old Age*. New York, NY: Springer Science, 2008.

Tourangeau, R., Rips L.J., and Rasinski, K. (2000) *The Psychology of Survey Response*, Cambridge: Cambridge University Press.

Trigg, R., Jones, R.W., and Skevington, S.W. (2007) Can people with mild to moderate dementia provide reliable answers about their quality of life? *Age Ageing*, **36**(6), pp. 663–9.

Vitaliano P.P., Zhang J., and Scanlan J.M. (2003) Is caregiving hazardous to one's physical health? A meta-analysis, *Psychol Bull*, **129**(6), pp. 946–72.

Ware, J.E. (1987) Standards for validating health measures: definition and content, *J Chron Dis*, **40**(6), pp. 473–80.

Ware, J.E., Kosinski, M.A., and Keller, S.D. (1994) *SF-36 Physical and Mental Component Summary Measures: A User's Mannual*. Boston, MA: New England Medical Center.

Whitehouse, P.J., Orgogozo, J.M., Becker R.E., *et al.* (1997) Quality of life assessment in dementia drug development: position paper from the International Working Group on Harmonization of Dementia Drug Guidelines, *Alzheimer Dis Assoc Disord*, **11**, pp. 56–60.

WHOQOL Group (1996) *WHOQOL-BREF: Introduction, Administration, Scoring and Generic Version of the Assessment*. Geneva: WHO.

Wilkin, D., Hallam, L., and Doggett, M. (1992) *Measures of Need and Outcome for Primary Care*. Oxford: Oxford University Press.

Wilson I.B., and Cleary, P.D. (1995) Linking clinical variables with health-related quality of life, *JAMA*, **273**(1), pp. 59–65.

Woods, B. (2011) Wellbeing and dementia: how can it be achieved? *Quality Ageing Older Adults*, **13**(3), pp. 205–11.

Woods, R.T. (1999) Promoting well-being and independence for people with dementia, *Int J Geriatr Psychiatry*, **14**(2), 97–109.

World Health Organization (WHO) (1947) *The Constitution of the World Health Organization*. Geneva: WHO.

World Health Organization (WHO) (1948) *Official Records of the World Health Organization*. Geneva: WHO.

World Health Organization (WHO) (1984) *Uses of Epidemiology in Aging: Report of a Scientific Group*. Geneva: WHO.

World Health Organization (WHO) (2001) *The World Health Report: Mental Health; New understanding, new hope*. Geneva: WHO.

CHAPTER 4

Socio-economic arguments for promoting living well with dementia

Economic, ethical, legal and public health arguments can all be proposed for pursuing an approach that prioritises 'living well' with dementia. The remaining chapters of this book, starting with **Chapter 5**, will examine how aspects of the person ('personhood') and his or her interaction to the environment can be analysed in greater detail.

The purpose of this chapter is to set the scene how it has come to be that wellbeing has taken 'pole position' in a multidisciplinary approach to dementia care.

AN ECONOMIC AS WELL AS A SOCIAL CASE FOR PROMOTING WELLBEING IN HEALTH POLICY?

According to the the International School for Communities, Rights and Inclusion and the University of Central Lancashire (2010), there are **four** principal drivers for promoting positive mental health and wellbeing: the economic case, the equalities case, the ethical case, the legal case and the public health case.

1. *The economic case*: promoting population mental health and wellbeing and illness prevention will reduce costs for the NHS and local authorities – in fact, for society in general over the next 2–5 years. With health and local authority colleagues commissioning well-evidenced programmes strategically there is a good likelihood this will lead to lower demand on primary care, hospital and community services, and that it will achieve improvements in overall population health.
2. *The ethical case*: everyone has the right to the best physical and mental health that society can afford, to enable them to enjoy their capabilities to the full and to contribute to society. Focusing on holistic wellbeing and emphasising

strengths and abilities (rather than 'deficits') offers a positive alternative to the illness and disability focus of much health and social care provision.

3. *The legal case*: reducing health inequalities using the evidence that mental wellbeing can play is critical to promoting positive mental health and wellbeing and to reducing the impact of 'prior discrimination' among minority groups.

4. *The public health case*: there is very good evidence that (1) mental health status affects a broad range of health and social outcomes and (2) a range of interventions can promote mental wellbeing and prevent poor mental health.

Local authorities and health services have a major rôle to play in raising the awareness of the factors that influence mental wellbeing and can take practical action through the proposed health and wellbeing boards, local partnerships and multi-agency plans.

The economic impact of mental illness is both serious and substantial. The cost of mental ill health in England is now approximately £100 billion a year: this includes the costs of health and social care, lost output in the economy and the human costs of reduced quality of life (Friedli and Parsonage, 2007). Preventive strategies not only reduce levels of mental distress (depression especially) in the general population but also reduce significantly the most damaging consequences of mental disorder for the individual. This is shown in Table 4.1.

TABLE 4.1 Costs of and inequalities in mental health

Cost of mental illness
Annual economic costs of mental health problems in England were estimated at £77.4 billion in 2003, rising to £105.2 billion in 2009/2010 Mental illness costs the NHS and local authorities £22.5 billion a year; lost earnings cost the economy a further £26.1 billion. In 2008 this represented 5.3% of gross domestic product and is predicted to double to 10.1% of gross domestic product in 2026.
Inequalities in mental health
Contribution to wider health inequalities. People with mental health problems are also likely to have a poor diet, take less exercise, smoke more, and misuse drugs and alcohol.
Inequalities for those with serious mental illness. People with a diagnosis of serious mental illness die on average 25 years earlier than the general population, largely because of physical health problems. Depression at age 65 is linked with a 70% increased risk of dying early.

Source: adapted from the International School for Communities, Rights and Inclusion and the University of Central Lancashire (2010).

Anticipated upward trends in the number of people with dementia will have to lead to substantial increases in health and social care spending unless provision is altered or there are major breakthroughs in prevention or disease course (Comas-Herrera *et al.*, 2007). One final driver for research and development of new methods to assist in the care of people with dementia is the relative decline in the numbers of people available to care for the older population. As the balance shifts towards the older population, there will be fewer and fewer people under the age of 60 available to care for the older person.

People over the age of 85 are now the fastest-growing demographic group in the UK. The Office for National Statistics estimates there are currently 1.5 million people in the UK over the age of 85; by 2050 this will have grown to 5 million. Age UK's report *Improving Later Life: Understanding the Oldest Old* (2013) brought together international expert opinion to identify the trends, challenges and opportunities presented by this diverse group of people. That report provided evidence of a relationship between levels of physical and mental activity throughout a lifetime and incidence of frailty and poor health in later life. The research found that most 85-year-olds have between three and six long-term conditions, yet the majority rate their health and quality of life as good. For these frail older people, the report found there to be significant health benefits to tailored exercise and physical activity, which led to improvements in participants' cardiovascular fitness, muscle strength and balance. This exercise didn't just benefit participants' physical wellbeing; mood and cognitive functions also received a boost. Finally, the research showed that older people who do not smoke, who are more physically fit and active, and who are generally healthier tend to have better thinking skills. **(It has increasingly been recognised that leisure activities are important for living well with dementia, and these are considered in Chapter 7.)**

This research adds to a growing awareness that social relationships are just as important as not smoking, exercising and having a healthy diet in maintaining physical and mental health and determining a longer life. Social loneliness can speed up cognitive decline and memory problems, and for individuals with dementia in particular it is important for people to maintain friendships. The growing awareness of the impact of loneliness has indeed been a substantial advance in health policy (see, for example, Tomlinson, 2013). Finally, people in late old age reported that a self-deprecating sense of humour, optimism, adaptability and a feisty sense of independence helped them to tackle the challenges thrown up by this stage of life.

Sharon Allen, chief executive of Skills for Care, writing in the *Guardian* on 14 March 2013, observed the following:

> The indirect effects of spending on goods and services provided by suppliers to our sector [social care] plus the induced effect of the wages being spent by workers in our sector contributes a further spend of £22.4bn. Much of that figure will be spent through local suppliers with the social care setting being the hub of a myriad of services.

These figures are a powerful argument for seeing adult social care providers as not only as players in the lives of their communities, but also as key contributors to the prosperity of these same communities.

When we consider the economic impact across the sector's workforce, throughout the supply chain and as a result of workers' spending, the adult social care sector supports a total of 2.8m full-time equivalent jobs.

> We also know that the ageing population in England means that the range and scale of services offered by the adult social care sector needs to be expanded in future, to keep up with demand.

THE WORLD'S ECONOMY AND DEMENTIA OF THE ALZHEIMER TYPE

Organisation for Economic Co-operation and Development (2011) data suggest that in 2009 the proportion of the gross domestic product spent on healthcare varied between 6.4% in Mexico and 17.4% in the United States, with the UK at 9.8% and Germany, Switzerland and Canada around 11%. These are considerable amounts of money and they are growing, and in many cases, exemplified by the United States, growing fast.

Dementia is exemplary of such an illness and public health challenge. The estimated annual incidence (rate of developing disease in one year) of dementia of the Alzheimer type (DAT), at the time of writing, appears to increase dramatically with age, from approximately 53 new cases per 1,000 people age 65 to 74, to 170 new cases per 1,000 people age 75 to 84, to 231 new cases per 1,000 people age 85 and older (the 'oldest-old') (Alzheimer's Association, 2013). In the UK and Europe the numbers with dementia are set to double in the next generation, with no likelihood that the disability and costs inherent in dementia will do anything other than continue.

Importantly, however, this is not just 'a First World problem'. The same trend is happening worldwide. In an attempt to measure the current and future burden of disease, Alzheimer's Disease International (ADI), the international umbrella group for national Alzheimer's societies commissioned the World Alzheimer Reports of 2009 and 2011 (ADI, 2009, 2011). First, data on the epidemiology of dementia are systematically reviewed to generate an estimate of the numbers with the illness and likely growth in the next decades. Second, the economic impacts of dementia are subject to similar review. Their best estimate is that dementia currently affects 35.6 million people, 0.5% of the global population, with the numbers set to double in the next 20 years. In the 2010 report (ADI, 2010), ADI estimate the global economic impact of dementias to be US$604 billion. The report illustrates this in terms of comparisons with the turnover of companies in that year. If this level of cost were income, this would make dementia the world's largest company by turnover, bigger than Walmart and ExxonMobil. If dementia were a company it would be the world's eighteenth largest economy.

Domestically, the National Audit Office's report on the value for money of this high spending on dementia was called *Improving Services and Support for People with Dementia* (NAO, 2007). The National Audit Office is the external auditor of UK government spending.

That report was profoundly critical of the quality of care received by people with dementia and their families, with findings including:

- too few people being diagnosed or being diagnosed early enough
- early diagnosis and intervention needed to improve quality of life
- GP confidence in spotting the symptoms of dementia poor
- deficiencies in caregiver support
- services not currently delivering value for money to taxpayers or people with dementia and their families
- services in the community, care homes and at the end of life not delivering consistently or cost-effectively against the objective of supporting people to live independently
- the need for a *'spend to save'* approach, with upfront investment in services, for early diagnosis and intervention and improved specialist services, community services and in general hospitals resulting in long-term cost savings from prevention of transition into care homes and decreased length of hospital stay.

Contrary to popular social perception, there is a very great deal that can be done to help people with dementia (NICE–SCIE, 2006; ADI, 2011). The problem as detailed later in the book with respect to the UK and confirmed internationally by the 2011 World Alzheimer Report is that services need to be re-engineered so that dementia is diagnosed in a timely fashion. The consequence of this is potentially a win-win scenario where persons with dementia and their family caregivers can receive the treatment, care and support following diagnosis that will enable them to live as well as possible with dementia, but also where harms and costs are prevented and contained at a societal level.

Memory services are designed to enable early intervention in dementia to address the fact that only a third of people with dementia receive a formal diagnosis or have contact with specialist services at any time in their illness. Banerjee and Wittenberg (2009) modelled the impact of national provision of memory services in preventing admissions to care homes. They estimated the overall savings to society including savings accruing to public funds and private individuals. The savings increase as the numbers of people prevented from entering care homes increases over a 10-year period. Total annual savings to society from a 6%, 10% and 20% reduction in the numbers of people with dementia entering care homes would amount to £150 million, £245 million and £490 million, respectively, by year 10 from the nationwide introduction of the early diagnosis and intervention service.

IMPORTANT COST-EFFECTIVE INTERVENTIONS

Knapp, Iemmi and Romeo (2012) famously reviewed the evidence on the *cost-effectiveness* of prevention, care and treatment strategies in relation to dementia. They identified 56 literature reviews and 29 single studies offering economic evidence on dementia care. There is more cost-effectiveness evidence on pharmacological therapies than other interventions. Acetylcholinesterase inhibitors for mild to moderate disease and memantine for moderate to severe disease were found to be cost-effective. Regarding non-pharmacological treatments, cognitive stimulation therapy, tailored activity programme and occupational therapy were found to be more cost-effective than usual care. There was some evidence to suggest that respite care in day settings and psychosocial interventions for carers could be cost-effective. Coordinated care management and personal budgets held by carers have also demonstrated cost-effectiveness in some studies.

Earlier reviews had reached slightly different conclusions. For instance, the literature review underpinning the 2006 National Institute for Health and Clinical Excellence guideline was unable to reach a conclusion on the cost-effectiveness of acetylcholinesterase inhibitors for mild to moderate **dementia of the Alzheimer type** or memantine for severe **dementia of the Alzheimer type** (Loveman *et al.*, 2006). The literature review by the Belgian Health Care Knowledge Centre (Hulstaert *et al.*, 2009) was similarly cautious because of the quality of available studies. Hulstaert and colleagues also highlighted that the difference in outcome and cost measures across studies made it difficult to pool evidence. They also made the well-known point that it is difficult to generalise the cost-effectiveness results of a study conducted in one country to the context of another. Finally, they noted the pervasive lack of long-term data. Geldmacher (2008) highlighted these same weaknesses in a brief review.

In terms of cost-effectiveness, in its tenth year of the service's operation, its estimated cost would be £265 million (in 2007/08 prices) taking account of real rises in care costs. If quality of life is factored in, the estimated net present value over 10 years would be positive, with a gain of around 6250 quality-adjusted life years (QALYs) in the tenth year, where a QALY is valued at £40 000, or 12 500 QALYS if a QALY is valued at £20 000. A gain of 12 500 QALYS would amount to only around 0.02 QALYs per person-year. These relative small improvements seem very likely to be achievable with ease in view of the rise of 4% achieved in the pilot of the Croydon Memory Service (Banerjee *et al.*, 2007). This intervention would therefore meet stringent accepted definitions of cost-effectiveness (NICE, 2004; Rawlins and Culyer, 2004). Two other cost-benefit analyses provide confirmatory evidence of the potential economic benefits associated with earlier diagnosis and intervention. Both analyses are based on screening programmes in primary care, with savings estimated of a similar order of magnitude at US$4000 and US$7700 per person (Getsios *et al.*, 2012; Weimer and Sager, 2009).

Cognitive stimulation therapy

Cognitive stimulation therapy offers 'activities involving cognitive processing; usually in a social context and often group-based, with an emphasis on enjoyment of activities' (NICE–SCIE, 2006). **Cognitive stimulation therapy** has been shown to be effective as primary prevention for older people with good cognitive functioning and as secondary prevention for older people with mild to moderate dementia (Medical Advisory Secretariat, 2008).

Occupational therapy

A randomised controlled study in the Netherlands found that **occupational therapy** at home for community-dwelling people with mild to moderate dementia was not only cost-effective but also cost saving when compared with usual care (Graff *et al.*, 2008). The study found that cost savings mainly accrued as a result of reductions in informal care and that occupational therapy 'yielded significant and clinically relevant improvements in daily functioning in patients and sense of competence in carers' (Graff *et al.*, 2008). The study has limitations: like many studies in this area, it was not possible to make it double blind, the follow-up period was short (3 months) and there were questions about representativeness of study participants.

INTERVENTIONS TARGETED ON CARERS

Given the key rôle that unpaid family and other carers play in supporting people with dementia, a breakdown in that relationship can often lead to short- or long-term admission into a care home or hospital, both of which generate high costs for funding bodies, the family or the person with dementia themselves.

Psycho-educational support

The Belgian Health Care Knowledge Centre identified only two literature reviews on cost-effectiveness of caregiver support (Hulstaert *et al.*, 2009).

The first was produced by the Swedish Council on Technology Assessment in Health Care and based on one short-term study and two long-term economic models of non-pharmaceutical interventions for carers (Knapp, Iemmi and Romeo, 2012). Support was broadly defined as programmes of counselling, education, emotional support and contact provided to carers. No significant change in cost or outcomes was reported when comparison was made with standard care.

The second review was produced by the National Institute for Health and

Clinical Excellence in collaboration with Social Care Institute for Excellence: it reached no conclusion on the cost-effectiveness of interventions for caregivers of individuals with dementia in comparison with usual care because of the scarcity of evidence and the heterogeneity of the five available economic evaluations (NICE–SCIE, 2006).

Psychosocial intervention

A quasi-experimental study of a psychosocial intervention for family carers in Sweden found that counselling sessions and conversation groups resulted in significant delays in nursing home placements for people with dementia when compared with standard care arrangements (Andren and Elmstahl, 2008).

A randomised trial was conducted in the United States, evaluating a multi-component intervention that included 'modules focusing on information, safety, caregiver health and wellbeing, and behaviour management for the care recipient' (Nichols *et al.*, 2008). Twelve individual sessions were delivered in the caregivers' home (nine sessions) and through telephone (three sessions) and supplemented by five telephone-administered support group sessions of five or six carers. The study highlighted a significant difference in caregiving hours, each additional hour of care-free time for carers costing just under US$5 per day or an extra US$893 over the 6-month period. However, the authors highlighted the short duration of their study (6 months) compared with the Brodaty and Peters (1991) study in Australia that demonstrated cost savings over 39 months from a multi-component residential training programme for carers.

THE ECONOMIC CASE FOR ASSISTIVE TECHNOLOGY

Many factors are combining to suggest that the adaptation of the home and provision of assistive technology (AT) are becoming increasingly important issues. Coupled with the incentives arising from the increasing costs of older people's care, research shows that the majority of older people wish to stay in their own homes, not least those who live alone and with chronic illness (Cowan and Turner-Smith, 1999; Tinker and Lansley, 2005).

It is important to remember that not all people with dementia are old. However, older people, some of whom are very old, display a readiness to use new technology if it addresses their needs. The Royal Commission on Long Term Care (Cowan and Turner-Smith, 1999; Tinker and Lansley, 2005) highlighted the rôle of adaptations and AT in enabling people to remain in their own home, and policy documents have increasingly emphasised this fact (e.g. Audit Commission, 2002).

UK research into well-established adaptations such as stairlifts, level-access showers and door-entry phones reports substantial consumer satisfaction (Heywood, 2005). Newer developments in alarm technology are mostly confined to a minority of older people and 'smart housing' developments have only reached an experimental stage (Pragnell, Spence and Moore, 2000). There has been little systematic research into the implications of a more pronounced policy focus in terms of feasibility and cost.

The scope for an individual older person to remain in his or her own home depends on many issues, but the most relevant are concerned with the following:

- extent of the person's capacities, his or her needs and his or her view of those needs
- how far these needs can be met through adapting the home and providing AT and other specialist equipment, and the cost
- availability of formal and informal care.

Home adaptations (environmental improvements) and AT provision are an increasingly attractive means of helping older people to maintain their independence and enhancing their quality of life. Although it is widely held that developments in AT will be capable of widespread adoption, will address consumer needs and may yield expenditure savings in health and social care, there has been little systematic research into the feasibility and cost of pursuing such a policy (e.g. Lansley, McCreadie and Tinker, 2004).

Lansley, McCreadie and Tinker (2004) completed and published detailed design studies to benchmark the adaptability of 82 properties against the needs of seven notional users, in the social rented housing sector. The adaptability of properties varies according to many design factors and the needs of occupiers. The most adaptable properties were ground-floor flats and bungalows; the least were houses, maisonettes and flats in converted houses. Purpose-built sheltered properties were generally more adaptable than corresponding mainstream properties, but the opposite was the case for bungalows. Adaptations and AT can substitute for and supplement formal care, and in most cases the initial investment in adaptations and AT is recouped through subsequently lower care costs within the average life expectancy of a user.

Lansley, McCreadie and Tinker (2004) concluded that increasing the input of adaptations and AT leads to savings, which are sometimes significant. In terms of practice, the successful achievement of this desirable outcome depends on the sensitive specification of care, and adaptations and AT requirements arising from a user's needs and ensuring that these are appropriately matched to the user's home and his or her individual preferences. Of course, properties vary greatly. Some can be very easy to adapt for all users, resulting in significant savings, whereas others can be difficult to adapt for most users and yield no saving, although adaptation may still be worthwhile through supporting the independence of the user. Given this, adaptations and AT can both enhance quality of life and do this in a cost-effective way. The findings suggest that adapting the homes of older people and providing AT 'pays for itself'.

In another study, Lansley and colleagues (Lansley *et al.*, 2004) reviewed a diverse range of existing publications, technical literature, policy documents, legislation and regulations relating to older people, health, housing provision, adaptations and AT. They found that the industry could make an important contribution to improving the quality of life of older people. The market for adaptations, which is already strong, will continue to develop in response to both demographic trends and the rising expectations of older people and society, and will be given a further impetus by the development of cheap and reliable smart home technologies. However, it is a challenging market, and one that relies on approaches to design and redesign of homes in a manner sensitive to the individual's needs as well as to the constraints and possibilities offered by a property, where site work has to be very well organised and sympathetic to the user – indeed, where good customer relationships are at a premium – and yet offer services that are clearly cost-effective. More important, the type of adaptation service implied in this paper is that where timeliness not only should bear heavily on developing a suitable business approach but also is critical to the quality of the lives of those who could benefit from it.

In summary, appropriately selected assistive technologies can lead to important improvements in independence and potential savings in formal care services. This research may lead to a more informed choice by organisations when they are making decisions about both the current and the future needs of their older tenants (Tinker and Lansley, 2005).

CONCLUSION

Forecasting and budgeting for how much should be put aside for effective care in the future is clearly unpredictable, even factoring in prevalence estimates and the anticipated cost of technological or pharmacological interventions. Therefore, there is considerable inbuilt uncertainty in information around which to build an economics of living well with dementia, and, indeed, the 'bounded rationality' of strategy formation for managers in this jurisdiction and beyond is full of a plethora of variables. Add on top of this a debate about the extent society should actively 'seek out' a diagnosis of dementia and you can see a narrative developing with considerable professional, moral and resource allocation implications. The following chapter (**Chapter 5**) focuses on 'screening' for dementia, and how the discussion of that has been conducted thus far in this jurisdiction.

REFERENCES

Age UK (2013) *Improving Later Life: Understanding the Oldest Old.* London: Age UK, available at: www.ageuk.org.uk/Documents/EN-GB/For-professionals/Research/Improving%20 Later%20Life%202%20WEB.pdf?dtrk=true

Allen, S. (2013) Adult social care worth £43bn to English economy, survey shows, *Guardian*, 14 March, available at: www.guardian.co.uk/social-care-network/2013/mar/14/adult-social-care-worth-43bn

Alzheimer's Association (2013) '2013 Alzheimer's disease: facts and figures', available at: www.alz.org/downloads/facts_figures_2013.pdf

Alzheimer's Disease International (ADI) (2009) *World Alzheimer Report 2009*. London: ADI.

Alzheimer's Disease International (ADI) (2010) *World Alzheimer Report 2010*. London: ADI.

Alzheimer's Disease International (ADI) (2011) *World Alzheimer Report 2011*. London: ADI.

Andren, S., and Elmstahl, S. (2008) Effective psychosocial intervention for family caregivers lengthens time elapsed before nursing home placement of individuals with dementia: a five-year follow-up study, *Int Psychogeriatr*, **20**(6), pp. 1177–92.

Audit Commission (2002) *Assisting Independence – Fully Equipped 2*, Audit Commission, 2002.

Banerjee, S. (2012) The macroeconomics of dementia: will the world economy get Alzheimer's disease? *Arch Med Res*, **43**(8), pp. 705–9.

Banerjee, S., Willis, R., Matthews, D., *et al.* (2007) Improving the quality of dementia care: an evaluation of the Croydon Memory Service Model, *Int J Geriatr Psychiatry*, **22**(8), pp. 782–8.

Banerjee, S., and Wittenberg, R. (2009) Clinical and cost effectiveness of services for early diagnosis and intervention in dementia, *Int J Geriatr Psychiatry*, **24**(7), pp. 748–54.

Brodaty H, and Peters K. (1991) Cost-effectiveness of a training program for dementia carers, *Int Psychogeriatr*, **3**(1): 11–22.

Comas-Herrera, A., Wittenberg, R., Pickard, L., *et al.* (2007) Cognitive impairment in older people: the implications for future demand for long-term care services and their costs, *Int J Geriatr Psychiatry*, **22**(10), pp. 1037–45.

Cowan, D., and Turner–Smith, A. (1999) The role of assistive technology in alternative models of care for older people. In: Tinker, A., *et al.* (eds.) *Alternative Models of Care for Older People: Royal Commission on Long Term Care Research Volume 2*. London: The Stationery Office. pp. 325–46.

Friedli, L., and Parsonage, M. (2007) *Mental Health Promotion: Building an Economic Case*. Belfast: Northern Ireland Association for Mental Health.

Geldmacher, D.S. (2008) Cost-effectiveness of drug therapies for Alzheimer's disease: a brief review, *Neuropsychiatr Dis Treat*, **4**(3), pp. 549–55.

Getsios, D., Blume, S., Ishak, K.J., *et al.* (2012) An economic evaluation of early assessment for Alzheimer's disease in the United Kingdom, *Alzheimers Dement*, **8**(1), pp. 22–30.

Graff, M.J., Adang, E.M., Vernooij-Dassen, M.J., *et al.* (2008) Community occupational therapy for older patients with dementia and their care givers: cost effectiveness study, *BMJ*, **336**(7636): 134–8.

Heywood, F. (2005) Adaptation: altering the house to restore the home, *Housing Studies*, **20**(4), available at: www.tandfonline.com/doi/abs/10.1080/02673030500114409#.UlUzbBY4Tww

Hulstaert F, Thiry N, Eyssen M, *et al.* (2009*) Pharmaceutical and Non-pharmaceutical Interventions for Alzheimer's Disease, a Rapid Assessment*. Brussels: Belgian Health Care Knowledge Centre.

International School for Communities, Rights and Inclusion, and University of Central

Lancashire (2010) *Commissioning Mental Wellbeing: A Leadership Brief for Boards and Senior Managers; The role of wellbeing and mental health promotion in achieving whole system improvement.* Preston, Lancashire: University of Central Lancashire, available at: www.nmhdu.org.uk/silo/files/commissioning-for-wellbeing-and-population-mental-health.pdf

Knapp, M., Iemmi, V., Romeo, R. (2012) Dementia care costs and outcomes: a systematic review, *Int J Ger Psychiatr*, **28**(6), pp. 551–561, text available at: http://eprints.lse.ac.uk/45540/1/Knapp_Dementia_care_costs.pdf

Knapp, M., Iemmi, V., and Romeo, R. (2012) Dementia care costs and outcomes: a systematic review, *Int J Geriatr Psychiatry*, Epub Aug 12.

Lansley, P., McCreadie, C., and Tinker, A. (2004) Can adapting the homes of older people and providing assistive technology pay its way? *Age Ageing*, **33**(6), pp. 571–6.

Lansley, P., McCreadie, C., Tinker, A., *et al.* (2004) Adapting the homes of older people: a case study of costs and savings, *Build Res Inf*, **32**(6), pp. 468–83.

Loveman, E., Green, C., Kirby, J., *et al.* (2006) The clinical and cost-effectiveness of donepezil, rivastigmine, galantamine and memantine for Alzheimer's disease, *Health Technol Assess*, **10**(1), pp. iii–iv, ix–xi, 1–160.

Medical Advisory Secretariat (2008) Caregiver- and patient-directed interventions for dementia: an evidence-based analysis, *Ont Health Technol Assess Ser*, **8**(4), pp. 1–98.

National Audit Office (NAO) (2007) *Improving Services and Support for People with Dementia: Report by the Comptroller and Auditor General; HC 604 Session 2006–2007.* London: The Stationery Office.

National Institute for Clinical Excellence (NICE) (2004) *National Institute for Clinical Excellence Guide to the Methods of Technology Appraisal.* London: NICE.

National Institute for Health and Clinical Excellence (NICE) and Social Care Institute for Excellence (2006) *CG42: Dementia. A NICE–SCIE Guideline on supporting people with dementia and their carers in health and social care*, available at: www.nice.org.uk/CG42

Nichols, L.O., Chang, C., Lummus, A., *et al.* (2008) The cost-effectiveness of a behavior intervention with caregivers of patients with Alzheimer's disease, *J Am Geriatr Soc*, **56**(3), pp. 413–20.

Organisation for Economic Co-operation and Development (OECD) (2011) *Health at a Glance 2011: OECD Indicators.* OECD Publishing, available at: www.oecd.org/health/health-systems/49105858.pdf

Pragnell, M., Spence, L., Moore, R. for the Joseph Rowntree Foundation (2000) *The Market Potential for Smart Homes*, available at: www.jrf.org.uk/publications/market-potential-smart-homes

Rawlins, M.D., and Culyer, A.J. (2004) National Institute for Clinical Excellence and its value judgments, *BMJ*, **329**(7459), pp. 224–7.

Tinker, A., and Lansley, P. (2005) Introducing assistive technology into the existing homes of older people: feasibility, acceptability, costs and outcome, *J Telemed Telecare*, **11**(Suppl. 1), pp. 1–3.

Tomlinson, J. (2013) *Loneliness*, available at: http://abetternhs.wordpress.com/2013/05/04/loneliness/

Weimer D.L., and Sager M.A (2009) Early identification and treatment of Alzheimer's disease: social and fiscal outcomes, *Alzheimers Dement*, **5**(3), 215–26.

A public health perspective on living well with dementia, and the debate over screening

As of 1 April 2013, dementia has become part of the 'public health health-check', and Public Health England is working very closely with NHS England. Clearly, giving somebody a 'label' of dementia, if that individual has no further benefit from such a label, is totally counterproductive. It appears that almost three-quarters of people in residential homes have dementia (Macdonald *et al.*, 2002), and yet reports still exist of individuals with dementia being 'refused' access to care homes. A correct diagnosis of dementia may allay uncertainty and allow individuals to access the appropriate services. Clinicians, patients and carers or advocates clearly must be in charge, and one of the priorities in English policy is to ensure adequate support is available.

THE IMPACT OF DEMENTIA: WHY IT IS A PUBLIC HEALTH ISSUE AT ALL

According to the UK Government website (25 March 2013), the cost of dementia is relatively enormous, and likely to get bigger.

> There are around 800,000 people with dementia in the UK, and the disease costs the economy £23 billion a year. By 2040, the number of people affected is expected to double – and the costs are likely to treble.

Dr Shekhar Saxena, Director of the World Health Organization's Department of Mental Health and Substance Abuse, and Mr Marc Wortmann, Executive Director of Alzheimer's Disease International, writing in the *Dementia: A Public*

Health Priority report published by Alzheimer's Disease International and the World Health Organization (WHO and ADI, 2012), explain categorically that **dementia is an important public health priority**.

> Dementia is seriously disabling for those who have it and is often devastating for their caregivers and families. With an increasing number of people being affected by dementia, almost everyone knows someone who has dementia or whose life has been touched by it. The number of people living with dementia worldwide is currently estimated at 35.6 million. This number will double by 2030 and more than triple by 2050.
>
> The high global prevalence, economic impact of dementia on families, caregivers and communities, and the associated stigma and social exclusion present a significant public health challenge. The global health community has recognized the need for action and to place dementia on the public health agenda.

The *Dementia: A Public Health Priority* report indeed cites that the current challenges are formidable, to improve the wellbeing of individuals with dementia and their carers.

> The challenges to governments to respond to the growing numbers of people with dementia are substantial. A broad public health approach is needed to improve the care and quality of life of people with dementia and family caregivers. The aims and objectives of the approach should either be articulated in a stand-alone dementia policy or plan or be integrated into existing health, mental health or old-age policies and plans. Some high-income countries have launched policies, plans, strategies or frameworks to respond to the impact of dementia.
>
> There are several key issues that are common to many national dementia policies and plans, and these may be necessary to ensure that needs are addressed in an effective and sustainable manner. These include: scoping the problem; involving all the relevant stakeholders, including civil society groups; identifying priority areas for action; implementing the policy and plan; committing resources; having intersectoral collaboration; developing a time frame; and monitoring and evaluation.
>
> The priority areas of action that need to be addressed within the policy and plan include raising awareness, timely diagnosis, commitment to good quality continuing care and services, caregiver support, workforce training, prevention and research.

As the cost of caring for the increasing number of people with dementia continues to rise, accurate estimates of dementia prevalence are needed. Recent systematic reviews of epidemiological studies have provided comprehensive estimates of dementia prevalence. Brayne and Davis (2012) previously argued that a need for standardised definitions of dementia has led to the development of diagnostic criteria that are based on clinical measures of symptoms and observations. However, even in fairly homogeneous cultural settings, these criteria had the potential to be interpreted differently by individual clinicians and researchers. Strandberg and O'Neill (2013) have latterly emphasised in the *Lancet* that designing *'multicomponent trials for dementia in predominantly older and more frail patients will clearly pose more of a challenge than single-component trials in younger and fitter patients, but it is not an insuperable task: it is also imbued with a strong moral and scientific imperative, strengthened by the observations of Brayne and Davis.'*

Ten years previously, according to the **Global Burden of Disease** estimated for the 2003 World Health Report (WHO, 2003) that dementia contributed 11.2% of years lived with disability in people aged 60 years and older – more than stroke (9.5%), musculoskeletal disorders (8.9%), cardiovascular disease (5.0%) and all forms of cancer (2.4%). The disability weight for dementia, estimated by an international and multidisciplinary expert consensus, was higher than for almost any other health condition, apart from spinal cord injury and terminal cancer. Although people with dementia are heavy consumers of health services, direct costs in developed countries arise mostly from community and residential care. It is estimated that,in the UK, 224 000 of the 461 000 elderly people with cognitive impairment live in institutions at a cost of £4.6 billion (US$8.2 billion) every year, or 0.6% of the UK gross domestic product (Comas-Herrera *et al.*, 2002). Family caregivers remain the cornerstone of support for people with dementia, experiencing substantial psychological, practical and economic strain (Schneider *et al.*, 1993; 10/66 Dementia Research Group, 2004). Dementia care is particularly time intensive, and many caregivers need to cut back on work. In the United States, the annual cost of informal care was US$18 billion per year in 1998 dollars (Langa *et al.*, 2001).

Ferri and colleagues (Ferri *et al.*, 2005) published a paper in the *Lancet* that they believed included detailed estimates that constituted the best currently available basis for policymaking, planning, and allocation of health and welfare resources. Twelve international experts were provided with a systematic review of published studies on dementia and were asked to provide prevalence estimates for every World Health Organization world region, for men and women combined, in 5-year age bands from 60 to 84 years, and for those aged 85 years and older. United Nations population estimates and projections were used to estimate numbers of people with dementia in 2001, 2020 and 2040. Evidence from well-planned, representative epidemiological surveys is scarce in many regions, but Ferri and colleagues (Ferri *et al.*, 2005) estimated that 24.3 million people have dementia today, with approximately 4.6 million new cases of dementia every year (one new case every 7 seconds). They estimated that the number of people affected will double every 20 years, to 81.1 million by 2040. They anticipated that most people with dementia live in developing countries (60% in 2001, rising to 71% by 2040). They also predicted that rates of increase will not be uniform; numbers in developed countries are forecast to increase by 100% between 2001 and 2040, but by more than 300% in India, China, and their south Asian and western Pacific neighbours.

BEHAVIOURAL AND PSYCHOLOGICAL SYMPTOMS

Behavioural and psychological symptoms (BPS) include depressive symptoms, anxiety, apathy, sleep problems, irritability, psychosis, wandering, elation and agitation. They are common in people with dementia, but they are not restricted to this group (Savva *et al.*, 2009). BPS have public policy implications, as they affect quality of life of older people and their carers, and they influence prescribing and use of services (Department of Health, 2009).

In nursing home patients with cognitive impairment, BPS were associated with the psychosocial environment, in addition to dementia type and stage and medication use (Zuidema, Koopmans and Verhey, 2007). In dementia patients, psychosis has been associated with age, illness duration and functional impairment, whereas results are weak or inconsistent for sociodemographic variables (Ropacki and Jeste, 2005). In two 'moderate quality' reviews of the older population by Huang and colleagues (Huang *et al.*, 2010), depression was reported to be common in those with poor self-rated health, disability and chronic disease, including stroke, sensory impairment, cardiac disease or chronic lung disease. Depression is more common in women, and has been associated with many risk factors, including other diseases, low social support, cognitive impairment, disability, prior depression and bereavement (e.g. Meeks *et al.*, 2011). Vink and colleagues (Vink, Aasten and Schoevers, 2008) report that health factors were less clearly related to anxiety than to depression. Psychosocial associations of other BPS have not been reviewed. Finally, Van der Linde and colleagues (Van der Linde *et al.*, 2012) recommend, on the basis of their systematic reviews on behavioural and psychological symptoms in the older or demented population, that more research is recommended on risk factors for depression and randomised controlled trials to investigate if manipulation of risk factors reduces the onset of BPS.

RISK FACTORS FOR DEMENTIA OR DEMENTIA OF THE ALZHEIMER TYPE

As reviewed by Reitz, Brayne and Mayeux (2001), various risk factors have been found to be associated with dementia and/or dementia of the Alzheimer type (DAT). Of note, many recognised vascular risk factors for ischemic heart disease and/or stroke are also risk factors for dementia. Diabetes, hypertension, smoking and obesity have all been found to increase dementia risk. Nevertheless, while vascular risk factors and cerebrovascular disease clearly underlie vascular dementia, an etiological rôle for vascular changes in amyloid-beta deposition and, hence, Alzheimer's disease remains unclear. Diets high in fish, fruit and vegetables appear high in antioxidants and polyunsaturated fatty acids, and in some observational population-based studies, people who had a high intake of vitamins E and C (both antioxidants) were less likely to show cognitive decline and had a lower DAT risk than individuals with a low intake of these vitamins (Morris *et al.*, 2002; Engelhart *et al.*, 2002; Masaki *et al.*, 2000).

The EClipSE Collaborative Members and colleagues (EClipSE Collaborative Members *et al.*, 2010) in the journal *Brain* have produced an authoritative paper on the impact of education in dementia. The potential protective rôle of education for dementia is an area of major interest. Almost all older people have some pathology in their brain at death but have not necessarily died with dementia. The authors have explored these two observations in large population-based cohort studies (Epidemiological Clinicopathological Studies in Europe, or EClipSE) in an investigation of the relationships of brain pathology at death, clinical dementia and time in education, testing the hypothesis that greater exposure to education reduces the risk of dementia. EClipSE harmonised longitudinal clinical data and neuropathology from three long-standing population-based studies that included *post-mortem* brain donation.

These three studies started, in fact, between 1985 and 1991. The number of years of education during earlier life was recorded at baseline. Incident dementia was detected through follow-up interviews, complemented by retrospective informant interviews, death certificate data and linked health/social records (dependent on study) after death. Dementia-related neuropathologies were assessed in each study in a comparable manner based on the Consortium to Establish a Registry for Alzheimer's Disease protocol. Eight hundred and seventy-two brain donors were included, of whom 56% were demented at death. Longer years in education were associated with decreased dementia risk and greater brain weight but had no relationship to neurodegenerative or vascular pathologies. The associations between neuropathological variables and clinical dementia differed according to the 'dose' of education, such that more education reduced dementia risk largely independently of severity of pathology. More education did not protect individuals from developing neurodegenerative and vascular neuropathology by the time they died but it did appear to mitigate the impact of pathology on the clinical expression of dementia before death. The findings suggest that an understanding of the mechanisms leading to functional protection in the presence of pathology may be of considerable value to society.

ENGLISH PUBLIC HEALTH STRATEGY
Health and wellbeing boards will be established as committees of upper-tier local authorities. The way they will be structured is different from previous

joint working or partnership arrangements. As well as the intention to further develop effective working between upper-tier local authorities and health partners, it is hoped there will be opportunities for greater joint working across the tiers of local government as a result of the new system. Recognising the complexity of the system will be important to ensure that it is able to function effectively. Health and wellbeing boards should not be considered islands cut off from other areas. They will need to work with other health and wellbeing boards regionally and with the national structures such as the NHS Commissioning Board and Public Health England. They will also need to build credibility and trust with local communities.

Tackling health inequalities is a major priority for health and wellbeing boards. An approach that identifies needs and assets in the Joint Strategic Needs Assessment and the Joint Health and Wellbeing Strategy may be more effective in treating or preventing illness than one that focuses solely on needs (Local Government *et al.*, 2010). Addressing the structural, material and relational barriers to individuals and communities achieving their potential will significantly contribute towards tackling health inequalities. Health and wellbeing boards can lead this. The factors driving both material and psychosocial wellbeing are not equally distributed among local populations. Some individuals or population groups live in better-quality housing than others. Some have fewer money concerns. Some have stronger support networks. Some feel valued, respected and included in a way that others do not. Some have the time and facilities they need to engage in activities to promote their wellbeing. It seems that wellbeing is highly dependent on the distribution of social, economic and environmental resources in any population. The prevalence of social or cultural discrimination (on grounds of social class, gender or ethnicity, for example) impedes equality in the distribution of social determinants of wellbeing.

Under the Health and Social Care Act 2012, responsibility for local public health is transferred from primary care trusts to local authorities and a new organisation, Public Health England. Local authorities are required jointly to appoint a director of public health with Public Health England. A key part of the director of public health's rôle is to formulate the Joint Strategic Needs Assessment and Joint Health and Wellbeing Strategy, which are legal requirements for all health and wellbeing boards.

SCREENING

Screening is a public health service in which members of a defined population, who do not necessarily perceive they are at risk of, or are already affected by, a disease or its complications, are asked a question or offered a test, to identify those individuals who are more likely to be helped than harmed by further tests or treatment to reduce the risk of a disease or its complications. It is, however, easy to lose sight of the fact the National Dementia Strategy in 2009 itself argued that, '*A strong and consistent message emerged from DH's consultation process that the diagnosis of dementia, and in particular mild dementia where the diagnosis is more complex, should be carried out by a clinician with specialist skills.*'

The idea of treating a disease earlier is easier to understand for conditions such as breast cancer, but there is as yet no 'treatment' for dementia that, say, is a 'magic bullet' for preventing dementia in all cases. The National Screening Committee criteria for appraising the viability, effectiveness and appropriateness of a screening programme are based on the criteria developed by Wilson in 1968 and address the condition, the test, the treatment and the screening programme (Wilson and Jungner, 1968).

WILSON AND JUNGNER CRITERIA FOR SCREENING (WILSON AND JUNGNER, 1968)

Knowledge of disease

The condition should be important. This may mean that it is a common disease, or that it has very serious consequences, even if relatively rare. There must be a recognisable latent or early symptomatic stage. The natural course of the condition, including development from latent to declared disease, should be adequately understood, and there should be an adequate time period in which this progression from the early stages takes place.

Knowledge of test

There should be a suitable test or examination, and this test acceptable to the population. Case finding should be ideally continuous (not just a 'once and for all' project).

Treatment for disease

There should be an accepted treatment for patients with recognised disease. Facilities for diagnosis, follow-up investigation and subsequent treatment should be available. There should be an agreed policy concerning whom to treat as patients. This brings into question: who are the borderline cases? Does the treatment actually confer benefit?

Cost considerations

Costs of case finding (including diagnosis and treatment of patients diagnosed) economically should be balanced in relation to possible expenditures on medical care as a whole. This is likely to be an increasing problem, as many economies face some extent of austerity.

CURRENT UK CRITERIA FOR SCREENING

The condition

The condition should be an important health problem. The epidemiology and natural history of the condition, including development from latent to declared disease, should be adequately understood and there should be a detectable risk factor, disease marker, latent period or early symptomatic stage. All the cost-effective primary prevention interventions should have been implemented as far as practicable. If the carriers of a mutation are identified as a result of screening, the natural history of people with this status should be understood, including the psychological implications. This might be a valid approach – for example, for tau mutations in certain families of dementia of the Alzheimer type or frontotemporal dementia.

There also needs to be a practical consideration of defining the targeted population accurately – that is, there is a need to identify people most 'at risk'. Finally, members of the public should ideally be clearly informed about the possible benefits of screening, but also about the risks.

The test

There should be a simple, safe, precise and validated screening test.

By validity it is meant the test's ability to measure or discover what the investigator wants to know. The distribution of test values in the target population should be known and a suitable cut-off level defined and agreed. The test should be acceptable to the population.

There should be an agreed policy on the further diagnostic investigation of individuals with a positive test result and on the choices available to those individuals. If the test is for mutations, the criteria used to select the subset of mutations to be covered by screening, if all possible mutations are not being tested, should be clearly set out.

Validity is usually expressed in terms of *sensitivity* and *specificity*. The main concern is people who, despite having the disease, are classified as healthy by the screening test (*false negatives*) and healthy people who are classified by the screening test as diseased (*false positives*).

The treatment

There should be an effective treatment or intervention for patients identified through early detection, with evidence of early treatment, rather than late treatment, leading to better outcomes. There should be agreed evidence-based policies covering which individuals should be offered treatment and the appropriate treatment to be offered. Clinical management of the condition and patient outcomes should be optimised in all healthcare providers prior to participation in a screening programme. There should be a plan for managing and monitoring the screening programme and an agreed set of quality assurance standards. Treatments will vary across the type of dementia being treated (e.g.

copper chelation for a dementia in Wilson's disease, or anti-HIV medication in HIV dementia), but the rest of this particular section on treatment considers the most common type of dementia in the senium and presenium, dementia of the Alzheimer type.

In the case of DAT, there are legitimate concerns that the impact of cholinesterase inhibitors has been overstated. For example, in a study with large power published in the prestigious jounal *Lancet*, in a sample of 565 patients with DAT, Courtney and colleagues (Courtney *et al.*, 2004) found that donepezil is not cost-effective, with benefits below minimally relevant thresholds. The authors advised that more effective treatments than cholinesterase inhibitors are needed for Alzheimer's disease. The sample of 565 community-resident patients with mild to moderate Alzheimer's disease entered a 12-week run-in period in which they were randomly allocated donepezil (5 mg/day) or placebo. The 486 who completed this period were rerandomised to either donepezil (5 or 10 mg/day) or placebo, with double-blind treatment continuing as long as judged appropriate. Cognition averaged 0.8 MMSE (Mini-Mental State Examination) points better and functionality 1.0 Bristol Activities of Daily Living Scale points better with donepezil over the first 2 years. No significant benefits were seen with donepezil compared with placebo in institutionalisation (42% versus 44% at 3 years; $p = 0.4$) or progression of disability (58% versus 59% at 3 years; $p = 0.4$). There has never been a robust body of evidence in humans that cholinesterase inhibtors delay progression of Alzheimer's disease, and certainly no evidence at all that this evidence points to an improvement in 'many'.

Thus far, very few and not conclusive comparative clinical trials have been performed with the different cholinesterase inhibitors currently used to treat Alzheimer's disease. In fact, elegant studies in a model based on the human neuroblastoma line suggest that the cholinesterase inhibitors differ in their cellular mechanism of any neuroprotection, which may in any case be independent of cholinesterase inhibition (Arias *et al.*, 2005). The study by Aguglia and colleagues (Aguglia *et al.*, 2004) was the first study to compare the effects of the three most commonly used cholinesterase inhibitors on a handful of key measures of cognition screening and activities of daily living. Limitations included its small population size, its open-label design, and the fact that patients were randomised only after the introduction of galantamine. There were no statistically significant differences between the three drugs at 3 months. While numerical trends were observed suggesting the effect of rivastigmine > donepezil > galantamine, it is conceded larger, longer-term prospective studies are needed to confirm whether there are important differences in the long-term efficacy of the three drugs. One suspects that much longer neuroimaging results – for example, using radio-ligand binding or functional explorations – might be needed to see whether there are any meaningful protective effects on individuals treated with cholinesterase inhibitors.

The screening programme

For a reliable description of screening in general, the reader is strongly advised to refer to 'Essential Public Health' by Donaldson and Scally (2009).

Ideally, there should be evidence from high-quality randomised controlled trials that the screening programme is effective in reducing mortality or morbidity. Where screening is aimed solely at providing information to allow the person being screened to make an informed choice (e.g. Down's syndrome, cystic fibrosis carrier screening), there must be evidence from high-quality trials that the test accurately measures risk. The information that is provided about the test and its outcome must be of value and readily understood by the individual being screened.

There should be evidence that the complete screening programme (test, diagnostic procedures, treatment/intervention) is clinically, socially and ethically acceptable to health professionals and the public. The benefit from the screening programme should outweigh the physical and psychological harm (caused by the test, diagnostic procedures and treatment). The opportunity cost of the screening programme (including testing, diagnosis and treatment, administration, training and quality assurance) should be economically balanced in relation to expenditure on medical care as a whole (i.e. value for money).

Adequate staffing and facilities for testing, diagnosis, treatment and programme management should be available prior to the commencement of the screening programme. All other options for managing the condition should have been considered (e.g. improving treatment, providing other services), to ensure that no more cost-effective intervention could be introduced or current interventions increased within the resources available. Evidence-based information, explaining the consequences of testing, investigation and treatment, should be made available to potential participants to assist them in making a valid choice.

Limitations of screening

Screening can reduce the risk of developing a condition or its complications, but it cannot offer a guarantee of protection. In any screening programme, there is an irreducible minimum of false-positive and false-negative results.

Potential dangers of screening

Although drug treatment can help to improve the symptoms of dementia, the World Health Organization's document *Dementia: A Public Health Priority* states, '*No treatments are currently available to cure or even alter the progressive course of dementia*', reflecting the lack of evidence that early drug treatment alters the course of the disease (WHO, 2012). There is a danger that screening for dementia would result in patients simply being treated for longer, at extra cost to the NHS, but with no benefit to the patient, and possibly even distress. Although screening programmes may benefit populations, not all participants will benefit and some will even be harmed by participation (Raftery and Chorozoglou, 2011).

False negatives also can occur, as no test is 100% sensitive, which can then lead to false reassurance by both patients and doctors. This may even dis-suade patients from returning for future screening tests. It is well known, for example, that individuals with behavioural variant frontotemporal dementia can perform within 'normal limits' on standard screening tests (Leyton and Hodges, 2010). False positives can occur too, and some examples of this, with reference to potential screening tests, are mentioned in **Chapter 18**, the final chapter of this book. According to Tripathi and Vibha (2009), the most fre-quently observed potentially reversible conditions identified in patients with cognitive impairment or dementia are depression, adverse effects of drugs, drug or alcohol abuse, space-occupying lesions, normal pressure hydroceph-alus, and metabolic and endocrinal conditions such as hypothyroidism and nutritional conditions such as vitamin B_{12} deficiency. Depression is by far the most common of the potentially reversible conditions. These false positives can produce substantial psychological cost. Costs to society can be substantial too – for example, actual costs of equipment, services, treatment – also, the time taken off work for people to attend the screening test and for the treat-ment. Implementing screening tests may mean that funds are diverted away from other services.

CONCERNS OF GPs AT THE END OF 2012

Screening for dementia in primary care in the UK has been a 'hot potato' for several years now (Brayne, Fox and Boustani, 2007). Things, nonetheless, have come at a head with the 'Prime Minister's Dementia Challenge' with genuine concern that there may be 'mission creep' in policy (Brunet *et al.*, 2012).

A significant group of GPs in the English NHS wrote to the *BMJ* at the end of December 2012 to express concerns about the potential consequences of the recent announcement by the health secretary of a 'dementia case finding scheme'. The proposal is that doctors should 'proactively' ask patients at risk of dementia – including all those aged 75 or over – about their memory, and offer a screening test (Kmietowicz, 2012; Department of Health, 2012).

They reported a *'mission creep'* of going beyond the raising of awareness about dementia that amounts to a clear intention to screen a section of the population for the condition, without the articulation of any evidence that it fulfils the established criteria for screening. They warned that this could lead to overtreatment, harm to patients, unnecessary expense, and diversion of pre-cious resources away from other services, including support for people who are seeking help for a timely diagnosis of dementia or who have already been given a diagnosis. They argued that before any screening programme is introduced it must be shown that the benefits outweigh any potential harm (Brayne, Fox and Boustani, 2003). Screening for dementia, arguably, must be assessed in the same way as any other screening intervention.

They provided that, although they welcomed the government's emphasis in the NHS mandate on improving care of people with dementia (Department of Health, 2012) the proposal to assess a prescribed section of the population for memory problems amounted effectively to a non-evidenced population screening programme that has not been subjected to the same scrutiny as other such programmes. In fact, in June 2010 the UK National Screening Committee, whose remit is to advise the government on all screening programmes, advised very clearly that screening for Alzheimer's disease 'should not be offered' (UK National Screening Committee, 2010). The full report (Public Health Resource Unit, 2009) analysed the case for screening against the widely accepted Wilson and Jungner screening criteria published by the World Health Organization. It concluded, 'The analysis of the literature against the above criteria indicates that the implementation of an evidence based routine screening programme for Alzheimer's disease that will reduce mortality and morbidity is not yet a possibility.' However, carers and patients themselves report themselves wishing to have a diagnosis.

The GPs furthermore argued that screening, in fact, could be **unethical**:

Unlike in most other NHS screening programmes, patients are not to be invited for screening for dementia; instead healthcare professionals would have to screen opportunistically, such as when patients were admitted to hospital or visited their general practitioner. This means that patients, or their relatives or carers, would not have prior warning of the screening test or an opportunity to be informed of the potential benefits or harms of screening. The lack of provision of information and of choice to patients in this proposal are major concerns. Of course, where general practitioners or other healthcare professionals had reason to believe that the patient's symptoms might be due to dementia they could still carry out an assessment of memory and refer appropriately. However, this is very different from 'screening' asymptomatic individuals identified just by virtue of attending the surgery.

While the healthcare profession needs to work together to help reduce the stigma associated with dementia, the diagnosis remains a frightening one, and one of which the public, thanks to the success of awareness campaigns, is now very mindful. We should not underestimate the potential negative effects of such a diagnostic label.

The NHS mandate itself states, 'Dementia is the illness most feared by people in England over the age of 55.' And a recent study on the impact of a dementia diagnosis concluded, 'Being told one had dementia had a big impact on a patient's identity and often caused feelings of loss, anger, fear, and frustration.

If patients became aware that a visit to their GP could result in their being 'examined' for a diagnosis of dementia, irrespective of the reason for their attendance, there would be a very real danger that some patients might avoid seeking help from their GP when it was needed.

The lack of effective treatment for dementia is indeed a consideration, but in a wide-ranging piece by Brunet (2013) in the *Journal of Dementia Care*, Brunet also casts doubt on the often proposed reason for 'crisis prevention' as a raison d'être for early diagnosis. Brunet feels that there are often other reasons that could prevent a crisis – for example, adequate addressing of factors such as social isolation – and even many individuals with a 'label' of diagnosis of dementia can experience crises anyway.

Brunet argues, conversely, that we should encourage planning for service provision of individuals regardless of a diagnostic label anyway. He articulates a very reasonable 'alternative':

> The alternative to proactive measures to drive up diagnosis rates is not nihilism, but it does involve trusting the patient, their families and even their doctor, to decide when to seek a diagnosis. As the Nuffield Council on Bioethics (2009) concludes: 'Early diagnosis has important benefits, but not every person with dementia will find that these advantages outweigh the possible disadvantages. A timely diagnosis is one which is at the right time for the person concerned, and for their family.'
>
> There is much that can be done to improve dementia care. Access to memory clinics needs to be improved so that waiting times are brought into line with the 4–6 week maximum recommended by the Memory Service National Accreditation Programme. Care for those diagnosed needs to focus more on actual hands-on support rather than just a decision on whether or not to prescribe medication.

FURTHER DISCUSSION BETWEEN PROFESSOR BRAYNE AND PROFESSOR BURNS AND THEIR COLLEAGUES IN THE *BMJ*

Early diagnosis

The **All-Party Parliamentary Group** (2012) had recommended that public health directors across the UK should make early dementia diagnosis a priority. They recommended that improving dementia diagnosis rates should be a key priority for local directors of public health, and that the Dementia Action Alliance action group on diagnosis should spearhead the creation of a clear and consistent message on the value of diagnosis, early in and throughout the course of the illness, for members to share and communicate.

The **National Council for Palliative Care** (2012) had made clear their concerns about delayed diagnosis clear.

> Anecdotal evidence suggests that often GPs do not diagnose dementia in their patients because they feel that 'nothing can be done' to help them. This can be for a number of reasons surrounding lack of good dementia care services in the area, lack of social care funding, severity of the condition, ignorance on the part of the GP or lack of general public awareness. However, regardless of any voids in current dementia services or awareness, we believe that the failure to diagnose a person suffering with dementia is fundamentally wrong.
>
> Failure to diagnose dementia is a human rights issue. If you have an illness, do you not have a right to know? Especially when that illness has a detrimental effect on your capability to reason, make decisions and care for yourself? The issue of failing to diagnose would simply not be tolerated if we applied it to conditions such as cancer, so why do we tolerate it with dementia? Often a person can feel a great amount of distress when suffering from dementia unknowingly, and can question their relationships, morals and spirituality. To know that there is an explanation for their confusion, memory problems, balance, coordination or lack of mental capacity can often be a great comfort or relief, not only to the sufferer, but also to their family and friends.
>
> We strongly believe that every person with dementia has the right to be diagnosed and to be offered all the relevant information and help, regardless of the severity of their condition. ' to be a void in dementia services, this is not an acceptable excuse for their not to be a thorough investigation and diagnosis and not to be told that you are suffering from a neurodegenerative condition. We recommend that more is done to encourage GPs to give an early diagnosis, regardless of what help they feel they can offer the person and to encourage people to present symptoms to their GP early on. Failure to make or communicate a diagnosis also deprives people of the window of opportunity to makes plans for their future whilst they have capacity.

Reproduced with kind permission of the National Council for Palliative Care from National Council for Palliative Care (NCPC) Response, All-Party Parliamentary Group on Dementia 2012 Inquiry: Improving dementia diagnosis rates in the UK, 1 March 2012. Retrieved from www.ncpc.org.uk/sites/default/files/NCPC_response_APPG_Dementia_diagnosis_inquiry.pdf, December 2013.

A striking concern from Professor Carol Brayne, Chair of Public Health at the University of Cambridge, and colleagues (Brayne *et al.*, 2012) was about the language of the discourse:

> Our first point is around the use of the term 'early' diagnosis, which appears to have entered public discourse without discussion of what it actually means. The prevailing view from many patients, their representatives and professionals is that a diagnosis should be made

as soon as possible in every individual case. This is understandably driven by personal and professional experiences of delays in access to diagnosis and appropriate support. But timely diagnosis for that person in their particular setting is undeniably current good clinical practice, if not universally available. This 'timely' diagnosis is not necessarily the same as 'early'. There is currently no high quality evidence that diagnosis before the usual point of clinical presentation leads to long term improvements for people with dementia and their families. Early diagnosis is driven by the ambition to 'close' the gap between those people estimated to have dementia without a diagnosis and those in contact with services who have a diagnosis. This has implicit acceptance that all these people would benefit from earliest possible diagnosis. The Nuffield Bioethics Report from 2009 provides a useful moral argument in this area; the report stated that there is a 'distinction between early and timely diagnosis' and that if a person's wellbeing is not enhanced by receiving a diagnosis, it should not be forced upon them.

Reproduced from Brayne, C., Bayer, A., Boustani, M., *et al.* (2013) Rapid response to 'There is no evidence base for proposed dementia screening' (27 February 2013): 'A rallying call for an evidence based approach to dementia and related policy development', available at: www.bmj.com/content/345/bmj. e8588/rr/633370 with permission from Prof Brayne (and the BMJ Publishing Group Ltd).

Professor Alistair Burns and colleagues (Burns *et al.*, 2013) responded appropriately, arguing that *'timely* diagnosis' was a better way of describing the situation than 'early diagnosis'. This emphasises a person-centred approach (*see* **next chapter**), and not making the diagnosis at a particular stage arbitrarily. This precise use of language is later resumed as a theme in **Chapter 18**, the final chapter.

The issue of the terminology of early or timely diagnosis of dementia is important. Most people now agree that 'timely' is a better way of describing what is trying to be achieved – it suggests a person centred approach, does not tie the diagnosis to any particular disease stage and encompasses the fact that the person (and/or their families and carers) will gain benefit from the process. Family carers cite lack of diagnosis as the greatest unmet need. The need for people to be able to ask about memory concerns is enshrined in the All Party Parliamentary Group's recent report on Unlocking Diagnosis (www.alzheimers.org.uk/appg). We would extend this to say specifically that there needs to be support after diagnosis, an aspiration captured in the NHS Mandate (http://mandate.dh.gov.uk) which sets out the objectives for the NHS.

Reproduced from Burns, A., Alessi, C., Banerjee, S., *et al.* (2013) A rallying call for an evidence based approach to dementia and related policy development. Rapid response to 'There is no evidence base for proposed dementia screening' (21 March 2013), available at: www.bmj.com/content/345/bmj. e8588?tab=responses, with permission from Prof Burns (and the BMJ Publishing Group Ltd).

In fact, this language of 'timely' has been reflected in the newest version of Scotland's National Dementia Strategy (2013):

Timely diagnosis enables people to plan ahead while they still have capacity to do so and means they can get early and effective access to drug and other interventions which can sustain their cognition, mental wellbeing and quality of life.

Nonetheless, the UK Government website (2013) continues with the term 'early diagnosis', establishing the following 'targets'.

If it's diagnosed early enough, a lot can be done to help people cope with the symptoms of dementia. But at the moment, the diagnosis rate in England is only 45% – lower than Scotland and Northern Ireland.
We want to increase diagnosis rates so that they're among the best in Europe by:
- making sure that doctors give 65 to 74 year olds information about memory services as part of the NHS health check programme, and refer them for assessment if they need it (from April 2013)
- making £1 million available for innovative NHS projects to increase diagnosis rates through the Innovation Challenge Prize for Dementia (prize winners will be announced in March 2014)
- launching a new toolkit to help GPs provide better support.

Chapman and colleagues (Chapman *et al.*, 2006) argue that, to promote cognitive functioning and independence among older adults, public health interventions need to facilitate both early detection and treatment of dementia. The availability of adult day care and respite services is important in maintaining the health and quality of life of individuals caring for older adults with dementia. Recent advances in the treatment of dementia may slow the course of cognitive decline, thereby enhancing the quality of life of older individuals as well as decreasing costs associated with institutional care. Despite the growing availability of pharmacological and psychosocial interventions that are potentially helpful to people with dementia and their caregivers, the majority of older adults with dementia do not receive appropriate treatment.

Harm

A genuine concern from Professor Carol Brayne and colleagues (Brayne *et al.*, 2012) is about the potential **harm** of such an approach:

Of particular concern is the lack of acknowledgement in current policy development and implementation of potential harms of premature diagnosis. The usual argument in favour of very early diagnosis is the apparently self-evident question 'Why would you not do this?' However, there are potential adverse effects, many of which have been articulated by others (and are familiar to those who work in screening). They include: diversion of resources from activities of proven value; misclassification of substantial numbers of people through application of screening tests which cannot have 100% sensitivity and 100% specificity; introduction of testing in unprepared settings to people – who do not fully understand what screening means, have had no chance to consider the benefits or harms of being tested, which must include possibility of overdiagnosis and overtreatment (viz. the breast cancer screening discussions), and have not therefore had the opportunity to give informed consent; raising expectations of support and services that cannot be provided and may be of limited benefit; and raising further the levels of anxiety in the population, particularly among older people.

Reproduced from Brayne, C., Bayer, A., Boustani, M., *et al.* (2013) Rapid response to 'There is no evidence base for proposed dementia screening' (27 February 2013): 'A rallying call for an evidence based approach to dementia and related policy development', available at: www.bmj.com/content/345/bmj. e8588/rr/633370 with permission from Prof Brayne (and the BMJ Publishing Group Ltd).

However, critically, they did not appear to rule out a rôle for 'screening' in the future:

This not to say that screening for dementia in one or more guises should not be introduced at some point in the future. Our concern is that we do not know and will not know what is appropriate and better than current practice unless these changes are made within an evaluative and research based approach. To address the current gaps in knowledge requires rigorous research of different types: formal trials, experimental roll out with evaluation, implementation research and qualitative research, all of which play unique and complementary roles and which must be integrated to create a sound evidence base.

Reproduced from Brayne, C., Bayer, A., Boustani, M., *et al.* (2013) Rapid response to 'There is no evidence base for proposed dementia screening' (27 February 2013): 'A rallying call for an evidence based approach to dementia and related policy development', available at: www.bmj.com/content/345/bmj. e8588/rr/633370 with permission from Prof Brayne (and the BMJ Publishing Group Ltd).

Professor Alistair Burns and colleagues (Burns *et al.*, 2013), indeed, argued firstly that the intention was not to introduce screening, or to impose a diagnosis on individuals:

However, the lack of evidence does reflect the decision not to support population screening for dementia, something which is plainly, according to any definition of population screening, not being advocated. It is misleading to suggest that what is being consulted upon is tantamount to a diagnosis being 'forced' on people and absolute respect must be given to anyone not wishing to know. We must be aware of the dangers of being overtaken by events and the availability of online tests, the success of awareness campaigns and the interest in dementia means that the public are much more informed and willing to talk about dementia and symptoms of memory loss.

Reproduced from Burns, A., Alessi, C., Banerjee, S., *et al.* (2013) A rallying call for an evidence based approach to dementia and related policy development. Rapid response to 'There is no evidence base for proposed dementia screening' (21 March 2013), available at: www.bmj.com/content/345/bmj. e8588?tab=responses, with permission from Prof Burns (and the BMJ Publishing Group Ltd).

However, Professor Alistair Burns, National Clinical Lead for Dementia and Professor of Psychiatry at the University of Manchester, did clearly advocate that people could be supported appropriately, and described that there might be harm by not diagnosing individuals appropriately.

We accept that the issue of potential harm is crucial, would contend that a definitive view on this should be subject to an evidence base, and by putting clinicians in the driving seat of any clinical assessment will protect individuals against any inappropriate intervention. Of course balanced with this, is the harm done to the estimated 400,000 people with dementia who do not have a diagnosis and who could benefit from the treatment and support which is available. As a group of clinical and applied researchers we urge governments, charities, the academic community and others to be more coordinated in order to put the policy cart after the research horse. Dementia screening should neither be recommended nor routinely implemented unless and until there is robust evidence to support it. The UK can play a unique role in providing the evidence base to inform the ageing world in this area, whilst making a positive difference to the lives of individuals and their families in the future.

Reproduced from Burns, A., Alessi, C., Banerjee, S., *et al.* (2013) A rallying call for an evidence based approach to dementia and related policy development. Rapid response to 'There is no evidence base for proposed dementia screening' (21 March 2013), available at: www.bmj.com/content/345/bmj. e8588?tab=responses, with permission from Prof Burns (and the BMJ Publishing Group Ltd).

THE SCREENING 'TEST'

A **screening test** for dementia, however it is executed, is supposed to be inexpensive, easily done, and able to reliably identify those people who need further investigations for dementia. Current screening texts for dementia have been extensively reviewed elsewhere, and this remains a very intense area of work. The dementias have diverse presentations, and a screening test ideally should not 'load' too heavily on any particular structure or function of the brain overduly. Lischka and colleagues (Lischka *et al.*, 2012) recently used 10 databases in identifying relevant articles, yielding 751 papers. Of these, 12 met relevance criteria for inclusion, and screening tools were assessed for test accuracy, cognitive domain coverage, predictive ability and feasibility. Four screening tools were recommended. Addenbrooke's Cognitive Examination (ACE) was considered to be the ideal tool. A revised version of this tool is now used in clinical practice but the psychometric properties of the ACE-R remain to be established. The ACE (Mioshi *et al.*, 2006) incorporates five sub-domain scores (orientation/attention, memory, verbal fluency, language and visuospatial). Conceptually, a screening test does not have to be simply taking a history or doing a focused examination. It could conceivably be a finding on a computed tomography report, but Dr John Stevens and Professor Nick Fox (2001) from the National Hospital for Neurology and Neurosurgery have warned specifically about the problems about the visual assessment of atrophy in regard to DAT:

> The overlap with normal ageing, and the relative insensitivity of visual inspection, limit the usefulness of atrophy assessment when applied to the individual patient. The overlap with age-related atrophy is less in early onset DAT but nonetheless in the early stages of AD [Alzheimer's disease] scans are ofren reported as normal for age. The difficulties inherent in assessing atrophy have been recognized [sic] in clinical criteria which state that 'the diagnosis of PROBABLE Alzheimer's disease is supported by evidence of clinical atrophy' …. but a 'normal for age' scan is consistent with this diagnosis.

Therefore, the danger is that a diagnosis of 'incipient dementia' is made on the basis of a computed tomography scan, without referring to the history or examination of a patient, and, at worst, not even communicated to the patient him- or herself. A GP is of course is incredibly busy. It is possibly the hardest job in medicine. In asking patients in a general practice whether they are aware of memory problems, it's like to looking for any horses once they have bolted. In terms of English policy, at least an attempt to find these bolted horses is presumably welcome, given that the general impression is that we are missing many horses bolting under our very eyes.

> The question which Prof Burns proposes that doctors in passing might ask is, 'Do you think you have any problems with your memory?'

GPs consistently have warned that they are terrified about their patients being 'scared' to see their GP, in case this question pops up 'on the sly' and the possibility of dementia is raised publicly in the 'confidential' medical notes. In theory, any of the disease processes can affect any parts of the brain, affecting any number of the cognitive functions of the brain, behaviour and personality according to the precise distributed neuronal networks affected. This means that memory might not be the presenting feature of a dementia at all; it could be visuospatial difficulties or apraxia, behavioural problems or isolated problems with planning. This question of course assumes that the patient can communicate the answer, and it is possible even that the method in which the answer is executed, even if it is nothing to do with memory, reveals a substantial language impairment (e.g. the progressive primary aphasias – see Savage *et al.*, 2013). A patient with early Alzheimer's disease is very likely to report memory problems, in anterograde memory, and the purpose of a brief question of a GP in a busy clinic is to detect at an unrefined way possible glaring 'diagnoses' of Alzheimer's disease. Loss of cognitive function in the elderly population is a common condition encountered in general medical practice, and fairly precise clinical diagnosis is feasible (e.g. Knopman, Boeve and Petersen, 2003). An unfortunate theoretical problem exists that a patient does indeed have memory problems but the patient is unaware of them. In a seminal paper by Starkstein and colleagues (Starkstein *et al.*, 2006), the authors reported on how unawareness of cognitive deficits in Alzheimer's disease might be related to the severity of intellectual impairment, a phenomenon known as 'anosognosia'.

The ideal is that a patient might report memory problems, when probed, but the question suffers from a lack of specificity. In other words, all sorts of people, even if they don't have dementia, might at first answer *yes*! This inevitably will include what used to be called 'the worried well'. Real memory problems could be caused by a whole manner of other conditions, as well as dementia, such as stroke, depression or an underactive thyroid. It could conceivably be an epilepsy affecting the memory circuits, such as transient global amnesia. A mild cognitive impairment (MCI) is a clinical diagnosis in which deficits in cognitive function are evident but not of sufficient severity to warrant a diagnosis of dementia (Nelson and O'Connor, 2008). In addition to presentations featuring memory impairment, symptoms in other cognitive domains (e.g. executive function, language or visuospatial) have been identified. Indeed, in humans, heterogeneity in the decline of hippocampal-dependent episodic memory is observed during ageing, and animal models now exist for this phenomenon (Foster, 2012).

There is also a problem that individuals with a dementia syndrome sometimes do not exhibit **any** memory problems. Indeed, as reviewed by Hornberger and Piquet (2012), over the last 20 years or so, however, the clinical view has been that episodic memory processing is relatively intact in the frontotemporal dementia syndrome; but these authors also note that recent evidence questions the validity of preserved episodic memory in frontotemporal dementia, particularly in behavioural variant frontotemporal dementia, a progressive syndrome characterised in its early stages by changes in personality and behaviour, and which indeed gets confused with common adult psychiatric conditions (Pose *et al.*, 2013). It is of course theoretically possible that individuals may have a subclinical form of dementia, where there are no florid memory symptoms for example, but there is an underlying cause (e.g. Morvan's syndrome, a rare complex syndrome with antibodies to the potassium-channel gated complex producing a dementia involving cognitive problems (Loukaides *et al.*, 2012)), or a paraneoplastic limbic encephalitis producing a dementia (Gultekin *et al.*, 2010). Indeed, in the paraneoplastic dementias, mild cognitive deficits may present before a florid dementia or before the presentation even of the underlying malignancy, for which a full hunt might later then be instigated.

Full-blown screening on a national scale would fundamentally depend on finding a cheap test for finding individuals at risk of later developing the disease. Any quick question is immediately going to run into problems in that dementia is such a wide diagnostic group. Certainly, the question is not sufficient on its own. For example, in an appropriate patient, it might be sensible to ask if the patient has seen things that are not there (in the hope of identifying visual hallucinations as in diffuse Lewy body dementia, e.g. Gaig *et al.*, 2011). Even for the most common type of dementia, there is a very active debate whether there might be a reliable prodromal or preclinical phase of Alzheimer's disease, when changes are taking place even without overt symptoms. Molineuvo and colleagues (Molinuevo *et al.*, 2012), consistent with previous findings, indeed suggest that the preclinical stage is biologically active and that there may be structural changes when amyloid is starting its deposition, reflected in changes in concentrations of markers in cerebrospinal fluid or cortical thickness.

Clearly, investing a lot of time, money and effort in using such techniques currently would be considered impractical in any booming economy (which we do not have), especially given that the cost-impact implications of managing patients with dementia in the community are unclear (Brilleman *et al.*, 2013), and the very modest effects of treatments to improve memory such as the cholinesterase inhibitors have in fact been well known for some considerable time (Holden and Kelly, 2002). It might be attractive to think that MCI is a preclinical form of dementia of the Alzheimer type, but unfortunately the evidence is not there to back this claim up at present: only approximately 5%–10% and most people with MCI will not progress to dementia even after 10 years of follow-up (Mitchell and Shiri-Feshki, 2009). If one takes the point of view in that the existence of memory symptoms above a certain age might cause 'alarm bells' about the need for further investigation, such as specialist opinion about neuroimaging, cognitive psychometry, or even cerebrospinal fluid or brain biopsy (the latter conceivably in the case of cerebral vasculitis or prion disease), such an approach might be worthwhile. However, such a strategy is hugely dependent on the quality of clinicians in primary care and beyond in the NHS, where quality is not a function of economic competition. Quality of dementia care depends on a clinician's aptitude in taking a targeted history, examination, investigations and management plan.

So, to all intents and purposes, this simple question is dirt cheap, but fails somewhat on specificity and sensitivity. and it all might be pretty innocent enough, if individuals with a genuine diagnosis of dementia are able to access routes enabling them to live well through person-centred care. However, as it is presented, this is potentially a *'huge ask'* if politicians raise expectations, and do not allocate resources in primary care and specialist dementia and cognitive disorders clinics to match. While the reported underreporting of dementia in the community is not a trivial issue, the demands concerning adequate care of individuals successfully found to be identified with a dementia are likely to be substantial, and for which, curiously, no convincing impact assessment data have ever been published. Diagnosing lots of dementia might become somebody else's problem for management if there are inadequate resources; and by that stage this current government and key personnel might have even moved on, of course.

'OPPORTUNISTIC SCREENING' AND PRIMARY CARE INVOLVEMENT

In guidance from the NHS Commissioning Board from 2013, *Enhanced Service Specification: Facilitating Timely Diagnosis and Support for People with Dementia*, following changes to the GP contract for 2013/14, the Secretary of State for Health directed the NHS Commissioning Board to establish an **enhanced service** to provide timely diagnosis and support for patients known to be at risk of dementia. The original design of this policy was widely considered to have complicated ethical and professional concerns.

'Improving the diagnosis and care of patients with dementia' was therefore prioritised by the Department of Health through its mandate to the NHS Commissioning Board and by the NHS Commissioning Board through its planning guidance for clinical commissioning groups. It was argued that a 'system-wide integrated approach' is required to enable patients with dementia and their families to receive a timely diagnosis and to access appropriate treatment, care and support.

According to their specification, national action to support local system-wide improvements include:

- a national dementia calculator, which has been made available to support GP practices to understand prevalence of dementia in their registered population
- the national Commissioning for Quality and Innovation scheme, which

provides incentives for providers of healthcare services commissioned through the NHS Standard Contract (including hospital, community and mental health services) to improve identification, prompt referral on to specialist services for diagnosis and support, and improved dementia care

- commissioning guidance for memory assessment services currently being produced by the Royal College of Physicians.

This enhanced service is designed to support GP practices in contributing to these system wide improvements by supporting timely diagnosis, supporting individuals and their carers, and supporting integrated working with health and social care partners. For the purposes of this enhanced service, an opportunistic offer means an offer made during a routine consultation with a patient identified as at risk and where the attending practitioner considers it appropriate to make such an offer. Once an offer has been made there is no requirement to make a further offer during any future attendance.

For the purposes of this enhanced service, 'at-risk' patients are:

- patients aged 60 and over with cardiovascular disease, stroke, peripheral vascular disease or diabetes
- patients aged 40 and over with Down's syndrome
- other patients aged 50 and over with learning disabilities
- patients with long-term neurological conditions that have a known neuro-degenerative element (e.g. Parkinson's disease).

These assessments would be in addition to other opportunistic investigations carried out by the GP practice (e.g. anyone presenting raising a memory concern). The assessment for dementia offered to at-risk patients can only be undertaken following establishing patient consent to an enquiry about their memory. The assessment for dementia offered to consenting at-risk patients shall be undertaken following initial questioning (through appropriate means) to establish whether there are any concerns about the attending patient's memory (GP, family member, the person themselves).

Therefore, in this new policy scheme, GPs are encouraged to make opportunistic offers of dementia assessment where the attending practitioner considers it appropriate to make such an offer. The NHS England specification for the dementia-enhanced service notes that a system-wide approach is required to enable patients with dementia to access appropriate treatment. The British Medical Association has warned government of the risk of increasing dementia diagnosis without the requisite support services available locally (BMA, 2013). Other views are that the Quality and Outcomes Framework component has been 'overplayed', and the 'dementia prevalence calculator' is not particularly helpful for individual clinical care

Finally, the issue of 'opportunistic screening' in primary care throws up the accusation made by some people who have influence and power in policy circles that GPs are somehow 'colluding' in not disclosing the diagnosis to patients, and this accusation is a tricky one. Patients who may be candidates to receive a 'timely' diagnosis may or may not have legal capacity at the time at which the diagnosis is given, but there is no objective evidence, currently, that GPs as a professional body are withholding this information *en masse*. The general professional regulatory guidance has been that patients' views should be respected, if a patient does not wish to know in detail about their condition, but information should be given in relation to any proposed treatment. Patients may still wish to decline this information, but this is supposed to be recorded in the medical notes, and the risks explained concerning non-disclosure of this information should be explained. However, the precise relationship between autonomy, capacity, consent, beneficence and non-maleficence needs careful consideration on legal/regulatory and ethical dimensions, in any individual, and appropriate professional bodies can be asked for advice if necessary. Notwithstanding, the idea that GPs are 'colluding' in withholding the diagnosis shows a failure to appreciate the professional duties of doctors in this jurisdiction, and does not particularly take the discussion forward in a constructive way.

THE GROWING IMPORTANCE OF 'WELLBEING'

Instead of giving false promises about neuropharmacological agents that have been evidenced to have modest effects, it is more justifiable to focus resources fulfilling Bentham's famous axiom, 'it is the greatest happiness of the greatest number that is the measure of right and wrong' (Bentham, 1776). 'Wellbeing' is a term that has cropped up increasingly frequently over recent years, in politicians' speeches, in policy documents, in mental and physical health strategies and in the names of local strategic partnership subgroups all over England. It was also given prominence in legislation: the **Local Government Act** 2000 granted local authorities the power to promote social, economic and environmental wellbeing in their areas.

In view of this it is worth recalling the various existing policy definitions of wellbeing to inform how it can be defined and improved upon in a local government context. They share some key characteristics.

- Wellbeing is **about how people experience their own lives**, so, for example, people must feel able to achieve things or feel they have a sense of purpose to have wellbeing.
- Wellbeing is **more than the absence of problems or illness**. This requires a shift in focus from what can go wrong in people's lives to what makes them go well.
- Wellbeing is **about the personal and the social**, so improving the wellbeing of local populations needs to involve a strengthening of local social connections, support networks and the sense of belonging that make up the social fabric of communities.

- **Wellbeing is more than happiness.** The aim of local government, therefore, should not be to set out to make people happy, but, rather, to create the conditions that enable citizens and communities to do well in life, to flourish.

COMMUNICATING THE PUBLIC HEALTH MESSAGE: AVOIDING 'MORAL PANIC'

The whole use of language surrounding the diagnosis of dementia matters, not least in the general context of how risk is communicated with the general public. A further problem is that medical terms often get adopted by more general media such as tabloids in a fairly non-discriminatory way. Take for example, the formal definition of an '**epidemic**':

> The occurrence in a community or region of cases of an illness, specific health-related behavior, or other health-related events clearly in excess of normal expectancy. (Greenland, Last and Porta, 2008)

According to Professor Paradis at Stanford University (2012), presented later by Paradis and colleagues (Paradis *et al.*, 2012) in a public presentation, there has been an apparent '**epidemic of epidemics**', with no apparent restriction on the type of disease, on frequency or rates of affliction; there was no growth or contagion threshold. In the forthcoming decades, it is predicted that large numbers of people will enter the ages when the incidence rates of forms of dementia are the highest. People 60 years and over make up the most rapidly expanding segment of the population: in the year 2000, there were over 600 million persons aged 60 years or over worldwide, making up just over 10% of the world population, and, by the year 2050 it is estimated that this figure will have tripled to nearly 2 billion older persons, making up 22% of the world population (United Nations, 2007).

Stephan and Brayne (2008) from the University of Cambridge state specifically that, 'this ageing **epidemic**, while once limited to developed countries, is expected to become more marked in developing countries.' Supporting this, Sosa-Ortiz, Acosta-Castillo, and Prince (2012) propose that 'global population aging has been one of the defining processes of the 20th century, with profound economic, political and social consequences. It is driving the current **epidemic of dementia**, both in terms of its extent and global distribution.' It could be that stakeholders in the research community, as Paradis (2011) proposes, are effectively competing for 'social capital' (*after* Bourdieu, 1986). Bourdieu's definition of 'capital' extends far beyond the notion of material assets to capital that may be social, cultural or symbolic (Bourdieu, 1986, cited in Navarro, 2006).

In professional circles, the diagnosis of dementia enmeshes a plethora of ethical issues, as reviewed elegantly by Strech and colleagues (Strech *et al.*, 2013):

- risk of making a diagnosis too early or too late because of reasons related to differences in age- or gender-related disease frequencies
- risk of making inappropriate diagnoses related to varying definitions of MCI
- underestimation of the relatives' experiences and assessments of the person with dementia
- adequate point of making a diagnosis
- risk of disavowing signs of illness and disregarding advanced planning
- respecting psychological burdens in breaking bad news
- underestimation of the relatives' experiences and assessments of the person with dementia reasonableness of treatment indications
- overestimation of the effects of current pharmaceutical treatment options
- considering challenges in balancing benefits and harms (side effects)
- not considering information from the patient's relatives
- adequate appreciation of the patient
- insufficient consideration of the patient as a person
- insufficient consideration of existing preferences of the patient
- problems concerning understanding and handling of patient autonomy.

A correct early diagnosis may be clarifying, and appreciated by patients even without disease-modifying treatment, and a diagnosis could be valuable since it allows informed planning for the future (Kaduszkiewicz, Bachmann and van den Bussche, 2008). A 'positive test result' indicating DAT will almost certainly lead to extended follow-up, and that individual being plugged into the system. However, at worst, the diagnosis could lead to stigmatisation resulting in feelings of hopelessness, agony and despair. The rôle of the clinician and support, such as family members, relatives, friends and other members of the 'dementia-friendly community', will be to mitigate against this risk. From a legal perspective, a test result indicating DAT could potentially affect insurance premiums and the right for an individual to hold a driver's licence, depending on the jurisdiction in question. Certainly, the ethical consequences in *falsely diagnosed cases* could be grave. Furthermore, as Matthson and colleagues explore (Matthson, Brax and Zetterberg, 2008), if a false-positive diagnosis results in treatment, any harmful side effect is a serious infringement on the basic medical ethics principle of non-maleficience, accurately summarised in the Latin phrase *primum non nocere* (**'first, do not harm'**).

A salutory warning is provided by the well-documented discussions of the communication of obesity as a public health issue. The very fast increase in mass media attention to obesity in the United States and beyond seems to have many of the elements of what social scientists call a **'moral panic'**. Moral panics are typical during times of rapid social change and involve an exaggeration or fabrication of risks, the use of disaster analogies, and the projection of societal anxieties onto a stigmatised group (Cohen, 1972; Goode and Ben-Yehuda,

1994). Moral panic is a term usually used to describe media presentation of something that has happened that the public will react to in a panicky manner. Moral panic has a tendency to exaggerate statistics and to create a 'bogeyman', known as a 'folk devil' in sociological terms. In recent years moral panic and media presentation have covered a wide-ranging number of topics, from HIV/AIDS in the 1980s to immigrants into the UK in the 2000s. Moral panic goes back as far as World War I, when the wartime government used the media to portray the Germans in a certain manner in the hope of provoking a response. The conduct of the media is pivotal in all this.

Despite arguably the very weak evidence that obesity represents a health *crisis*, scientific studies and news articles alike continue to treat the population's weight gain as an 'impending disaster'. A content analysis of 221 press articles discussing scientific studies of obesity found that over half employed alarming metaphors such as 'time bomb' (Saguy and Almeling, 2005). The fundamental problem is that there is no adequate treatment for the commonest type of dementia, DAT, and yet authors still talk in a language suggesting that it is possible to treat this epidemic successfully. For example, Korczyn and Vakhapova (2007) in their article entitled, 'The prevention of the dementia epidemic', cite polio as an example of an epidemic that was successfully 'treated'.

> The last epidemic which has been fought with outstanding success is poliomyelitis. In order to win that war, the first step was to identify the cause, the polio virus. The next step, achieved within a few years, was to develop methods to cultivate the virus. Justifiably, J. Enders, T. H. Weller and F. C. Robbins were awarded the Nobel Prize in 1954 for this important discovery, which led to the development of immunization [sic] methods by A. B. Sabin and J. E. Salk.

This is nothing new. Even the Department of Health (2002) has referred to the **'obesity time bomb'**:

> The growth of overweight and obesity in the population of our country – particularly amongst children – is a major concern. It is a health time bomb with the potential to explode over the next three decades .... Unless this time bomb is defused the consequences for the population's health, the costs to the NHS and losses to the economy will be disastrous.

In a remarkable paper, Bethan Evans (2010) considered the characterisation of obesity as a 'threat to the future nation' through considering obesity as a biopolitical problem – which simultaneously addresses the individual body and the 'population' (Foucault, 1997) – and as a form of 'pre-emptive politics'.

An example of this use of language is seen in the report of Alzheimer's Disease International (ADI, 2012) on stigma in DAT. They clearly wish the reader to project to the future.

Our healthcare and financial systems are not prepared for this epidemic. Dementia is the main cause of dependency in older people and we will not have enough people to care for these large numbers of people with dementia. Globally, less than 1 in 4 people with dementia receive a formal diagnosis. Without a diagnosis, few people receive appropriate care, treatment and support.

The authors of that particular report cite numerous examples supporting their thesis that an early diagnosis is beneficial. For example, they state that Scotland's national dementia plan includes 'overcoming the fear of dementia' as one of its plan's five key goals. This plan seeks to improve access to diagnosis by providing general practitioners with information and resources. If the 'dementia epidemic' is a real one, according to Nepal and colleagues (Nepal *et al.*, 2008), policy strategies to deal with the dementia 'epidemic' could be informed in a number of ways. The prevalence depends upon interaction of age with other factors (e.g. co-morbidities, genetic or environmental factors) that in turn are subject to change. If the onset of a dementia could be postponed by modulating its risk factors, this could significantly affect its incidence (e.g. Treves and Korczyn, 2011). The need for longitudinal and population-based data that would enable analyses of resource allocation and cost implications has been identified (Wimo and Winblad, 2004). Conducting prospective intervention studies is an established approach to test alternative policy models in the field, but these studies require substantial investment in time and resources. Computer-based dynamic microsimulation models are an ideal alternative to these, as the computer simulations provide an opportunity to test a range of policy options in a virtual world in a shorter time frame.

Overall, this debate is better 'out than in', and should be conducted openly for the benefit of those individuals with dementia, and the most immediate people in their community, including partners, friends, relatives or family members. Even charities have been known to use terms such as 'epidemic' and 'time bomb' in common parlance, and the debate outline here could go some way into explaining why the word 'early' in dementia diagnosis has been replaced by 'timely' in most UK circles. As we are all relatively new to the dementia journey, some more than others, it is appropriate we stop to think before rushing at full speed into an uncontrollable situation about communication.

CONCLUSION

The current feeling is that a roll-out *'national screening programme'* for dementia would be a step too far. Dementia is a complex, heterogeneous condition, reflecting diverse aetiologies, and is not easily diagnosed in a simple clinical test in the same way ischaemic myocardial changes in the heart might be revealed by dynamic ECG changes, or troponin blood tests, for example. There is currently, however, an emerging situation where the numbers of people given an accurate diagnosis of dementia is unreasonably low, and the question is how might more individuals be diagnosed accurately, quickly and inexpensively. Producing any 'screening test' has proved to be notoriously difficult. The medications for early dementia have always been generally considered to have modest effects in rigorous placebo-controlled, double-blind trials, but some clinicians report some families who have experienced beneficial outcomes. However, an accurate diagnosis of dementia might be 'enabling rather than labelling', if an individual is able to access more services (and is not excluded from some). The patient's journey obviously must start with a diagnosis.

The following chapter (**Chapter 6**) considers what could be the next best management step – taking a whole person-centred perspective to an individual faced with a fresh diagnosis of dementia.

WEBSITES

- *Scotland's National Dementia Strategy 2013*, 3 June, available at: www.scotland.gov.uk/Resource/0042/00423472.pdf
- National Council for Palliative Care (NCPC) (2012) *National Council for Palliative Care (NCPC) response to the 'All-Party Parliamentary Group on Dementia 2012' Inquiry: Improving dementia diagnosis rates in the UK.* London: NCPC, 1 March, available at: www.ncpc.org.uk/sites/default/files/NCPC_response_APPG_Dementia_diagnosis_inquiry.pdf
- UK Government (2013) *Improving Care for People with Dementia.* 25 March, available at: www.gov.uk/government/policies/improving-care-for-people-with-dementia
- UK National Screening Committee (2010) *The UK NSC Policy on Alzheimer's Disease Screening in Adults*, available at: www.screening.nhs.uk/alzheimers
- NHS Commissioning Board (2013) *Enhanced Service Specification: Facilitating Timely Diagnosis and Support for People with Dementia*, available at: www.england.nhs.uk/wp-content/uploads/2013/03/ess-dementia.pdf
- British Medical Association (BMA) (2013) *Facilitating Timely Diagnosis and Support for People with Dementia.* London: BMA, available at: http://bma.org.uk/practical-support-at-work/contracts/gp-contract-survival-guide/survival-guide-des-dementia

REFERENCES

10/66 Dementia Research Group (2004) Care arrangements for people with dementia in developing countries, *Int J Geriatr Psychiatry*, **19**(2), pp. 170–7.

Aguglia, E., Onor, M.L., Saina, M., *et al.* (2004) An open-label, comparative study of rivastigmine, donepezil and galantamine in a real-world setting, *Curr Med Res Opin*, **20**(11), pp. 1747–52.

All-Party Parliamentary Group on Dementia (2012) *Unlocking Diagnosis: The Key to Improving the Lives of People with Dementia*. London: House of Commons All-Party Parliamentary Group on Dementia, available at: www.alzheimers.org.uk/site/scripts/download_info.php?downloadID=873

Alzheimer's Disease International (ADI) (2012) *World Alzheimer Report 2012: Overcoming the Stigma of Dementia*. London: ADI, available at: www.alz.co.uk/research/WorldAlzheimerReport2012.pdf

Alzheimer's Disease International and the World Health Organization (ADI and WHO) (2012) *Dementia: A Public Health Priority*. London: WHO.

Arias, E., Gallego-Sandín, S., Villarroya, M., *et al.* (2005) Unequal neuroprotection afforded by the acetylcholinesterase inhibitors galantamine, donepezil, and rivastigmine in SH-SY5Y neuroblastoma cells: role of nicotinic receptors, *J Pharmacol Exp Ther*, **315**(3), pp. 1346–53.

Banerjee, S., *et al.* (2013) A rallying call for an evidence based approach to dementia and related policy development [Rapid response to 'There is no evidence base for proposed dementia screening'], 21 March, available at: www.bmj.com/content/345/bmj.e8588/rr/637358

Bentham, J. (1776) (ed. Harrison, R., 1998) *Bentham: A Fragment on Government (Cambridge Texts in the History of Political Thought)*. Cambridge: Cambridge University Press.

Bourdieu, P. (1986) The forms of capital. In: Richardson, J. (ed) *Handbook of Theory and Research for the Sociology of Education*. New York, NY: Greenwood, pp. 241–58.

Brayne, C., Bayer, A., Boustani, M., *et al.* (2013). Rapid response to 'There is no evidence base for proposed dementia screening' (27 February 2013): 'A rallying call for an evidence based approach to dementia and related policy development', available at: www.bmj.com/content/345/bmj.e8588/rr/633370

Brayne, C., and Davis, D. (2012) Making Alzheimer's and dementia research fit for populations, *Lancet*, **380**(9851), pp. 1441–3.

Brayne, C., Fox, C., and Boustani, M. (2007) Dementia screening in primary care: is it time? *JAMA*, **298**(20), pp. 2409–11.

Brilleman, S.L., Purdy, S., Salisbury, C., *et al.* (2013) Implications of comorbidity for primary care costs in the UK: a retrospective observational study, *Br J Gen Pract*, **63**(609), pp. e274–82.

Brunet, M.D. (2013) Screening and early diagnosis, *J Dement Care*, **21**(3), pp. 22–4.

Brunet, M.D., McCartney, M., Heath, I., *et al.* (2012) Open letter to the prime minister and chief medical officer for England: there is no evidence base for proposed dementia screening, *BMJ*, 345, p. e8588, available at: www.bmj.com/content/345/bmj.e8588.

Burns, A., Alessi, C., Banerjee, S., *et al.* (2013) *A Rallying Call for an Evidence Based Approach to Dementia and Related Policy Development*. (Rapid response to: *There Is No Evidence Base for Proposed Dementia Screening*) 21 March 2013, available at: www.bmj.com/content/345/bmj.e8588/rr/637358.

Chapman, D.P., Williams, S.M., Strine, T.W., *et al.* (2006) Dementia and its implications for public health, Public health research, practice and policy, **3**(2), pp. 1–13, available at: www.cdc.gov/pcd/issues/2006/apr/05_0167.htm

Cohen, S. (1972) *Folk Devils and Moral Panics*. New York, NY: Routledge.

Comas-Herrera, A., Wittenberg, R., Pickard, L., *et al.* (2003) Cognitive impairment in older people: its implications for future demand for services and costs, *PSSRU Discussion Paper*, available at: www.pssru.ac.uk/pdf/dp1728_2.pdf

Courtney, C., Farrell, D., Gray, R., *et al.* (2004) Long-term donepezil treatment in 565 patients with Alzheimer's disease (AD2000): randomised double-blind trial, *Lancet*, **363**(9427), pp. 2105–15.

Department of Health (2002) *Annual Report of the Chief Medical Officer 2002: Health Check, on the State of the Public Health*. London: Department of Health, available at: http://webarchive.nationalarchives.gov.uk/+/www.dh.gov.uk/en/PublicationsAndStatistics/Publications/AnnualReports/DH_4006432

Department of Health (2009) *Living Well with Dementia: A National Dementia Strategy; Putting people first*. London: The Stationery Office, available at: www.gov.uk/government/uploads/system/uploads/attachment_data/file/168221/dh_094052.pdf

Department of Health (2012) *General Medical Services: Contractual Changes 2013–2014*. [Letter to chairman of General Practitioners Committee, British Medical Association], 6 Dec, available at: www.wp.dh.gov.uk/publications/files/2012/12/GMS-Contract-letter.pdf

Department of Health (2012) *The Mandate: A Mandate from the Government to the NHS Commissioning Board; April 2013 to March 2015*. London: The Stationery Office. available at: www.gov.uk/government/uploads/system/uploads/attachment_data/file/127193/mandate.pdf.pdf

Donaldson, L.J., and Scally, G. (2009) *Donaldson's Essential Public Health*. 3rd ed. Oxford: Radcliffe Publishing.

EClipSE Collaborative Members, Brayne, C., Ince, P.G., *et al.* (2010) Education, the brain and dementia: neuroprotection or compensation? *Brain*, **133**(Pt. 8), pp. 2210–16.

Engelhart, M.J., Geerlings, M.I., Ruitenberg, A., *et al.* (2002) Dietary intake of antioxidants and risk of Alzheimer disease, *JAMA*, **287**(24), pp. 3223–9.

Evans, B. (2010) Anticipating fatness: childhood, affect and the pre-emptive 'war on obesity', *Trans Inst Br Geogr*, **35**, pp. 21–38.

Ferri, C.P., Prince, M., Brayne, C., *et al.* (2005) Global prevalence of dementia: a Delphi consensus study, *Lancet*, **366**(9503), pp. 2112–17.

Foster, T.C. (2012) Dissecting the age-related decline on spatial learning and memory tasks in rodent models: N-methyl-D-aspartate receptors and voltage-dependent Ca2+ channels in senescent synaptic plasticity, *Prog Neurobiol*, **96**(3), pp. 283–303.

Foucault, M. (1997) *'Society Must Be Defended': Lectures at the Collège de France 1975–76*. Translated by Macey, D., London: Penguin.

Gaig, C., Valldeoriola, F., Gelpi, E., *et al.* (2011) Rapidly progressive diffuse Lewy body disease, *Mov Disord*, **26**(7), pp. 1316–23.

Goode, E., Ben-Yehuda, N. (1994) *Moral Panics: The Social Construction of Deviance*. Malden, MA: Blackwell Publishers.

Greenland, S., Last, J.M., and Porta, M.S. (2008) *A Dictionary of Epidemiology*. New York, NY: Oxford University Press.

Gultekin, S.H., Rosenfeld, M.R., Voltz, R., *et al.* (2010) Paraneoplastic limbic encephalitis: neurological symptoms, immunological findings and tumour association in 50 patients, *Brain*, **123**(Pt. 7), pp. 1481–94.

Holden, M., and Kelly, C. (2002) Use of cholinesterase inhibitors in dementia, *Advances in Psychiatric Treatment*, **8**, pp. 86–96, available at: apt.rcpsych.org/content/8/2/89.full

Hornberger, M., and Piguet, O. (2012) Episodic memory in frontotemporal dementia: a critical review, *Brain*, **135**(Pt. 3), pp. 678–92.

Huang, C.Q., Dong, B.R., Lu, Z.C., *et al.* (2010) Chronic diseases and risk for depression in old age: a meta-analysis of published literature, *Ageing Res Rev*, **9**(2), pp. 131–41.

Kaduszkiewicz, H., Bachmann, C., and van den Bussche, H. (2008) Telling 'the truth' in dementia: do attitude and approach of general practitioners and specialists differ?, *Patient Educ Couns*, **70**(2), pp. 220–6.

Kmietowicz, Z. (2012) Cameron launches challenge to end 'national crisis' of poor dementia care, *BMJ*, **344**, p. e2347. doi: 10.1136/bmj.e2347.

Knopman, D.S., Boeve, B.F., and Petersen, R.C. (2003) Essentials of the proper diagnoses of mild cognitive impairment, dementia, and major subtypes of dementia, *Mayo Clin Proc*, **78**(10), pp. 1290–308.

Korczyn, A.D., and Vakhapova, V. (2007) The prevention of the dementia epidemic, *J Neurol Sci*, **257**(1–2), pp. 2–4.

Langa, K.M., Chernew, M.E., Kabeto, M.U., *et al.* (2001) National estimates of the quantity and cost of informal caregiving for the elderly with dementia, *J Gen Intern Med*, **16**(11), pp. 770–8.

Leyton, C.E., and Hodges, J.R. (2010) Frontotemporal dementias: recent advances and current controversies, *Ann Indian Acad Neurol*, **13**(Suppl. 2), pp. S74–80.

Lischka, A.R., Mendelsohn, M., Overend, T., *et al.* (2012) A systematic review of screening tools for predicting the development of dementia, *Can J Aging*, **31**(3), pp. 295–311.

Local Government, nef, National Mental Health Development Unit (2010) *The Role of Local Government in Promoting Wellbeing Report: Healthy Communities Programmes*, available at: www.local.gov.uk/c/document_library/get_file?uuid=bcd27d1b-8feb-41e5-a1ce-48f9e70ccc3b&groupId=10180

Loukaides, P., Schiza, N., Pettingill, P., *et al.* (2012) Morvan's syndrome associated with antibodies to multiple components of the voltage-gated potassium channel complex, *J Neurol Sci*, **312**(1–2), pp. 52–6.

Macdonald, A.J., Carpenter, G.I., Box, O., *et al.* (2002) Dementia and use of psychotropic medication in non-'Elderly Mentally Infirm' nursing homes in South East England, *Age Ageing*, **31**(1), pp. 58–64.

Masaki, K.H., Losonczy, K.G., Izmirlian, G., *et al.* (2000) Association of vitamin E and C supplement use with cognitive function and dementia in elderly men, *Neurology*, **54**(6), pp. 1265–72.

Matthson, N., Brax, D., and Zetterberg, H. (2010) To know or not to know: ethical issues related to early diagnosis of Alzheimer's disease, *Int J Alzheimers Dis*, pii: 841941.

Meeks, T.W., Vahia, I.V., Lavretsky, H., *et al.* (2011) A tune in 'A minor' can be 'B major': a review of epidemiology, illness course, and public health implications of subthreshold depression in older adults, *J Affective Disord*, **129**(1–3), pp. 126–42.

Mioshi, E., Dawson, K., Mitchell, J., *et al.* (2006) The Addenbrooke's Cognitive Examination Revised: a brief cognitive test battery for dementia screening, *Int J Geriatr Psychiatry*, **21**(11), pp. 1078–85.

Mitchell, A.J., and Shiri-Feshki, M. (2009) Rate of progression of mild cognitive impairment to dementia: meta-analysis of 41 robust inception cohort studies, *Acta Psychiatr Scand*, **119**(4), pp. 252–65.

Molinuevo, J.L., Sánchez-Valle, R., Lladó, A., *et al.* (2012) Identifying earlier Alzheimer's disease: insights from the preclinical and prodromal phases, *Neurodegener Dis*, 10(1–4), pp. 158–60.

Morris, M.C., Evans, D.A., Bienias, J.L., *et al.* (2002) Dietary intake of antioxidant nutrients and the risk of incident Alzheimer disease in a biracial community study, *JAMA*, **287**(24), pp. 3230–7.

National Council for Palliative Care. (2012) *National Council for Palliative Care (NCPC) Response: All-Party Parliamentary Group on Dementia 2012 Inquiry; Improving dementia diagnosis rates in the UK*. London, NCPC, available at: www.ncpc.org.uk/sites/default/files/NCPC_response_APPG_Dementia_diagnosis_inquiry.pdf

Navarro, Z. (2006) In search of cultural intepretation of power, *IDS Bulletin*, **37**(6), pp. 11–22.

Nelson, A.P., and O'Connor, M.G. (2008) Mild cognitive impairment: a neuropsychological perspective, *CNS Spectr*, **13**(1), pp. 56–64.

Nepal, B., Ranmuthugala, G., Brown, L., *et al.* (2008) Modelling costs of dementia in Australia: evidence, gaps, and needs, *Aust Health Rev*, **32**(3), pp. 479–87.

Paradis, E. (2011) Changing meanings of fat: fat, obesity, epidemics and America's children, Stanford University unpublished dissertation.

Paradis, E., Albert, M., Byrne, N., *et al.* (2012) *Changing Meaning of Epidemic and Pandemic in the Medical Literature, 1900–2010*, American Sociological Association Conference, Denver, CO: August, available at: www.eliseparadis.com/files/EoE-DenverV1.pdf

Pose, M., Cetkovich, M., Gleichgerrcht, E., *et al.* (2013) The overlap of symptomatic dimensions between frontotemporal dementia and several psychiatric disorders that appear in late adulthood, *Int Rev Psychiatry*, **25**(2), pp. 159–67.

Public Health Resource Unit (2009) *Appraisal for Screening for Alzheimer's Disease*. Oxford, PHRU, available at www.screening.nhs.uk/alzheimers (*see* Key downloads: Last external review).

Raftery, J., and Chorozoglou, M. (2011) Possible net harms of breast cancer screening: updated modelling of Forrest report, *BMJ*, **343**, p. d7627.

Reitz, C., Brayne, C., and Mayeux, R. (2001) Epidemiology of Alzheimer disease, *Nat Rev Neurol*, 7(3), pp. 137–52.

Ropacki, S.A., and Jeste, D.V. (2005) Epidemiology of and risk factors for psychosis of Alzheimer's disease: a review of 55 studies published from 1990 to 2003, *Am J Psychiatry*, **162**(11), pp. 2022–30.

Saguy, A.C., and Almeling, R. (2005) *Fat Devils and Moral Panics: News Reporting on Obesity Science*. Presented at the SOMAH workshop, UCLA Department of Sociology, June 1.

Savage, S., Hsieh, S., Leslie, F., *et al.* (2013) Distinguishing subtypes in primary progressive aphasia: application of the Sydney language battery, *Dement Geriatr Cogn Disord*, **35**(3–4), pp. 208–18.

Savva, G.M., Zaccai, J., Matthews, F.E., *et al.* (2009) Prevalence, correlates and course of behavioural and psychological symptoms of dementia in the population, *Br J Psychiatry*, **194**(3), pp. 212–19.

Schneider, J., Murray, J., Banerjee, S., *et al.* (1999) EUROCARE: a cross-national study of co-resident spouse carers for people with Alzheimer's disease: I. Factors associated with carer burden, *Int J Geriatr Psychiatry*, **14**(8), pp. 651–61.

Sosa-Ortiz, A.L., Acosta-Castillo, I., and Prince, M.J. (2012) Epidemiology of dementias and Alzheimer's disease, *Arch Med Res*, **43**(8), pp. 600–8.

Starkstein S.E., Jorge R., Mizrahi R., *et al.* (2006) A diagnostic formulation for anosognosia in Alzheimer's disease, *J Neurol Neurosurg Psychiatry*, **77**(6), pp. 719–25. Epub 2006 Mar 20.

Stephan, B., and Brayne, C. (2008) Prevalence and projections of dementia. In: Downs, M., and Bowers, B. (eds) *Excellence in Dementia Care: Principles and Practice*. Maidenhead: Open University Press (McGraw-Hill Education).

Stevens, J.M., and Fox, N.C. (2001) Structural imaging. In: *Early Onset Dementia: A Multidisciplinary Approach*, Oxford: Oxford University Press.

Strandberg, T.E, and O'Neill, D. (2013) Dementia: a geriatric syndrome, *Lancet*, **381**(9866), pp. 533–4.

Strech, D., Mertz, M., Knüppel, H., *et al.* (2013) The full spectrum of ethical issues in dementia care: systematic qualitative review, *Br J Psychiatry*, **202**, pp. 400–6.

Treves, T.A., and Korczyn, A.D. (2012) Modeling the dementia epidemic, *CNS Neurosci Ther*, **18**(2), pp. 175–81.

Tripathi, M., and Vibha, D. (2009) Reversible dementias, *Indian J Psychiatry*, **51**(Suppl. 1), pp. S52–5.

United Nations Department of Economic and Social Affairs, Population Division (United Nations) (2007) *World Population Ageing 2000*, available at: www.un.org/esa/population/publications/publications.htm

UK Government. (2000) *Local Government Act 2000*, available at: www.legislation.gov.uk/ukpga/2000/22/contents

UK National Screening Committee. (2010) *The UK NSC Policy on Alzheimer's Disease Screening in Adults*, available at, www.screening.nhs.uk/alzheimers

Van der Linde, R.M., Stephan, B.C., Savva, G.M., *et al.* (2012) Systematic reviews on behavioural and psychological symptoms in the older or demented population, *Alzheimers Res Ther*, **4**(4), p. 28.

Vink, D., Aartsen, M.J., and Schoevers, R.A. (2008) Risk factors for anxiety and depression in the elderly: a review, *J Affective Disord*, **106**(1–2), pp. 29–44.

Wilson, J.M.G., and Jungner, G. (1968) *Principles and Practice of Screening for Disease*. Geneva: World Health Organization.

Wimo, A., and Winblad, B. (2004) Economic aspects on drug therapy of dementia, *Curr Pharm Des*, **10**(3), pp. 295–301.

World Health Organization (WHO) (2003) *World Health Report 2003: Shaping the Future*. Geneva: WHO.

World Health Organization and Alzheimer's Disease International (WHO and ADI) (2012) *Dementia: A Public Health Priority*. Geneva: WHO, available at: www.who.int/mental_health/publications/dementia_report_2012/en/

Zuidema, S., Koopmans, R., and Verhey F. (2007) Prevalence and predictors of neuropsychiatric symptoms in cognitively impaired nursing home patients, *J Geriatr Psychiatry Neurol*, **20**(1), pp. 41–9.

CHAPTER 6

The relevance of the person for living well with dementia

Statement 5. People with dementia are enabled, with the involvement of their carers, to maintain and develop relationships.

Statement 6. People with dementia are enabled, with the involvement of their carers, to access services that help maintain their physical and mental health and wellbeing.

Evidence for improved outcomes for people with dementia through provision of person-centred care had been largely observational. This one issue can make convincing pitches for wellbeing in dementia tricky. However, Chenoweth and colleagues have recently reported (Chenoweth *et al.*, 2009) a cluster randomised controlled trial, where urban residential sites were randomly assigned to person-centred care, Dementia Care Mapping (DCM), or usual care. The authors found that person-centred care and DCM both seem to reduce agitation in people with dementia in residential care. A brief description of DCM is provided later in this chapter.

Nonetheless, what has been striking is that relationships are important in wellbeing of individuals with dementia, and this is a recurrent theme indeed throughout this book. In general, 'social trust' (trust in other people) is strongly associated with high life satisfaction and happiness (e.g. Helliwell, 2003), and the number and strength of social connections are among the largest and most robust predictors of subjective wellbeing, including life satisfaction, overall happiness and decrease in depressive symptoms (e.g. Dolan, Peasgood and White, 2008; Helliwell and Putnam, 2004; Pichler, 2006).

Research traditionally focuses on how disease affects the brain of an individual with dementia, and it is hoped that results from animal models will inform on the neurobiology of health and disease. Through 'translationary

research', the ideal is that animal models, where medical and surgical interventions can be investigated, will lead to better treatments in human beings.
However, with animal models, while we arguably have a good understanding
of what happens in the brains of these animals – for example, through cellular
or histochemical, electrophysiological or neuroimaging techniques – we really
are unable to understand what is going on in the *minds* of non-human primates
and other non-human species. The focus in contemporary English health policy has been, however, to take the concept of a 'person' seriously, and a subtle
appreciation has been recently that that the mind and body are possibly not as
dissociable as previously thought. Notwithstanding the precise way in which
cognition, emotion and the body interact is as yet poorly understood, there is
certainly a wish to understand the 'whole person', and to think how aspects
of the wellbeing are related to its counterpart – illbeing. This approach is critical if we are to make sense of how carers can help to enhance the wellbeing of
individuals with dementia, where possible, and the importance of constructive social relationships in the environment of an individual with dementia.
Physical health can clearly affect mental wellbeing, as well, and therefore it is
essential that the 'needs' of pain management and nutrition for any individual
with dementia are addressed in full.

AN OVERVIEW OF THE IMPORTANCE OF PHYSICAL AND MENTAL HEALTH FOR LIVING WELL IN DEMENTIA

Treating an individual living well with dementia is a critical plank of policy.

Chapter 5 of the National Dementia Strategy (Department of Health, 2009)
explains early on that this is to be taken in the context of an individual living
well with dementia as part of a wider community, and that individuals including immediates need access to high-quality services.

> Access to flexible and reliable services, ranging from early intervention to specialist home
> care services, which are responsive to the personal needs and preferences of each indi-
> vidual and take account of their broader family circumstances. Accessible to people living
> alone or with carers, people who pay for their care privately, through personal budgets, or
> through local authority-arranged services.

The starting point is that individuals with dementia are not always in a position
to seek help or advice about other issues that could be affecting their health
and wellbeing. Therefore, it is important that they are enabled to access services
where further help can be given. People with dementia should be empowered,
with the involvement of their carers, to access services that help maintain their
physical and mental health and wellbeing.

Chapter 5 of the National Dementia Strategy (Department of Health, 2009) provides a helpful overview as follows.

A comprehensive community personal support service would provide:
- home care that is reliable, with staff who have basic training in dementia care;
- flexibility to respond to changing needs, not determined by rigid time slots that prevent staff from working alongside people rather than doing things for them;
- access to personalised social activity, short breaks and day services;
- access to peer support networks;
- access to expert patient and carer programmes;
- responsiveness to crisis services;
- access to supported housing that is inclusive of people with dementia;
- respite care/breaks that provide valued and enjoyable experiences for people with dementia as well as their family carers;
- flexible and responsive respite care/breaks that can be provided in a variety of settings including the home of the person with dementia;
- independent advocacy services; and
- assistive technologies such as telecare.

SERVICES THAT HELP MAINTAIN PHYSICAL AND MENTAL HEALTH AND WELLBEING

The National Institute for Health and Clinical Excellence (NICE) Quality Standard 30 quality statement 6 on the importance of physical and mental health for living well with dementia is relevant to different stakeholders.

- **People with dementia** can have routine check-ups of their physical and mental health and can see healthcare professionals when they have concerns.
- **Carers of people with dementia** are involved in helping the person they support have routine physical and mental health check-ups and see healthcare professionals when they have concerns. The Department of Health defines a 'carer' as someone who provides unpaid support to family or friends who couldn't manage without this help, whether they are caring for a relative, partner or friend who is ill, frail, disabled or has mental health or substance misuse problems.
- **Local authorities and others commissioning services** work with providers to ensure the services they commission enable people with dementia, with the involvement of their carers, to have routine check-ups of their physical and mental health and see healthcare professionals when they have concerns.
- **Organisations** providing care and support ensure people with dementia are enabled, with the involvement of their carers, to access services that help maintain their physical and mental health and wellbeing.

- **Social care and healthcare staff** enable people with dementia, with the involvement of their carers, to access services that help maintain their physical and mental health and wellbeing.

THE IMPORTANCE OF CARERS

Family carers are possibly the most important 'resource' available for people with dementia. Carers have a right to an assessment of their needs and can be supported through an agreed plan to support the important rôle they play in the care of the person with dementia. This clearly requires joined-up thinking in the benefits system, thinking what support carers might be entitled to on a statutory basis.

Independence is a pervasive critical feature in wellbeing in dementia. Most people want to remain living in their own homes for as long as possible. That message appears to be consistently communicated by the public, by older people generally and by people with dementia specifically, whether they are young or old. Indeed, while the effects of cholinesterase inhibitors in improving memory symptoms in **dementia of the Alzheimer type** are considered to be modest at best, the argument was advanced that even such modest effects might be beneficial in delaying the institutionalisation of individuals with dementia (e.g. Fillit and Hill, 2004). According to the National Dementia Strategy (Department of Health, 2009), most family carers want to be able to provide support to help the person with dementia stay at home, but they sometimes need more assistance than is currently routinely available. Residential care may be the most appropriate and effective way of meeting someone's needs and providing a service of choice.

Examples of services that help maintain physical and mental health and wellbeing include:
- general practice
- occupational therapy services
- Admiral Nurses
- community palliative care
- health promotion services, including smoking cessation
- mental health teams
- opticians
- hearing therapists
- dentists
- chiropodists
- physiotherapy services.

A PERSON-CENTRED CARE APPROACH

'Person-centred care' principles are a good starting point for high-quality care, laid out in the National Service Framework (Department of Health, 2001). These principles reflect the increasing evidence that individuals with dementia are able to continue with their emotional lives and experience pleasure and distress in response to things they enjoy or dislike (Kitwood, 1997).

Christine Bryden (2005), in her powerful story of her journey with dementia, talks of her fear of ceasing to be:

> We all believe the toxic lie of dementia; that the mind is absent and the body is an empty shell. Our sense of self is shattered with this new label of dementia. Who am I, if I can no longer be a valued member of society? What if I don't know who I am and who I was?

Loss of self is a persistent philosophy in everyday thinking about dementia, although increasingly, carers, practitioners, philosophers and academics are turning away from this view of 'identity', towards one in which interdependence and relationships contribute towards maintenance of self.

Person-centred care principles include:

- valuing the person and their family
- treating the person as an individual
- taking the perspective of the person when planning and providing care
- ensuring that a positive social environment exists in which the person can experience relative wellbeing.

For the late Tom Kitwood, an essential part of person-centred care was a focus on the *uniqueness* of individuals. This follows from his position that personhood is relational, in that each of our relationships is unique. Focusing on uniqueness requires us to focus on the differences between us (for, by definition, similarity is not unique). Kitwood's (1997) work was pivotal in implicating the interactions of caregivers in contributing to 'depersonalisation' and illbeing of people with dementia. He has been instrumental in calling for recognition of an enduring personhood and arguing for the centrality of the person within person-centred care. Kitwood, therefore arguing against the determinism of the biomedical model, proposed that the symptoms and behavioural changes associated with dementia do not arise purely from neuropathology, but from a dialectical interplay between neuropathology and the person's psychosocial environment.

Kitwood, who developed the Bradford Dementia Group at the University of Bradford in the UK, was the initial developer of person-centred care. Kitwood argued that viewing people with dementia only in medical terms leads them to be seen as objects and as having no subjectivity or personhood. Kitwood argued that people's experience of dementia not only arises from biomedical phenomena such as their degree of neurological impairment and their physical health but also from social and psychological factors such as their personal biography and day-to-day interaction with other people. Kitwood described the mutual contribution of biomedical and social/psychological on the development of dementia as a 'dialectical process' and expressed it as an equation:

$$D = NI + PH + B + MSP$$
D = dementia
NI = neurological impairment
PH = physical health
B = biography
MSP = malignant social psychology

Kitwood's approach is usually known as 'person-centred care', although his approach needs to be differentiated from **'person-centred approaches'** that merely highlight the need for individualised care. Kitwood's approach is more conceptually and theoretically developed, and it highlights the importance of the person with dementia rather than the disease process itself. Kitwood argued that people with dementia do not lose their personhood, but rather it can be maintained through relationships with other people. Thus, Kitwood defines personhood as 'a standing or a status that is bestowed on one human being, by another in the context of relationship and social being' (Kitwood, 1997). Within person-centred care therefore, the personal and social identity of a person with dementia arises out of what is said and done with them.

According to *Tom Kitwood on Dementia: A Reader and Critical Commentary* (2007), edited by Clive Baldwin and Andrea Capstick, Kitwood's work on illbeing and wellbeing in dementia appears to have unfolded in three main phases. In the earliest of these (from around 1987–1990), the emphasis is entirely on illbeing, which is considered to be an inevitable consequence of dementia and is frequently suggested by him as a precondition for its onset. In the mid-phase (1991–95), the emphasis shifts from both illbeing and wellbeing in the context of the interpersonal interaction with the person with dementia, largely in formal care settings. In the latest phase of Kitwood's work (1995–98), the focus moves again from a binary distinction between illbeing and wellbeing to a more detailed consideration of the psychological needs of people with dementia and the challenges of the equipping caregivers to meet these needs.

FACTORS CONTRIBUTING TO, AND INDICATORS OF, WELLBEING

In the *Brighter Futures* report by Kitwood, Buckland and Petre (1995), the authors set out factors contributing to 'wellbeing' (and illbeing). The **factors contributing to wellbeing** are summarised in **Table 6.1**.

TABLE 6.1 The factors contributing to wellbeing

Social setting	A measure of importance is engagement. This represents an active and conscious link with the outside world. There has been a great deal of work to show that providing a structure and opportunity for interaction does create engagement in people with dementia of all levels of activity.
Cognitive ability	There are many examples of people 'faring well', despite having impaired cognitive function. Wellbeing can be expressed in different ways, according to level of cognitive activity; wellbeing is never taken away simply because of cognitive decline. However, there is a strong link between cognitive impairment and lower wellbeing.
Dependency	For those who have forms of physical dependency that isolate (e.g. visual impairment), there is an especial need for help in maintaining contact with the outside world. A person who is isolated from social contact is deprived of nourishment for their wellbeing. A person who is open to new experiences is better able to fare well with their changing and confusing circumstances.
Quality of social contact	People who have any social contact, regardless of its quality, fare better than those who are isolated and ignored. In short, where there is wellbeing present, it should be promoted as far as possible. Keeping the person engaged will help promote wellbeing a great deal. Moreover, if this can include good quality social interaction, there is a strong chance that the person will maintain or improve in their level of wellbeing.
Staff	Most staff describe themselves as being motivated by caring, and pay is rarely cited as a cause of satisfaction or dissatisfaction. Homes that have staff who have a personal concern for their work have residents with higher levels of wellbeing.
Physical setting	The data suggest that measures of physical environment have little relationship with wellbeing. However, there is a very mild effect relating to the physical amenities measure. The inference is that homes that have facilities such as adequate or accessible toilets and a decent laundry are more able to enhance the wellbeing of residents.

Source: Kitwood, Buckland and Petre (1995).

Likewise, the **factors contributing to illbeing** are shown in **Table 6.2**. In Kitwood and Bredin (1992), the authors identified 12 indicators of wellbeing that are operationally defined. In 'Towards a theory of dementia care: the interpersonal process' (1993), Kitwood summarised it as follows:

> Behind this, we postulated 'four global states', grounded in the life of emotion and feeling rather than that of elaborate cognition. The states are self-esteeem, agency, social confidence and hope. … A communicative act was carried through successfully. The dementia suffered felt recognized [sic] as a person: self-esteem was enhanced. A gesture was transmuted into action: agency was confirmed. The dementia sufferer moved towards the Other and was welcomed: social confidence increased. Confusion and disorder within the psyche

were met with order and stability in the social world: hope was sustained. It is the repetition of the experience, we may hypothesize [sic], that can establish wellbeing even in the face of severe cognitive impairment.

TABLE 6.2 The factors contributing to illbeing

Social setting	One of the most important factors that lead to increased illbeing is for people to be left unattended, showing signs of illbeing, for long periods of time. The lack of attention, once over 30 minutes, very significantly contributes towards to a high state of illbeing. Apathy and loneliness are the most common forms of illbeing observative in those who are left unattended.
Dependency	Individual dependency varies greatly, and has a direct effect on the extent to which people can generate their own quality of life. Physical dependency can be extremely crippling, and loss of sight, hearing and language places the individual at risk of isolation, potentially leading to extreme anger, or withdrawal and despair.
Personality	Neuroticism, agreeableness and consciousness are three important dimensions of personality that discriminate between high and low illbeing.
Relationships	The data concerning this are not conclusive.
Staff	Higher levels of illbeing are observable where there is an emphasis of staff routines and procedures.

PERSONHOOD AS CENTRAL TO PERSON-CENTRED CARE

At the heart of Kitwood's conceptualisation of person-centred care was a sense of '**personhood**', meaning 'what it is like to be a person'. Kitwood argued that personhood depended not on ability or capacity, but it is a 'standing or status that is bestowed upon one human being, by others, in the context of relationship and social being.' It implies recognition, respect and trust (1997) and that personhood was the right of every human being regardless of capacity.

Kitwood drew attention to personhood as:

- **an essentially relational concept** – that is, one did not 'possess' personhood but personhood exists in the way one is treated
- **essentially dynamic** – that it could ebb and flow
- **to some extent situational** – the social and physical environment could support and uphold or undermine personhood
- **a unique encounter** between two individuals that could not be legislated for without using uniqueness.

Person-centred care for Kitwood thus flowed from a concept of personhood. Such was to be aimed at upholding the personhood of the individual threatened by the onset and progression of dementia (the dementia itself not being the factor that undermined personhood, but the individual and social responses to the dementia). Since Kitwood wrote, there has been much work that has demonstrated that, contrary to the popular perception, for those people with dementia, **the Self remains** (see, for example, Sabat and Harré, 1992; Klein *et al.*, 2003; Surr, 2006). Such a Self may be vulnerable but is nevertheless retrained in the face of dementia and the response of others to dementia.

MAINTAINING PERSONHOOD IN DEMENTIA CARE

As reviewed by the **National Care Forum** (2007) in their *Key Principles of Person-Centred Dementia Care*, in order for a person-centred approach to be embedded in an organisation, appropriate relationships have to be established.

This will be evidenced in areas such as:

- the philosophy of care
- the person with dementia being at the heart of all services
- the person with dementia being enabled to maintain the relationships with significant others as he or she chooses
- respect and value for human life
- communication will be open and honest, and presented in a way that is understood
- staff presenting a positive attitude.

PERSON-CENTRED CARE AND 'DEMENTIA CARE MAPPING'

As argued by Aveyard (2001), the concept of person-centred care, developed by Kitwood, has become a driving force in the philosophy of care for people with dementia, and could provide a valuable framework on which to base educational programmes. Person-centred care puts the needs of the person with dementia at the very heart of care provision. If those needs are also at the heart of education for people working in the field, then, arguably, the contents of an educational programme will reflect the needs of the person with dementia.

Person-centred care has been identified as a key factor for upholding dignity in health and social care (**SCIE Guide 9**), and **dementia care mapping (DCM)** is a method that has been specifically developed to improve person-centred care (Young and Sturdy, 2004; Bradford Dementia Group, 2005). Although other person-centred care tools exist (Nolan *et al.*, 2004; McCormack, 2004; McCormack and McCance, 2006), few are as well developed or as widely used as DCM.

DCM is a complex care improvement process whereby five to eight individuals within a care setting are continuously observed over 4–6 hours by a trained DCM practitioner (a 'mapper'). At 5-minute intervals, a record is made of what has happened to each individual being observed using two coding frameworks. *Behaviour Category Codes* capture the type of activity engaged in, and *Mood/Engagement Values* are a judgement of the state of affect and engagement experienced using a 6-point scale ranging from +5 (very positive mood or deep engagement) to –5 (very negative mood). Mood/Engagement Values are averaged over the mapping period to provide a summary Well/Illbeing score for an individual or group. A detailed set of operational coding rules informs decision-making.

Observations are undertaken, with the knowledge of patients, in communal places. The observation style is unobtrusive, and if it is seen to be increasing feelings of illbeing in patients, then the mapping is stopped. Observations are analysed and summarised, then fed back to the care team, and action plans for change can be developed at an individual, group or organisational level. After a suitable time period, the care setting is mapped again to evaluate whether the action arising from the initial evaluation has had any impact on the lived experience of care. A cycle of mapping, action planning and evaluation is therefore established.

DCM has face validity (Brooker *et al.*, 1998; Younger and Martin, 2000; Brooker, 2005), and there is some evidence to support its efficacy in long-term care (Martin and Younger, 2001). The latest version (DCM8) has been validated in psychiatric services (Brooker and Surr, 2006). Using the DCM method to develop person-centred care practice could apply equally well to people who have health conditions other than dementia (Jaycock, Persaud and Johnson, 2006), including older people receiving general hospital care.

WHOLE PERSON CARE

Whole person care is becoming an increasingly important policy strand. The Royal College of Psychiatrists in March 2013 produced a report, *Whole-Person Care: From Rhetoric to Reality; Achieving Parity Between Mental and Physical Health*, and introduced this by explaining the need for the 'parity' between physical and mental health:

The long-standing and continuing lack of parity between mental and physical health evidenced in this report is inequitable and socially unjust. This 'mental health treatment gap', exemplified by lower treatment rates for mental health conditions, premature mortality of people with mental health problems and underfunding of mental healthcare relative to the scale and impact of mental health problems, falls short of government commitments to international human rights conventions which recognise the rights of people with mental health problems to the highest attainable standard of health; yet it can be argued that this lack of parity is so embedded in healthcare and in society that it is tolerated and hardly remarked upon. It also affects people with physical health problems who also have mental health needs that may not be recognised in more physically healthcare-orientated settings. The poorer outcomes that result are considered by many, both within and outside mental healthcare, as all that can be expected.

There has been much consideration regarding what 'whole person care', a growing trend in healthcare, might be about. Tom Hutchinson (2011) writes as follows:

So, what does the 'whole person' in whole person care really mean? It is perhaps easiest to start with what it does not mean. Whole person care is not knowing all about the patient in all dimensions (biological, psychological, social, spiritual and many others that could probably be listed) and taking responsibility for taking care of all of them. Such an undertaking would be doomed to failure and would probably be perceived by patients as overstepping the bounds of the medical mandate and even seen as invasive. When a patient comes to see a doctor he does not expect a combination biological scientist, psychologist, social worker and spiritual guidance counselor [sic], all of them working full out at the same time. Within the context of the clinical interaction, he/she wants someone who will provide competent medical care and treat him/her seriously as a person, usually no more and no less. It sounds simple, and yet, there is more to it than first apparent. While not everything needs to be dealt with at the same time, nothing that comes up can necessarily be ruled out of bounds as a potential avenue for addressing the problem.

PHYSICAL HEALTH: NUTRITION AND 'DIGNITY IN CARE'

Social Care Institute for Excellence **Guide 15 on 'dignity in care'** describes also general principles regarding importance of nutrition and pain management.

Good nutrition, good hydration and enjoyable mealtimes can dramatically improve the health and wellbeing of older people. Mealtimes, therefore, should be considered a priority in terms of importance and dedication of staff time; systems within organisations should support this. Protected mealtimes have been introduced in many hospitals: this means that non-acute clinical activity stops, the ward is tidied and patients are made ready for their meals. It gives patients 'space' to eat and enjoy their meals. It also gives nurses time to give assistance to those who need it and raises staff awareness on the importance of good nutrition.

Water is vital to life, and there is increasing evidence of the benefits of good hydration in the promotion of health and wellbeing in older people. The evidence suggests that good hydration can help prevent falls, constipation, pressure ulcers, kidney stones, blood pressure problems and headaches. Furthermore, poor hydration has been shown to contribute to obesity, depression, inactivity and fatigue and to prolong healing and recovery.

It is interesting to note the perspective of a real '#dementiachallenger' (Beth Britton) on types of drinks that individuals with dementia might like. Beth writes passionately, based on her real experiences. Her blogs are very inspiring to read. This is a very short extract from a popular blogpost dated 8th May 2013.

First of all consider the sort of drinks being offered. Have you tasted them personally? Are they pleasant? It may seem obvious, but it's easy to ignore the fact that if what we are offering someone doesn't taste nice it is unlikely to be welcomed. When a person has dementia they may not be able to articulate their dislike for something, so they will just leave it or spit it out, causing immense frustration for them and their carer(s).

Many care providers are hooked on giving their residents squash – water flavoured with concentrated and often additive-packed so-called 'fruit'. This is about as far from real fruit juice as you can get – it is synthetic, can be metallic tasting and is full of preservatives that should be avoided. I certainly wouldn't want to drink it and we banned squash from being given to my dad, favouring real fruit smoothies that were a perfect consistency and a delicious taste.

Source: 'Hydrated and happy', a blogpost on Wednesday 8 May 2013, from Beth Britton's 'D4Dementia' blog: http://d4dementia.blogspot.co.uk/2013/05/hydrated-and-happy.html, © Beth Britton 2013, extract reproduced by kind permission of the author.

EQUALITY AND DIVERSITY CONSIDERATIONS

NICE clinical guideline 42 (CG42) recommendation 1.1.1.7 lists alternative and additional support that may be needed if language or acquired language impairment is a barrier to accessing or understanding support.

Social care and healthcare staff should identify the specific needs of people with dementia and their carers arising from diversity, including gender, sexuality, ethnicity, age and religion. These needs should be recorded in care plans and addressed (**NICE clinical guideline 42, recommendations 1.1.1.3 and 1.1.1.5**).

NICE clinical guideline 42 recommendation 1.1.1.1 highlights that people should not be excluded from services because of diagnosis, age or coexisting learning disabilities.

'THINK LOCAL, ACT PERSONAL'

The real challenge with the person-led initiatives is that such iniatives must be accessible for the wider public for them to succeed. Gill Phillips in her 'Whose Shoes' movement (*see* the Case Study later in this chapter) has made an outstanding contribution in this area. This idea embodies true innovation at its best, with a clear focus in user-adoption, protected in law by registered trademark and registered design right. It is striking that no one session using the 'Whose Shoes' board game or the electronic format can ever be the same, because there are different participants, different questions/themes, and different perspectives (e.g. person, carer, provider). One of the most important

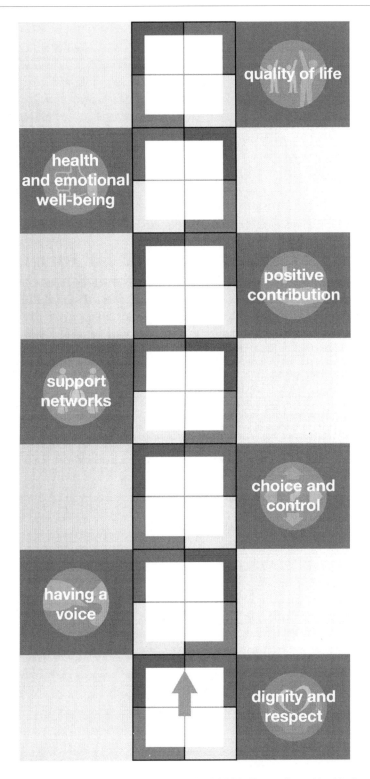

quality of life

health and emotional well-being

positive contribution

support networks

choice and control

having a voice

dignity and respect

aspects also is that it gently encourages participants to question their own assumptions, as this is essential for 'unfreezing' from a particular cultural set of beliefs (Lewin, 1951). This ultimately will be one of the biggest challenges as healthcare becomes integrated with social care in English health policy with time. The Foreword to this book written by Sally-Ann Marciano is a good example of how a medical model in its purest form, with all its rigid funding applications, can fail dismally the wellbeing of the person with dementia.

Phillips' '**path to personalisation**' was included in the original board game version 'Whose Shoes? Putting People First' to reflect the seven outcomes of *Putting People First: A Shared Vision and Commitment to the Transformation of Adult Social Care*. You will see that they match very closely some main themes of my thesis: quality of life (**whole book**), health and emotional wellbeing (some health aspects are discussed in **Chapters 6** and **8**), support networks (and dementia-friendly communities, **Chapter 17**), choice and control (decision-making, **Chapter 11**), having a voice (advocacy, **Chapter 11**, and communication, **Chapter 12**). It brings alive the collaborative nature of the tool as people add tiles to the board, representing contributions from all the key stakeholders. In the electronic tool, the wording on the pathway has been updated to align more closely with Think Local Act Personal's 'Making It Real' markers: the cross-cutting themes 'marking progress towards personalised, community based support', derived from work led by members of the National Co-Production Advisory Group, which is made up of people who use services and carers.

Gill has recently also collaborated with the **Think Local Act Personal** initiative, a sector-wide commitment to transform adult social care through personalisation and community-based support.

Case Study: The Whose Shoes? story

GILL PHILLIPS, 22 JUNE 2012

www.thinklocalactpersonal.org.uk/Blog/WhoseShoes/

'Whose Shoes?', like so many ideas that turn out to be successful, was born out of frustration. I was passionate about the possibilities offered by the emerging personalisation agenda. I had originally heard Caroline Tomlinson talking about the amazing differences a personalised approach had made to her disabled son Joseph and indeed to the whole family. Caroline had explained how Joseph became able to exercise choice and control over his support needs, assisted by his 'circle of support'. They moved away from a life of impersonal 'services' to one where Joe had a good quality of life – something that most of us take for granted. I had been totally inspired but asked 'But what if you don't have a Caroline? …'. I didn't expand but people knew what I meant – a wonderful, dedicated mother, able and willing to take on the system, to fight tooth and nail for what her son needed. I started to see the challenges and barriers that lay ahead in trying to 'make personalisaton real' for everyone.

I subsequently led the Research and Evaluation work of the Individual Budgets pilot in Coventry. In a booklet called 'Our stories' we collected the experiences of service users who received individual budgets. Great stories they were too, in many cases transforming lives. But again I was worried how people would fare outside and beyond the spotlight of the 'pilots' …

I attended conferences. I listened to what people were saying – service users, carers, care providers as well as the keynote speakers. I had a growing sense of unease as I heard presenters saying how 'vital' it was that people made progress with personalisation, often focusing on graphs and charts and targets. They said it was 'imperative' for people to engage with the agenda … but often seemed to miss the point that 'engagement' is a matter of hearts and minds, not sector leaders saying things a bit louder!

I became frustrated that people didn't seem to 'get' the fact that the new approach meant total transformation. It needed to evolve from grass-roots level. Nobody knew all the answers. People needed time to think things through, to work together and take ownership – all the different interest groups dropping their sometimes entrenched 'silo' positions. They needed to listen to 'people with lived experience', experts in their own lives and support needs. They needed to co-produce sustainable solutions, especially in the context of rapidly dwindling funds. The Whose Shoes? concept was born and much midnight oil was burned on R&D.

As the Whose Shoes? network grew, I adopted a very personalised approach, putting customers in touch with each other, co-producing and sharing facilitation ideas. We experimented together, pushing the boundaries. To begin with, people tended to use the tool to explore personalisation with their own staff. But then, as confidence grew, it became a genuine co-production tool to work with service users and carers; everyone contributing as equals.

Think Local Act Personal committed over 30 national organisations to work together and to develop, as one of the key priorities, a set of markers. These markers are being used to support all those working towards personalisation. This will help organisations check their progress and decide what they need to do to keep moving forward to deliver real change and positive outcomes with people.

Making It Real highlights the issues most important to the quality of people's lives. It helps the sector take responsibility for change and publicly share the progress being made.

Making It Real is built around 'I' statements. These express what people want to see and experience; and what they would expect to find if personalisation is really working well. I statements are an assertion about the feelings, beliefs and values of the person speaking. In the case of 'Making it Real', the I statements are what older and disabled people, carers and citizens expect to feel and experience when it comes to personalised care and support. They are grouped around six key themes:

1. information and advice
2. active and supportive communities
3. flexible integrated care and support
4. workforce
5. risk enablement *and*
6. personal budgets and self-funding.

There are in total twenty-six statements. Some examples of these statements are:

> *'I know the amount of money available to me for care and support needs, and I can determine how this is used (whether it is my own money, direct payment, or a council managed personal budget).'*
>
> *'I feel that my community is a safe place to live and local people look out for me and each other.'*
>
> *'I have good information and advice on the range of options for choosing my support staff.'*

CONCLUSION

There has been a recent shift from thinking about a 'patient' with a series of 'itemised problems' to be managed to a 'person' with his or her own individual issues. The past and present of that individual will shape that person's future, and approaches of person-centred care are pervasive in thinking about an individual may 'live well' with dementia. This book now progresses how elements of the physical environment can affect people with dementia – for example, assistive technologies and similar innovations (such as ambient assisted living devices) – as well as how parts of the home or ward can best be designed with an individual in mind. However, not all individuals with a clinical diagnosis of dementia will experience the same problems as result of their illness, and specific problems (such as in social dealings or wayfinding) may come to the fore as a result of the unique dementia process. Furthermore, it is clear that the community at large needs to be a welcoming one for an individual with dementia to live well in, and that will be the focus of the penultimate chapter of this book.

WEBSITE

- Think Local Act Personal: www.thinklocalactpersonal.org.uk

REFERENCES

Aveyard, B. (2001) Education and person-centred approaches to dementia care, *Nurs Older People*, **12**(10), pp. 17–19.

Baldwin, C., and Capstick, A. (eds) (2007) *Tom Kitwood on Dementia: A Reader and Critical Commentary*. Maidenhead: Open University Press.

Bradford Dementia Group (2005) *DCM 8 User's Manual*. Bradford: University of Bradford.

Brooker, D. (2005) Dementia Care Mapping (DCM): a review of the research literature, *Gerontologist*, **45 Spec No 1**(1), pp. 11–18.

Brooker, D., Foster, N., Banner, A., *et al.* (1998) The efficacy of Dementia Care Mapping as an audit tool: report of a 3-year British NHS evaluation, *Aging Ment Health*, **2**(1), 60–70.

Brooker D.J., and Surr C. (2006) Dementia Care Mapping (DCM): initial validation of DCM 8 in UK field trials, *Int J Geriatr Psychiatry*, **21**(11), pp. 1018–25.

Bryden, C. (2005) *Dancing with Dementia: My Story of Living Positively with Dementia*. London: Jessica Kinsley.

Chenoweth, L., King, M.T., Jeon, Y.H., *et al.* (2009) Caring for Aged Dementia Care Resident Study (CADRES) of person-centred care, dementia-care mapping, and usual care in dementia: a cluster-randomised trial, *Lancet Neurol*, **8**(4), pp. 317–25.

Department of Health (2001) *National Service Framework for Older People*. London: Department of Health.

Department of Health (2009) *Living Well with Dementia: A National Dementia Strategy; Putting people first*. London: The Stationery Office, available at: www.gov.uk/government/uploads/system/uploads/attachment_data/file/168221/dh_094052.pdf

Dolan, P., Peasgood, T., and White, M. (2008) Do we really know what makes us happy? A review of the economic literature on the factors associated with subjective wellbeing, *J Econ Psychol*, **29**(1), pp. 94–122.

Fillit, H., and Hill, J. (2004) The economic benefits of acetylcholinesterase inhibitors for patients with Alzheimer disease and associated dementias, *Alzheimer Dis Assoc Disord*, **18**(Suppl. 1), pp. S24–9.

Helliwell, J.F. (2003) How's life? Combining individual and national variables to explain subjective well-being, *Econ Model*, **20**, pp. 331–60.

Helliwell, J.F., and Putnam, R. (2004) The social context of well-being, *Philos Trans R Soc Lond B Biol Sci*, **359**(1449), pp. 1435–46.

Hutchinson, T.A. (2011) The challenge of medical dichotomies and the congruent phtsician-patient relationship. In: Hutchinson, T.A. (ed.) *Whole Person Care: A New Paradigm for the 21st Century*. New York, NY: Springer-Verlag. pp. 31–44.

Jaycock, S., Persaud M., and Johnson, R. (2006) The effectiveness of Dementia Care Mapping in intellectual disability residential services: a follow-up study, *J Intellect Disabil*, **10**(4), pp. 365–75.

Kitwood, T. (1993) Towards a theory of dementia care: the interpersonal process, *Ageing Soc*, **13**(1), pp. 51–67.

Kitwood, T. (1997) *Dementia Reconsidered: The Person Comes First*. Buckingham: Open University Press.

Kitwood, T., and Bredin, K. (1992) Towards a theory of dementia care: personhood and wellbeing, *Ageing Soc*, **12**, pp. 269–87.

Kitwood, T., Buckland, S., and Petre, T. (1995) Findings relating to wellbeing, and findings relating to illbeing'. In: *Brighter Futures: A Report into Provision for Persons with Dementia in Residential Homes, Nursing Homes and Sheltered Housing*, London: Anchor Housing Association.

Klein, S.B., Cosmides, L., Costabile, K.A. (2003) Preserved knowledge of self in a case of Alzheimer's disease, *Soc Cogn*, **21**(2), pp. 157–63.

Lewin, K. (1951) *Field Theory in Social Science: Selected Theoretical Papers*. Edited by Cartwright, D., New York, NY: Harper & Row.

Martin, G.W., and Younger, D. (2001) Person-centred care for people with dementia: a quality audit approach, *J Psychiatr Ment Health Nurs*, **8**(5), pp. 443–8.

McCormack, B. (2004) Person-centredness in gerontological nursing: an overview of the literature, *J Clin Nurs*, **13**(3a), pp. 31–8.

McCormack, B., and McCance, T.V. (2006) Development of a framework for person-centred nursing, *J Adv Nurs*, **56**(5), pp. 472–9.

National Care Forum (2007) *Key Principles of Person-Centred Dementia Care*. Coventry: National Care Forum, available at: www.guidepoststrust.org.uk/wp-content/uploads/2012/05/Key-principles-of-person-centred-dementia-care.pdf

National Institute for Health and Care Excellence (NICE) (2013) *Supporting people to live well with dementia (Quality Standard 30)*, statement 5, available at: http://publications.nice.org.uk/quality-standard-for-supporting-people-to-live-well-with-dementia-qs30/quality-statement-5-maintaining-and-developing-relationships

National Institute for Health and Care Excellence (NICE) (2013) *Supporting people to live well with dementia (Quality Standard 30)*, statement 6, available at: http://publications.nice.org.uk/quality-standard-for-supporting-people-to-live-well-with-dementia-qs30/quality-statement-6-physical-and-mental-health-and-wellbeing

Nolan, M.R., Davies, S., Brown, J., *et al.* (2004) Beyond person-centred care: a new vision for gerontological nursing, *J Clin Nurs*, **13**(13a), pp. 45–53.

Pichler, F. (2006) Subjective quality of life of young Europeans: feeling happy but who knows why? *Soc Indicat Res*, **75**, pp. 419–44.

Royal College of Psychiatrists (2013) *Whole-Person Care: From Rhetoric to Reality; Achieving Parity Between Mental and Physical Health*. London: Royal College of Psychiatrists.

Sabat, S.R., and Harré, R. (1992) The construction and deconstruction of self and Alzheimer's disease, *Ageing Soc*, **12**(4), pp. 443–61.

Social Care Institute for Excellence (SCIE) (2007) *Implementing the Carers (Equal Opportunities) Act 2004: SCIE Guide 9*. London, SCIE, available at: www.scie.org.uk/publications/guides/guide09/

Social Care Institute for Excellence (SCIE) (2009) *Dignity in Care: SCIE Guide 9*. London: SCIE, available at: www.scie.org.uk/publications/guides/guide15/

Surr, C.A. (2006) Preservation of self in people with dementia living in residential care: a socio-biographical approach, *Soc Sci Med Care*, **62**(7), pp. 1720–30.

UK Government/LGA/ADASS/NHS (2007) *Putting People First: A Shared Vision and Commitment to the Transformation of Adult Social Care*. London: The Stationery Office, available at: www.cpa.org.uk/cpa/putting_people_first.pdf

Young, J., and Sturdy, D. (2004) Senior moments, *Health Serv J*, **114**(5909), pp. 26–7.

Younger, D., and Martin, G. (2000) Dementia Care Mapping: an approach to quality audit of services for people with dementia in two health districts, *J Adv Nurs*, 32(5), pp. 1206–12.

CHAPTER 7

Leisure activities and living well with dementia

Statement 4. People with dementia are enabled, with the involvement of their carers, to take part in leisure activities during their day based on individual interest and choice.

Individuals with dementia, like other individuals, enjoy participating in a range of activities. There has been a renaissance in interest in '**leisure activities**'. Everyone has an inbuilt need to participate in activity, and, some might say, essentially what we do makes us who we are. Engaging in a balance of self-care, work and play activities is essential to our physical and mental wellbeing and thereby our quality of life. People with dementia are no exception – but dementia inevitably affects the ability to '*do*'. Leisure activities are the focus of this chapter, but other activities are considered in **Chapter 8**.

The specific effects of social and leisure activities on dementia have been investigated in only two known case-control studies (Broe *et al.*, 1990; Kondo *et al.*, 1994) and two follow-up studies (Fabrigoule *et al.*, 1995). As discussed by Wang and colleagues (Wang *et al.*, 2002), however, these studies found that an inactive life was related to a higher risk of dementia. However, case-control studies have been criticised because of the presence of selection and recall biases. Follow-up studies have been hampered by the fact that subjects in the early phases of dementia could reduce their activities because of initial cognitive impairment, depressive symptoms or other dementia-related conditions. However, the fundamental conclusion has been that, with respect to health-related behaviours, physical activity has a beneficial effect on subjective wellbeing (e.g. Biddle and Ekkekakis, 2005), and is also associated with fewer mental health problems (e.g. O'Connor, Smith and Morgan, 2000), though there is perhaps limited evidence on the exact direction of causality.

THE IMPORTANCE OF ACTIVITY AND SOCIAL NETWORKS

One of the most challenging aspects of providing care for someone with a dementing illness is to develop daily routines and activities that are interesting, meaningful, doable and valued by the person with the disease. Making sure there is a mix of activities to meet social, physical, mental and spiritual needs for each individual is a complex and ever-changing task. Also, social networks are becoming increasingly online, and this is an important consideration for care. According to Shirley Ayres in her excellent 'provocation paper' for the Nominet Trust (2013), social networks can be widened and enhanced by web-based tools and technology. The growth of online personal support networks strengthens the informal networks that already exist within communities. This paper has turned out to be a seminal contribution.

Studies related to older people with (or without) dementia have not been able to reach a consensus on the types and intensity of the exercise, nor the frequency and duration of the intervention to be most effective and efficient (Thom and Clare, 2011). Heyn and colleagues (Heyn, Abreu and Ottenbacher, 2004) carried out a meta-analysis of exercise in dementia and reported data on 30 trials of exercise. The authors reported on trials that included strength, cardiovascular or flexibility regimens, and analysed for functional, cognitive or behavioural outcomes. A significant positive effect of exercise on behavioural outcomes was reported. However, these trials do not provide a full picture of the effectiveness of exercise on behavioural and psychological symptoms of dementia for a number of reasons. There was considerable heterogeneity in terms of the interventions, and exercise was often combined with other behavioural interventions. Thus, it is difficult to isolate the effect that exercise has had on behavioural outcomes. Some regimens were quite complex and required a high degree of physical fitness that would preclude many older adults with complex physical problems and moderate or profound dementia from performing them. Moreover, they were potentially unsustainable without the support of trained therapists. Finally, the relatively high cost of delivery and specialist input required may prevent the interventions being used more widely. Most trials included in the analysis were relatively small, with only two of the eight studies that reported effects on behaviours having samples in excess of 100 participants.

Forbes and colleagues (Forbes *et al.*, 2008), on behalf of the Cochrane Collaboration, found that four trials met their inclusion criteria. However, only two trials were included in the analyses because the required data from the other two trials were not made available. Only one meta-analysis was conducted. The results from this review suggest that there is insufficient evidence of the effectiveness of physical activity programmes in managing or improving cognition, function, behaviour, depression and mortality in people with dementia. Few trials have examined these important outcomes. In addition, family caregiver outcomes and use of healthcare services were not reported in any of the included trials.

Some earlier studies had suggested that physical exercise might be beneficial in dementia. Physical activity and regular exercise training may slow down cognitive decline (Kramer, Erickson and Colcombe, 2006), and it has positive effects on cognition among those with cognitive decline (Heyn, Abreu and Ottenbacher, 2004). Physical exercise appears to alleviate depression and reduces behavioural symptoms in dementia patients (Teri *et al.*, 2003).

'Social activity' – specifically, activities that can broadly be seen as participation in society and between the generations – has been an important thrust of dementia wellbeing policy for some time. The World Health Organization (WHO, 2002) have defined active ageing as having not only physical and psychological dimensions but also as the capacity to participate in society. Social and cultural activities have also been shown to be beneficial in terms of wellbeing, functioning and survival (Glass *et al.*, 1999). What is clear is that successful ageing and wellbeing in dementia involve a complex interplay between personal and social factors – however, a common feature is 'activity', whether that is physical, cognitive or social.

A positive effect of physical activities on survival has long been recognised (Paffenberger *et al.*, 1993); more recently, a similar effect was also reported for social and productive activities (Glass *et al.*, 2006). Social disengagement has been suggested as a possible risk factor for cognitive decline in elderly persons (Bassuk, Glass and Berkman, 1999). In a Swedish community-based study, the Kungsholmen Project, a rich social network showed a protective effect against dementia (Fratiglioni *et al.*, 2000).

A FOCUS ON LEISURE ACTIVITIES

Some feel that there are essentially four categories of activities that fill our lives. They are work, self-care, leisure and rest activities. Maintaining a healthy balance among these activities helps us manage stress and optimise our positive sense of self and control in our lives.

Leisure activities are frequently seen as the highlight and most fun part of the day. These are the activities people do in their free time or when work is done and time permits. It is important to note, however, that some of the older generation we are now serving did not view leisure as a routine part of life or may in fact (wrongly) view leisure activities as 'wicked' or worthless. If this is the case, great care will need to be taken to provide leisure activities that are acceptable and mature, and perhaps deemed 'old-fashioned'. Some people may actually find 'working' leisure activities fun and rewarding. These might include setting up for or cleaning up after parties, participating in exercise groups, helping someone else complete a project or even helping to care for a pet.

Many practitioners in the dementia care field see activity and occupation as central to promoting wellbeing for people with dementia. Activities for people with dementia can be therapeutic, enhance quality of life, arrest mental decline and generate and maintain self-esteem (Marshall and Hutchinson, 2001). Activities can also create immediate pleasure, re-establish dignity, provide meaningful tasks, restore rôles and enable friendships.

NICE RECOMMENDATION AND QUALITY STANDARD

The National Institute for Health and Clinical Excellence (NICE) CG42 guidance on dementia (1.5.1.1) provides that *'Health and social care staff should aim to promote and maintain the independence'* and *'support for people to go at their own pace and participate in activities they enjoy'*.

Quality statement 4 provides that *'people with dementia are enabled, with the involvement of their carers, to take part in leisure activities during their day based on individual interest and choice'*.

People with dementia can choose to take part in leisure activities, during their day, which match their interests. Carers of people with dementia are involved in helping the person they support to choose and take part in leisure activities, during their day, which match the interests of the person with dementia. Local authorities and others commissioning services work with providers to ensure the services they commission enable people with dementia, with the involvement of their carers, to take part in leisure activities during their day based on individual interest and choice.

Social care staff enable people with dementia, with the involvement of their carers, to take part in leisure activities during their day based on individual interest and choice.

THE 'ROUGH-HEWN HYPOTHESIS' AND LEISURE ACTIVITIES

Unlike physical activity, there is no real guidance or measure for how much 'exercise' is needed to maintain wellbeing. Compared with the body of research on physical activity, there is relatively little research on the effects of intellectual activity on mental wellbeing. Where studies exist, they remain speculative and await further research into neurobiological and cognitive processes.

Published in 2001, a longitudinal analysis of leisure activities and intellectual functioning does establish a **'rough-hewn hypothesis'** (Schooler and Mulatu, 2001) that exposure to complex environments increases individuals' levels of intellectual functioning, while exposure to simple environments decreases them. As a result, the 'intellectual benefits for middle-ages and older adults of doing intellectually challenging things in their leisure time are significant and meaningful' (Schooler and Mulatu, 2001). These findings echo those of studies on the relationship between complex intellectual activities and dementia of the Alzheimer type where more research is available. One such study shows that patients with dementia of the Alzheimer type had reduced complexity of leisure time activities at least 5 years before the onset of the disease (Friedland *et al.*, 1997).

Evidence of the types of intellectual activities that are most beneficial for dementia wellbeing is notoriously difficult to find. Anecdotally, activities that involve some degree of complex mental processing – such as crosswords, bridge, Scrabble and sudoku – are valued by older people, but there is no evidence that demonstrates whether and how these activities have health benefits. That they have other benefits in terms of confidence seems likely. There is increasing interest in computer-based puzzles as a way of stimulating mental activity.

HOW TO PROMOTE 'CHOICE AND CONTROL'

Social Care Institute for Excellence (SCIE) guidance 15 gives practical advice on how to promote 'choice and control'. The following are some examples of this.

- Take time to understand and know the person, their previous lives and past achievements, and support people to develop 'life story books'
- Treat people as equals, ensuring they remain in control of what happens to them.
- Empower people by making sure they have access to jargon-free information about services when they want or need it.
- Don't assume that people are not able to make decisions.
- Value the time spent supporting people with decision-making as much as the time spent doing other tasks.

Rationale

It is important that people with dementia can take part in leisure activities during their day that are meaningful to them. People have different interests and preferences about how they wish to spend their time. People with dementia are no exception, but increasingly need the support of others to participate. Understanding this and how to enable people with dementia to take part in leisure activities can help maintain and improve quality of life.

Local arrangements

It is extremely important that local arrangements are in place to find out about the individual interests and preferences of people with dementia in order to ensure access to leisure activities of interest. People with dementia should be enabled to take part in leisure activities during their day based on individual interest and choice. Choices of activities during their day could be made under the **Mental Capacity Act** 2005 on behalf of people with dementia who lack capacity, provided that they are made in line with the 'code of practice' that accompanies the Act.

THE HIGH LEVEL OF INACTIVITY IN CARE HOMES

The National Dementia Strategy (Department of Health, 2009) clearly recognises that the policy of developing living well in dementia is relatively underdeveloped in care homes.

> One-third of people with dementia live in care homes and at least two-thirds of all people living in care homes have a form of dementia. This state of affairs has not been planned for, either through commissioning services or through workforce planning. The need for workforce development is profound, and training in this area is covered in the next chapter. This section focuses on: making dementia an explicitly owned priority within care homes; enabling a minimum standard level of input into care homes from specialist mental health services for older people; and using the inspection regimes to drive up care quality. Following the NICE/SCIE clinical guideline on dementia, SCIE work is now focusing on supporting the independent sector in its work on dementia care. More specifically, as part of the implementation of this Strategy, the Department will be discussing with SCIE and others how to promote best practice in dementia care in care homes.

Functional dependence in geriatric institutions raises important issues related to decline in overall health-related quality of life and professional caregivers' distress. Physical inactivity and disability in elderly institutionalised patients may negatively affect their ability to perform activities of daily living and worsen their health-related quality of life status (Andersen et al., 2004; Lazowski et al., 1999; Pham et al., 2003; Richardson, Bedard and Weaver, 2001).

Most busy people would probably admit to sometimes wishing they could just sit and do nothing for a few hours. Sadly, this is often the case for care home residents; the high level of inactivity in care homes has been documented since the 1950s and continues today. This is despite the evidence that participating in activity can reduce the levels of depression, challenging behaviour, falls and dependency in care home residents. A recent study assessed daytime activities as an unmet need for 76% of care home residents with dementia (Orrell et al., 2006). Many respondents were able to report their met and unmet needs despite having moderately severe dementia. The views of the person with dementia were commonly in agreement with the staff and family carers' views. In particular, respondents provided relatively higher unmet needs for psychological distress, company and information, and high unmet needs for daytime activities and eyesight or hearing problems.

Such issues have to be addressed, not least because the National Minimum

Standards for Care Homes for Older People (Department of Health, 2000) require care homes to provide 'opportunities for stimulation through leisure and recreational activities in and outside the home which suit the residents' needs, preferences and capacities'. A number of factors influence activity provision, for better or worse, including residents' abilities, interests and motivation; the physical environment; staffing levels and skills; and the organisational culture. The selection and provision of appropriate and personally meaningful activities requires staff to understand the nature of dementia and how it affects the ability to 'do'. It is, however, possible to utilise a range of skills and strategies in response to these difficulties.

COGNITION AND ACTIVITIES

Again, it is vital to appreciate that dementia is not a homogeneous condition, and the type of dementia of an individual as a working diagnosis is a vital consideration for leisure activities. The pivotal recognition that 'dementia' is a portmanteau term for a wide diversity of issues is an important theme of this book. It is important to understand how dementia affects the individual's ability to 'do', rather than the snapshot recorded in a photographic brain scan. Think about an activity that you thoroughly enjoy doing. Now, try to imagine doing this activity while experiencing any of the difficulties associated with dementia. For example, what if you forget (memory loss, a prominent symptom in dementia in the Alzheimer type) the sequence or goal halfway through? What if you cannot communicate with the other participants (language impairment or aphasia; this might be a prominent symptom in primary progressive non-fluent aphasia in the temporal variant of frontotemporal dementia). Perhaps you are disoriented in time, place and person; or perceptual problems affect your recognition of colours, shapes, objects – even your ability to use them (agnosia; this might be a prominent symptom in 'posterior cortical atrophy'); or you have difficulty learning.

As explained in the North West Dementia Centre (2005) fact sheet *Activities in Care Homes for People with Dementia*, most activities need a combination of skills to perform; therefore, it is useful to break down the activity into its component parts, as shown in Table 7.1.

TABLE 7.1 A breakdown of different competences needed for successful completion of activities (this analysis helpfully includes physical, sensory, cognitive, emotional and social domains)

Physical	Range of movement, strength, coordination, physical endurance, speed
Sensory	Enable us to interpret and interact with the world around us: smell, kinaesthetic, touch, sight, hearing, taste
Cognitive	Memory, problem-solving, logical thought processes, ability to organise oneself and time effectively, communication
Emotional	Internal drives and beliefs, motivate and enable us 'to do', borne out of culture, life experiences – in turn influence our choice of activities
Social	Interaction with other people and development of relationships influences and motivates our selection of, and participation, in activities

Source: North West Dementia Centre (2005).

It is impossible to be prescriptive about suitable activities. It can be difficult to distinguish precisely the stage a person is at, and activity preference is very individual. However, there are some useful general principles. In the early stages people can still follow the 'rules' and work towards a goal – for example, sports and board games (draughts, Scrabble, bowls and darts), group discussions and quizzes (about topics of interest or relevance); structured crafts (craft kits, knitting from a pattern). As thought processes and language are further impaired, it is difficult to follow such rules. However, familiar routines are retained, as is the ability to use familiar objects, so now offer music, dance and movement, reminiscence (using objects to prompt), painting and expressive crafts. As the

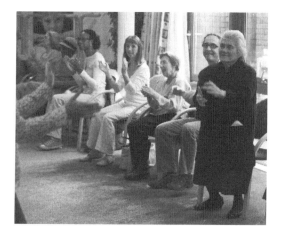

FIGURE 7.1 Individuals with dementia and their carers provide each other with much peer support, and contribute to the learning of the organisers of 'Healthy Living Club', with their understanding of their conditions. (Photograph by kind permission of the 'Healthy Living Club'.)

individual's world 'shrinks' further, activities need to stimulate the senses, encourage movement and be rhythmic and repetitive, one-step and simple. Examples include movement to music, dance, simple games using balls and balloons, folding, dusting, polishing, rummaging (using items with life history relevance – e.g. fabric, lace and buttons for a dressmaker), massage and multisensory stimulation, including the use of dolls, soft toys and animals.

As a glowing example of good practice, the **Healthy Living Club** is a self-directed community group in Lambeth (London) promoting the wellbeing of its members – people with dementia, their carers and friends – by giving them a strong sense of belonging, but also a sense of shared purpose: all members contribute to the functioning of the Club to the extent that they are able. The Club meets weekly at Lingham Court around a programme of activities designed to alleviate the symptoms of dementia and/or to help arrest, or reverse, cognitive decline.

The pioneer Simona Florio, coordinator of the 'Healthy Living Club at Lingham Court', explains as follows, quoted on the 'Whose Shoes' blog:

The decision to develop the 'product' collaboratively with the people for whom it was intended was wise in that the process of choosing the activities – with everybody expressing their likes and dislikes – turned out to be a community-building exercise in its own right, as it endowed participants with a strong sense of ownership. None of us refers to the people with dementia and the carers who participate as 'users' of a 'service' provided for them. It is experienced by all of us as our community. The fact that some of us have job or role descriptions (e.g. coordinator, workshop leader, support volunteer) does not necessarily mean that our input is greater than anybody else's and this is not just because the so called 'service users' also contribute to the group's functioning to the extent they are able (e.g. by helping serve lunch, fetching chairs, reciting poems and singing songs to the group). It is especially because our members with dementia and their carers contribute in ways we can't: they provide each other with peer support, and us with their insight into the disease. Through sharing their stories they very often also provide us with a source of inspiration, while improving our understanding of people from other generations, and of the past. In other words, our community produces relationships of exchange, with everybody being a giver as well as a beneficiary, and the currency which is exchanged the most is warmth. As a result, I can say, very confidently, that our meetings on Wednesdays are equally enjoyed by all.

Source: Phillips (2012) 'Whose Shoes' blog – see main references for citation. Quotation kindly reproduced by permission of Simona Florio and Gill Phillips.

There are undoubtedly challenges to developing more flexible and responsive services to make them more culturally and ethnically sensitive and inclusive, and to ensure that they are being integrated into the fabric of the community.

The Healthy Living Clubs demonstrate a powerful policy commitment for a focus on individuals with dementia to be in contact with others, and to enjoy daily activities.

INTERGENERATIONAL ACTIVITIES

Since its formation in 1999, Age Concern Kingston has pioneered intergenerational practice, purposefully bringing together older and younger generations to promote greater understanding between them.

An intergenerational programme in West Leeds that connects older people in the early stages of dementia with primary school children from two local schools has been an impressive initiative (Leeds City Council, 2012). The programme is based on a 'circle-time' model, where intergenerational conversation is encouraged in weekly sessions, plus a range of activities including board games, craft sessions, word games, quizzes and bell-ringing. Initially, the conversations have a reminiscence theme, such as World War II. The programme has now been running for 2 years and there are approximately 30 sessions per year with, on average, 10 older and younger participants each time.

The programme takes place in the school. The evaluation tools used were project diaries, participant feedback after each session (using *'my word about today is …'*), participant and carer feedback overall, and project worker/teacher feedback. The nature of failing memory means it is difficult to get people involved in any activity (e.g. I do not want to try anything new, I like to keep to a routine, I do not want to go out) let alone an intergenerational one (e.g. I am not interested in spending time with children, I find children too noisy). Once involved, failing memory brings additional difficulties. For instance, despite telephone reminders on the morning of the activity, people are not always in when transport arrives to pick them up.

WEBSITE

● Age Concern Kingston, Intergenerational project: www.ageconcernkingston.org/who/intergenerational-project/

REFERENCES

Andersen, C.K., Wittrup-Jensen, K.U., Lolk, A., *et al.* (2004) Ability to perform activities of daily living is the main factor affecting quality of life in patients with dementia, *Health Qual Life Outcomes*, 2, pp. 52.

Ayres, S. (2013) *Can Online Innovations Enhance Social Care?* Oxford: Nominet Trust, available at: www.nominettrust.org.uk/sites/default/files/Enhancing%20social%20care_PP_0113.pdf

Bassuk, S.S., Glass, T.A., and Berkman, L.F. (1999) Social disengagement and incident cognitive decline in community-dwelling elderly persons, *Ann Intern Med*, **131**(3), pp. 165–73.

Biddle, S.J.H., and Ekkekakis, P. (2005) Physically active lifestyles and well-being. In: Huppert, F.A., Baylis, N., and Keverne, B. (eds) *The Science of Well-Being*, Oxford: Oxford University Press, pp. 141–68.

Broe, G.A., Henderson, A.S., Creasey, H., *et al.* (1990) A case-control study of Alzheimer's disease in Australia, *Neurology*, 40(11), pp. 1698–707.

Department of Health (2000) *Care Homes for Older People: National Minimum Standards; Care Home Regulations*. Third edition. London: The Stationery Office, available at: www.dignityincare.org.uk/_library/Resources/Dignity/OtherOrganisation/CSCI_National_Minimum_Standards.pdf

Department of Health (2009) *Living Well with Dementia: A National Dementia Strategy; Putting people first*. London: The Stationery Office, available at: www.gov.uk/government/uploads/system/uploads/attachment_data/file/168221/dh_094052.pdf

Fabrigoule, C., Letenneur, L., Dartigues, J.F., *et al.* (1995) Social and leisure activities and risk of dementia: a prospective longitudinal study, *J Am Geriatr Soc*, 43(5), pp. 85–90.

Forbes, D., Forbes, S., Morgan, D.G., *et al.* (2008) Physical activity programs for persons with dementia, *Cochrane Database Syst Rev*, 16(3), CD006489.

Fratiglioni, L., Wang, H.X., Ericsson, K., *et al.* (2000) The influence of social network on the occurrence of dementia: a community-based longitudinal study, *Lancet*, **355**(9212), pp. 1315–19.

Friedland R.P., Smyth, K., Esteban-Santillan, C., *et al.* (1997) Premorbid environmental complexity is reduced in patients with Alzheimer's disease (AD) as compared to age and sex matched controls: results of a case-control study. Proceedings of the Fifth International Conference on Alzheimer's Disease and Related Disease. In: Iqbal, K., Winblad, B., Wisniewski, H. (eds) *Neurobiology of Aging*, New York, NY: John Wiley & Sons, pp. 33–7.

Glass, T.A., De Leon, C.F., Bassuk, S.S., *et al.* (2006) Social engagement and depressive symptoms in late life: longitudinal findings, *J Aging Health*, **18**(4), pp. 604-28.

Glass, T.A., de Leon, C.M., Marottoli, R.A., *et al.* (1999) Population-based study of social and productive activities as predictors of survival amongst elderly Americans, *BMJ*, 319(7208), pp. 478–83.

Heyn, P., Abreu, B.C., and Ottenbacher, K.J. (2004) The effects of exercise training on elderly persons with cognitive impairment and dementia: a meta-analysis, *Arch Phys Med Rehabil*, 85(10), pp. 1694–704.

Kondo, K., Niino, M., and Shido, K. (1994) A case-control study of Alzheimer's disease in Japan-Significance of life-styles, *Dementia*, 5(6), pp. 314–26.

Kramer, A.F., Erickson, K.I., and Colcombe, S.J. (2006) Exercise, cognition, and the aging brain, *J Appl Physiol*, **101**(4), pp. 1237–42.

Lazowski, D.A., Ecclestone, N.A., Myers, A.M., *et al.* (1999) A randomized outcome evaluation of group exercise programs in long-term care institutions, *J Gerontol A Biol Sci Med Sci*, **54**(12), pp. M621–8.

Leeds City Council (2012) *Living Well with Dementia in Leeds: Our Local Strategy 2012–15.* available at: www.tenfold.org.uk/downloads/publications/Living-well-with-dementia-in-Leeds-draft-strategy.pdf

Marshall, M.J., and Hutchinson, S.A. (2001) A critique of research on the use of activities with persons with Alzheimer's disease: a systematic literature review, *J Adv Nurs*, **35**(4), 488–96.

National Institute for Health and Care Excellence (NICE) (2013) *Supporting people to live well with dementia (Quality Standard 30)*, statement 4, available at: http://publications. nice.org.uk/quality-standard-for-supporting-people-to-live-well-with-dementia-qs30/ quality-statement-4-leisure-activities-of-interest-and-choice

North West Dementia Centre (2005) *Activities in Care Homes for People with Dementia*. London: Personal Social Services Research Unit, available at: www.pssru.ac.uk/pdf/ MCpdfs/Activities_factsheet.pdf

O'Connor, P.J., Smith, J.C., and Morgan, W.P. (2000) Physical activity does not provoke panic attacks in patients with panic disorder: a review of the evidence, *Anxiety Stress Coping*, **13**, pp. 333–53.

Orrell, M., Hancock, G.A., Woods, R., *et al.* (2006) The needs of older people with dementia in residential care, *Int J Geriatr Psychiatry*, **20**(5), pp. 941–51.

Paffenbarger, R.S. Jr, Hyde, R.T., Wing, A.L., *et al.* (1993) The association of changes in physical-activity level and other lifestyle characteristics with mortality among men, *N Engl J Med*, **328**(8), pp. 538–45.

Pham, M., Pinganaud, G., Richard-Harston, S., *et al.* (2003) Prospective audit of diabetes care and outcomes in a group of geriatric French care homes, *Diabetes Metab*, **29**(3), pp. 251–8.

Phillips, G. (2012) In the shoes of ... Simona Florio | Co-ordinator | The Healthy Living Club A blogpost on the 'Whose Shoes' blog, September 12, available at: http:// whoseshoes.wordpress.com/2012/09/12/in-the-shoes-of-simona-florio-co-ordinator-the-healthy-living-club/

Richardson, J., Bedard, M., and Weaver, B. (2001) Changes in physical functioning in institutionalized older adults, *Disabil Rehabil*, **23**(15), pp. 683–9.

Schooler, C., and Mulatu, M.S. (2001) The reciprocal effects of leisure time activities and intellectual functioning in older people: a longitudinal analysis, *Psychol Aging*, **16**(3), pp. 466–82.

Social Care Institute for Excellence (SCIE). *Guide 15: Dignity factors – Choice and control*. London: SCIE, available at: www.scie.org.uk/publications/guides/guide15/files/ guide15.pdf

Teri, L., Gibbons, L.E., McCurry, S.M., *et al.* (2003) Exercise plus behavioural management in patients with Alzheimer disease: a randomized controlled trial, *JAMA*, **290**(15), pp. 2015–22.

Thom, J.M., and Clare, L. (2011) Rationale for combined exercise and cognition-focused interventions to improve functional independence in people with dementia, *Gerontology*, **57**(3), pp. 265–75.

UK Government. *Mental Capacity Act 2005*, available at: www.legislation.gov.uk/ ukpga/2005/9/contents

Wang, H.X., Karp, A., Winblad, B., *et al.* (2002) Late-life engagement in social and leisure activities is associated with a decreased risk of dementia: a longitudinal study from the Kungsholmen project, *Am J Epidemiol*, **155**(12), pp. 1081–7.

World Health Organization (WHO) (2002) *Active Ageing: A Policy Framework*. Geneva: WHO.

CHAPTER 8

Maintaining wellbeing in end-of-life care for living well with dementia

The figures are staggering. For any given disorder, people with dementia have four to six times the mortality than the cognitively intact (Morrison and Siu, 2000). People with dementia often live for many years after their diagnosis. It is considered sensible to make end-of-life care plans well in advance of some-one entering the end-of-life phase, but effective end-of-life care is essentially focused person-centred care. This was considered in **Chapter 6** for all aspects of living well with dementia. Effective communication is also critical, and this will be considered in **Chapter 12** for all aspects of living well with dementia. Many people have a rôle to play in end-of-life care – a GP, district nurses, care staff, speech and language therapists, to name a few – so the network can be large. One of the most critical aspects to good end-of-life care is making sure that each member of the care team communicates reliably with others in the team. Without good information-sharing across explicit and implicit 'barriers to communication', a person is less likely to receive the care they need, and this inevitably is going to have an impact on their quality of care.

End-of-life care provides support for those people with an irreversible pro-gressive form of dementia, so they are able to live as well as possible until their death. This ideally provides support for those closest too. Care can be provided at home, in a hospice, a care home or hospital. Everyone who has been diagnosed with dementia should have a care plan drawn up with health-care professionals (NHS Choices, last reviewed February 2013). End-of-life care should be a key part of this dementia care plan, according to the National Institute for Health and Clinical Excellence (**NICE-SCIE guidance** 42). Having end-of-life care covered in the care plan means the person with dementia will hopefully be able to specify where he or she would like to die and to ensure that the person is treated with dignity in the way he or she would wish. The dementia care plan should also provide some support for carers of people with dementia who will experience feelings of bereavement and grief around the time of death. There is strong evidence to suggest that people with dementia receive poorer end-of-life care than those who are cognitively intact, in terms of provision of palliative care (Sampson *et al.*, 2006). For example, few people with dementia have access to hospice care.

People are very bad at discussing end-of-life issues. For example, Tessa Richards, in the *BMJ*'s '**A better way to die**' (2007), writes:

> Birth and death are rites of passage for which preparation is important. In rich countries, information and support during pregnancy and childbirth are available in spades from a vast range of professional and lay sources. Choice of venue for the birth is often on offer too. The risk is not so much of entering uncharted territory unprepared as entering it overwhelmed by a deluge of advice.
>
> Are we equally well prepared for dying and death? Speaking for myself, the answer is no. I dodged the issue before my own life threatening surgery and floundered as I witnessed my father's slow decline from dementia. Practising medicine conferred familiarity but not understanding, competence, or even compassion. I learnt a lot through following his journey. Not from the half dozen doctors he was nominally under, but from his nursing auxiliaries, who without exception came from poor countries. They tried, as we did, to bring meaning into a life that had been truncated by unexpected loss as well as disease.

During the later stages of dementia most people will become increasingly frail because of the progression of the illness. They will also gradually become dependent on others for all of their care. Knowing what to expect can help everyone to prepare. It can enable the person with dementia to think about the kind of treatment and care he or she might want, and allows them to write an informed advance decision before they reach this stage so they can have input into how they will be cared for. It also allows carers and family to think about these aspects too.

The later stages of dementia can be a distressing time for carers and relatives.

SUPPORT FOR CARERS

One of the best things we can do is to support carers to be able to talk about their feelings, and this is particularly true at the end of life. There are many possible sources for this emotional support for carers: perhaps a valued professional (e.g. a mental health nurse), a carers' group, a religious organisation, or even a close personal friend.

Another useful avenue for support is the '**Admiral Nurse service**'. Admiral Nurses are mental health nurses who specialise in dementia. They work in the community with families, carers and other supporters or paid carers of people with dementia throughout the illness and offer information, practice advice and emotional support. The charity '**Dementia UK**' works in partnership with NHS providers and commissioners, social care authorities and voluntary sector organisations to promote and develop new Admiral Nursing services. The charity is responsible for upholding standards, sustaining service and supporting Admiral Nurses in practice.

The Department of Health's *End of Life Care Strategy* (2008) emphasises that the wellbeing of families and carers also needs to be safeguarded with care. This strategy made clear the need for the development of end-of-life pathways that draw on the good practice. The National Dementia Strategy (Department of Health, 2009) later argued:

> local work on end of life care needs to focus on the large numbers of people who will die with dementia. In addition, in workforce development for end of life care, commissioners and providers need to consider how to ensure that effective end of life care for people with dementia can be made real, including the effective use of specialist liaison with palliative care providers and skilled training in pain detection, pain relief and end of life nursing care.

Sadly, however, this report described that support for family and carers both during a person's illness and into bereavement is often inadequate. This poor level of support can have an adverse impact on the carer's health and wellbeing and on his or her ability to provide care. Deficiencies in services can have a severe adverse impact on the wellbeing of patients and carers. There is now increasing evidence that the lack of well-coordinated community-based care leads to avoidable admissions and to prolonged hospital stays. However, there is also increasing evidence that these deficiencies in care can be rectified through the introduction of innovative service models and approaches to practice.

SYMPTOMS IN THE LATER STAGES

Each person with dementia experiences the illness in his or her own individual way. The symptoms described in this section do not necessarily indicate that a person is in the later stages of the disease, as several of them can also be experienced in the earlier stages. However, these symptoms are very likely to occur in the later stages of most dementias. Most of the symptoms experienced by frail older people with dementia at the end of life, such as pain or swallowing difficulties, do not require specialist palliative intervention but, rather, just good general care. They often experience symptoms similar to people with cancer, such as pain, pressure ulcers, agitation, eating problems and loss of appetite, constipation, breathing difficulties and low mood.

Memory loss

Memory loss is likely to be very severe in the later stages of dementia. People may be unable to recognise those close to them, or even their own reflection. They may no longer be able to find their way around familiar surroundings or identify everyday objects. However, they may occasionally experience sudden flashes of recognition. The person may believe that they are living in a time from their past, and may search for someone or something from that time. It can be helpful for those around them to use this as an opportunity to talk about the past and try to reassure the person. Even if a person has severe memory loss, they may still be able to appreciate or respond to stimuli such as music, scent and touch. It is important to continue to talk to the person, even if he or she can't respond.

Problems with communication

The person with dementia will experience increasing problems understanding what is being said to them and what is going on around them. They are likely to find it difficult to communicate with other people. They may gradually lose their speech, or they may repeat a few words or cry out from time to time.

Communication issues are discussed in further detail in **Chapter 12**.

Loss of mobility

Many people with dementia gradually lose their ability to walk as well as before; a stroke, a form of arthritis or the effects of a fall may also affect a person's mobility. Some people with dementia eventually become confined to a bed or chair. Those who are caring for the person should seek advice from a physiotherapist or community nurse on how best to help the person to move without injuring the person or themselves. An occupational therapist can also give advice about equipment and adaptations to aid mobility.

Sleep disorders and 'sundowning'

Sleep disorders or disruptive nocturnal behaviours are commonly reported in people with dementia, and can present as both a significant clinical problem and a cause of increased stress for caregivers. In later stages of the dementia of Alzheimer type, in a phenomenon known as '**sundowning**', behavioural symptoms can occur or become exacerbated in the afternoon and evening (Volicer et al., 2001). The neurobiological substrate of this phenomenon continues to spark substantial academic interest (for example, Klaffke and Staedt, 2006). In extreme cases, persons with dementia in the late stages may have a complete reversal of the usual daytime wakefulness-night sleep pattern. The area of sleep and wellbeing, in general, is likely to be a fertile area of research in forthcoming years.

Eating and weight loss

It is important to ensure that the person is getting enough food and liquid. He or she may need help and encouragement with eating and drinking. Problems with chewing and swallowing are common in the later stages of dementia because of the person's muscles and reflexes no longer working properly. These problems can cause the individual with advanced dementia to choke on food or to develop chest infections, and an occupational therapist may help. Furthermore, as the disease process of dementia might affect the central brain centres for satiety (such as the ventromedial hypothalamus), an individual with dementia might have a change in food preferences, such as a preference for sugary drinks, and, indeed, a specialist cognitive neurologist or dietitician can provide particular help.

Problems with continence

Persons may lose control of their bladder in the later stages of dementia. Some also lose control of their bowels. This may happen all or most of the time, or it may just be a case of occasional leakage.

Incontinence is not an inevitable symptom of dementia, but there are a number of reasons why someone with dementia could become incontinent. These include various medical conditions, a number of which are treatable. Possible causes include:

- urinary tract infection
- respiratory infection
- severe constipation
- side effects of medication
- prostate gland trouble
- forgetting to go to the toilet or forgetting where the toilet is
- not recognising the need to go to the toilet.

If a person develops problems with continence, their GP should refer them to a community nurse or local continence adviser, who can give advice and help with getting incontinence pads and other aids.

HEALTH RISKS

There are a number of factors common during the later stages of dementia that can cause problems for the person's health. These include immobility, the side effects of medication and illness or discomfort.

Pressure ulcers

If the person with dementia remains in the same position for too long – for example, in a bed or chair – he or she may develop pressure ulcers. Pressure ulcers need immediate attention, as they can easily become infected and painful. Persons in the later stages of dementia can be at increased risk of pressure ulcers for a number of possible reasons such as frailty, difficulties in mobility, incontinence, poor diet and dehydration.

A **pressure ulcer** can be described as *'localised, acute ischaemic damage to any tissue caused by the application of external force (either shear, compression, or a combination of the two)'* (review, Ebhardt, 2002). Pressure ulcers occur when soft tissues (most commonly the skin) are distorted in a fixed manner over a long period. It is important to understand that the application of pressure, *per se*, does not cause damage. The combined skills of a doctor, nurse, physiotherapist or occupational therapist may contribute to effective care to improve the well-being with a person with a pressure ulcer (NICE Clinical Guidance 29, 2005).

Adverse effects of medication

All drugs can have adverse effects, and some of the drugs that are frequently prescribed for behavioural symptoms in people with dementia can have severe side effects and may increase the person's confusion.

Illness and discomfort

Infections can increase confusion in people with dementia, and exacerbate existing cognitive and emotional dysfunction. It is therefore important that if a person with dementia develops an infection it is quickly diagnosed and treated.

OVERVIEW OF PRINCIPLES OF MANAGEMENT
Medication

It is reported that the anti-dementia drug **memantine** can help stabilise the condition and maintain important skills such as feeding and walking, and may improve symptoms of aggression and restlessness.

In a review, Lyseng-Williamson and McKeage (2013) have recently described that, in the European Union, once-daily memantine 20 mg is an option for the management of patients with moderate to severe Alzheimer's disease. In pooled clinical trials and studies in the clinical practice setting, memantine 20 mg/day improved cognition, functional ability and behavioural symptoms in this patient population.

The cost-effectiveness of memantine has already been introduced in this book in **Chapter 4**. Lyseng-Williamson and McKeage (2013) also reported that the beneficial effects of memantine are associated with delays in the need for full-time care, which were predicted to result in cost savings relative to standard care in recent cost-utility analyses in patients with moderate to severe dementia of the Alzheimer type conducted in European Union countries. Memantine is well tolerated, with an adverse event profile that is similar to that with placebo.

In 2011, the National Institute for Health and Clinical Excellence recommended memantine as part of NHS care for the treatment of severe Alzheimer's or moderate disease where drugs such as donepezil cannot be taken. Access to the medication may still vary across the country. Finally, it is worth noting that Mossello and Ballini (2012) have warned possible drug-related adverse events can affect quality of life and should always be weighed against expected benefits from the patient's perspective.

What care or treatment may be offered?

If someone in the later stages of dementia becomes seriously ill, there may be a discussion about whether to try to prolong the person's life or to allow him or her to die naturally. Only the doctor can make the final decision about whether to give or withhold treatment in the final stages of dementia. However, the views of relatives and of the person with dementia should always be taken into account where possible.

If a lasting power of attorney has been set up, the doctors must consult with the attorney before initiating or withdrawing any treatment. It may also be helpful if the person with dementia has put his or her wishes in writing at an earlier stage in the illness.

End-of-life treatments may include:
- resuscitation after a heart attack
- antibiotic treatment for pneumonia
- oxygen therapy for shortness of breath.

Resuscitation may be unsuccessful in people in the final stages of dementia, and even when it is successful, there is a risk of causing further brain damage.

What may be most likely to cause an individual's eventual death?

The life expectancy of a person with dementia is unpredictable, and the disease can progress for up to around 10 years. It is estimated that a third of people with dementia at any one time will be in the later stages of the disease. Another condition or illness (such as pneumonia – an infection in the lung) may actually cause a person's death. This other condition or illness will most likely be listed as the cause on the person's death certificate. Pneumonia is often cited as the ultimate cause of death in up to two-thirds of people with dementia.

The person's ability to cope with infections and other physical problems will be impaired because of the progression of the disease, and the person may die because of a clot on the lung or a heart attack. However, in some people no specific cause of death is found other than dementia. If the person is over 70, ageing may also be given as a contributing factor. Alternatively, the death of a person with dementia might be caused by a condition that is completely unrelated to his or her dementia. Depending on the circumstances and the practices of the doctor, dementia may be entered on the death certificate as the sole or main cause of death, or as a contributing factor. If it has not been mentioned, you can ask the doctor to include it if you wish.

DYING WELL IN DEMENTIA

There are 700 000 people with dementia in the UK (Knapp *et al.*, 1997), and at least 100 000 of these die each year (Bayer, 2006). National policy is clear that people should receive good end-of-life care, irrespective of the condition in which they die (Department of Health, 2008). However, problems exist on provision of care towards the end of the lives of individuals with dementia. Reported problems include underdiagnosis and poor treatment of pain (Scherder *et al.*, 2005), painful and unnecessary investigations (Mitchell *et al.*, 2004), and inappropriate use of aggressive treatments (Evers *et al.*, 2002). It is argued that failure to recognise dementia as a terminal condition, and the costs attached to accommodating non-cancer patients, may preclude access to palliative care (Sampson *et al.*, 2006). In fact, the majority of deaths of people with dementia occur in institutional settings such as care homes and hospitals (Mitchell *et al.*, 2005), where unmet needs and concerns about care quality appear most pervasive (Teno *et al.*, 2004).

In an attempt to pre-specify the content of end-of-life care, advance care planning has emerged (Department of Health, 2009). In the United States, advance directives, in which a person with dementia can indicate his or her wish to refuse medical treatment, have been associated with reduced family stress (Engel, Kiely and Mitchell, 2006). Lawrence and colleagues (Lawrence *et al.*, 2011) completed a study of 'Dying well with dementia': this was a qualitative examination of end-of-life care. The study's primary finding was that there is a need to 'dementia-proof' end-of-life care for people with dementia. If end-of-life care does not take into account the unique circumstances and needs of people with dementia, it is likely to fail them. This requires service providers and care professionals to ensure that the environments in which people live and die – be they at home, in a care home, in NHS continuing care or in a general hospital – do three things: (1) use knowledge of dementia to identify and respond to physical care needs; (2) go beyond task-focused care; and (3) prioritise planning and communication with the family.

These data support the general suggestion that NHS continuing care units might act as a model for meeting the complex needs of people with advanced dementia (Hughes, Robinson and Volicer, 2005). The units in this study provided valuable examples of good end-of-life care, whereby care plans were carefully formulated with the family and services worked to ensure that they were followed, including the avoidance of transfer to acute hospitals. The care homes within this study were in an intermediate position with respect to quality; some homes, where basic and palliative care needs had been identified and met and staff had got to know the individual, provided positive end-of-life experiences equivalent to those in NHS continuing care units. However, where there was less communication with the family or where plans were not followed and there were admissions to acute hospitals, individuals had poor experiences. For individuals with dementia, death in general hospital tended to be almost invariably associated with poor quality, with staff appearing to provide inadequate assistance with eating and drinking, and failing to manage pain, to seek information from carers about the individual or to discuss treatment options with families at the end of life. A high proportion of people with dementia in the UK die in general hospitals, and improvement in end-of-life care and in general hospital care are both priorities in the National Dementia Strategy (Department of Health, 2009), but the data indicate that little as yet has been achieved.

NATIONAL COUNCIL FOR PALLIATIVE CARE RECOMMENDATIONS FOR AN EARLY DIAGNOSIS

The National Council for Palliative Care's (NCPC) response (from 1 March 2012) concentrated on three key areas.

- Section 1 – the common failure of GPs to give a diagnosis 'because nothing can be done'.
- Section 2 – early diagnosis is essential in ensuring people are able to plan ahead for their care, including palliative and end of life care.

Early diagnosis is essential in ensuring that people with dementia are able to plan ahead for their future care, including palliative and end of life care. The progressive nature of dementia and its impact on cognition faces people with dementia, their family and friends with major losses that make the journey very difficult for those involved. However, these challenges can be made easier through early planning. Early diagnosis enables people with dementia to engage in Advance Care Planning (ACP), allowing them to discuss and record their wishes so that decisions can be made on the basis of the person's best interests at a future time when they have lost capacity. If a person with dementia is offered the opportunity early enough, through the Mental Capacity Act, to appoint a Lasting Power of Attorney (LPA), make an advance decision to refuse treatment (ADRT) or express a preference on where/what end of life care they would like to receive, then they have a much higher chance of experiencing a good death. Early diagnosis allows people with dementia the time to think about these important decisions and communicate their wishes with their family and friends.

If they are not able to do this, then their wishes may not be carried out and they might not receive the end of life care or death that they desired. This can influence their experience of care throughout their life with dementia, not just at the end.

NCPC and the Dying Matters coalition have produced a volume of work which encourages conversations to be held about the end of life. Difficult Conversations: for dementia for example, deal with different ways in which discussing end of life care can be approached.

This work showed that more needs to be done to ensure that at the time of diagnosis, GPs are giving people with dementia the correct information and advice regarding planning for palliative and end of life care. While these discussions may be difficult for a GP to initiate, they are vital to ensure that planning can occur while a person with dementia still has the capacity to express their wishes. NCPC and Dying Matters are running a series of GP training projects to help build the confidence of GPs to have these difficult conversations. A late diagnosis or delayed information can mean that people with dementia miss out on the opportunity to have some control over their future and death.

Reproduced with kind permission of the National Council for Palliative Care from National Council for Palliative Care (NCPC) Response, All-Party Parliamentary Group on Dementia 2012 Inquiry: Improving dementia diagnosis rates in the UK, 1 March 2012. Retrieved from www.ncpc.org.uk/sites/default/files/NCPC_response_APPG_Dementia_diagnosis_inquiry.pdf, December 2013.

- Section 3 – the direct relationship that diagnosis has on the experience of carers.

DEALING WITH PAIN IN ADVANCED DEMENTIA

Pain is one of the most common symptoms that people with dementia experience in the advanced stages. However, often it is poorly recognised and undertreated in dementia. People with dementia are usually older and therefore many of the causes of pain will be the same as those for older people in general – for example, osteoarthritis, a disease that can affect some or all of the bones and joints, pressure ulcers skin tears, leg ulcer dressings, muscle rigidity and excessive constipation. Therefore, it will be essential that due clinical attention is given to these domains by professionals. One can ask a range of professionals for advice on pain management: a tissue viability nurse, palliative care or district nurse, physiotherapist or massage therapist, or a GP or local pain specialist team.

As dementia progresses, the person's ability to communicate his or her needs becomes more difficult. The National Dementia Strategy (Department of Health, 2009) is very clear on the necessity for optimally managed pain control in advanced dementia.

The subject of pain illustrates the discriminatory care provided for people with dementia. In the last year of care giving, 63% of family carers reported that the patient had been in pain either 'often' or 'all the time'. Yet people with dementia receive less analgesia than other older people for a given illness. Dementia may impair the ability of an individual to make themselves understood, and at least some of the agitated and aggressive behaviours seen in late-stage dementia may be an expression of pain. People with dementia admitted to hospital for hip fracture with the same surgical intervention received less than half the pain relief of those who were cognitively intact. The majority of those with dementia were in severe pain post operatively and this pain was not actively managed. However, communication problems in dementia may lead staff to 'surmise that pain not expressed is pain

> not experienced', and that pain expressed as aggression or confusion may lead to labelling and management as 'difficult'.

The *How Would I Know? What Can I Do?* leaflet was a guide published by the NCPC in December 2012 for carers. It provides advice on how to help with pain and distress in people with dementia, and it has been published as part of the Prime Minister's Dementia Challenge.

Pain is a *very personal, subjective perception*, fundamentally because the brain processes pain entirely in its overall emotional context.

The NCPC advise that there are simple things one can do:

- ask the person what the matter is
- listen to him or her
- observe the individual's behaviour and what's going on
- act on what you've seen and heard.

Communication problems can lead to problems in ascertaining that an individual with dementia may be in discomfort or in pain. According to the Social Care Institute for Excellence 'End of life for people with dementia' resource (see the list of websites at the end of this chapter), the best thing to do is to ask the person directly. Many people with moderate or even advanced dementia may still be able to provide information on their pain. This resource advises people to keep questions simple, as some people may not understand what you mean when you use the word 'pain'. Furthermore, when a person has poor short-term memory, the person may only be able to tell you if he or she is in pain at that moment – the person may not remember if he or she had pain 5 minutes or 5 hours ago.

However, the following points could be important clues about such patients:

- What does the person's face look like? Is he or she grimacing or grinding or clenching his or her teeth?
- Is the person rubbing, pointing or pulling at a particular part of his or her body?
- Is the person irritable? Crying or tearful? Or groaning? Is he or she shouting or screaming?
- What is the person's body language like? I she or she stiff, or rocking or perhaps guarding part of his or her body?
- What happens when the person moves? Is he or she less mobile, or moving differently? Is he or she pacing, unable to settle for long, restless or fidgeting?
- Is the person looking fearful? Does he or she seem to be seeing things or to be frightened?
- Has his or her appetite changed?
- Has his or her breathing pattern changed?

Individuals with dementia can feel pain, and there are things you can do to treat it. It depends on the severity of the pain, but things that might help include the following:

- changing the person's position
- touch, massage, presence and reassurance
- cool compress, or warmth
- using easily available painkillers such as paracetamol if not contraindicated.

However, individuals are advised that sometimes this may not be enough, and it may be necessary to speak to a doctor or a dentist, to ask for expert help with pain management.

EATING AND DRINKING

Eating and drinking issues cannot be underestimated either in advancing dementia.

People with dementia can develop problems with swallowing food or fluids in any stage of their illness, although it is most common to see this at the advanced stage. Dysphagia, or swallowing impairment, is a growing concern in dementia and can lead to malnutrition, dehydration, weight loss, functional decline and fear of eating and drinking, as well as a decrease in quality of life. Alagiakrishnan, Bhanji and Kurian (2013) recently completed an electronic literature search of five electronic databases from 1990 to 2011. A total of 1010 records were identified and 19 research articles met the authors' inclusion criteria. The authors reported a number of useful findings. Prevalence of swallowing difficulties in patients with dementia ranged from 13% to 57%. Dysphagia developed during the late stages of frontotemporal dementia, but it was seen during the early stage of dementia of the Alzheimer type. Limited evidence was available on the usefulness of diagnostic tests, effect of postural changes, modification of fluid and diet consistency, behavioural management and the possible use of medications. Use of percutaneous endoscopic gastrostomy tubes in advanced dementia did not show benefit with regard to survival, improvement in quality of life or reduction in aspiration pneumonia. Significant gaps exist regarding the evidence for the evaluation and management of dysphagia in dementia.

When a person with advanced dementia takes in only a very limited amount of food and fluids or can no longer swallow safely, it may seem that they are starving to death. In fact, they are not. Even so, medical professionals may consider using tube feeding at this time. This can be an extremely difficult and emotional time for family and care staff as they try to work out how to best respond and care for the person with dementia. In the end stages of dementia, the person's food and fluid intake tends to decrease slowly over time. The body adjusts to this slowing-down process and the reduced intake. It is thought that by this stage the hunger and thirst part of the brain has now stopped functioning for most people. Furthermore, an individual with dementia may be immobile and so not need the same amount of calories to sustain his or her energy levels. Having reduced food and fluid intake and decreased interest in this can be thought of as a 'natural part' of the end of life and dying.

The discussion of artificial nutrition and hydration in end-of-life care is beyond the scope of this chapter, but please consult a professional clinician if this aspect of living well with dementia interests you at all.

WEBSITES

- 'The Dementia Challenge: Fighting back against dementia', Department of Health: http://dementiachallenge.dh.gov.uk
- Social Care Institute for Excellence Dementia Gateway: *End of Life Care for People with Dementia* with excellent sections on pain in advanced dementia, eating and drinking at end of life, end of life and carers' needs, and care in the last days and final hours of life (www.scie.org.uk/publications/dementia/endoflife/)
- Dementia UK: *Admiral Nurses* (www.dementiauk.org/what-we-do/admiral-nurses/)
- NHS Choices: *Dementia and End of Life Planning* (www.nhs.uk/Conditions/dementia-guide/Pages/dementia-palliative-care.aspx#careathome) (last reviewed 18 February 2013; next review due 18 February 2015)
- The National Council for Palliative Care website is particularly useful here and is strongly recommended.
  - ○ *National Council for Palliative Care (NCPC) Response. All-Party Parliamentary Group on Dementia 2012 Inquiry: Improving Dementia Diagnosis Rates in the UK* (1 March 2012) (www.ncpc.org.uk/sites/default/files/NCPC_response_APPG_Dementia_diagnosis_inquiry.pdf)
  - ○ The *How Would I Know? What Can I Do?* leaflet was a guide for carers that was published on 5 December 2012 and which provides advice on how to help with pain and distress in people with dementia. It has been published by the NCPC as part of the Prime Minister's Dementia Challenge, available at: www.ncpc.org.uk/news/how-would-i-know-what-can-i-do

REFERENCES

Alagiakrishnan, K., Bhanji, R.A., and Kurian, M. (2013) Evaluation and management of oropharyngeal dysphagia in different types of dementia: a systematic review, *Arch Gerontol Geriatr*, **56**(1), pp. 1–9.

Bayer, A. (2006) Death with dementia: the need for better care, *Age Ageing*, **35**(2), pp. 101–2.

Department of Health (2009) *Living Well with Dementia: A National Dementia Strategy; Putting people first*. London: The Stationery Office, available at: www.gov.uk/government/uploads/system/uploads/attachment_data/file/168221/dh_094052.pdf

Department of Health (2008) *End of Life Care Strategy: Promoting High Quality Care for All Adults at the End of their Life*. London: Department of Health, available at: www.gov.uk/government/publications/end-of-life-care-strategy-promoting-high-quality-care-for-adults-at-the-end-of-their-life

Ebhardt, K.S. (2002) *Nursing Times: Causes of Pressure Ulcers*, available at: www.nursing times.net/part-1-causes-of-pressure-ulcers/206473.article

Engel, S.E., Kiely, D.K., and Mitchell, S.L. (2006) Satisfaction with end-of-life care for nursing home residents with advanced dementia, *J Am Geriatr Soc*, **54**(10), pp. 1567–72.

Evers, M.M., Purohit, D., Perl, D., *et al.* (2002) Palliative and aggressive end-of-life care for patients with dementia, *Psychiatr Serv*, **53**(5), pp. 609–13.

Hughes, J.C., Robinson, L., and Volicer, L. (2005) Specialist palliative care in dementia: specialised units with outreach and liaison are needed, *BMJ*, **330**, pp. 57–8.

Klaffke, S., Staedt, J. (2006) Sundowning and circadian rhythm disorders in dementia, *Acta Neurol Belg*, **106**(4), pp. 168–75.

Knapp, M., Prince, M., Albanese, E., *et al.* (1997) *Dementia UK*. London: Alzheimer's Society.

Lawrence, V., Samsi, K., Murray, J., *et al.* (2011) Dying well with dementia: qualitative examination of end-of-life care, *Br J Psychiatry*, **199**(5), pp. 417–22.

Lyseng-Williamson, K.A., and McKeage, K. (2013) Once-daily memantine: a guide to its use in moderate to severe Alzheimer's disease in the EU, *Drugs Aging*, **30**(1), pp. 51–8.

Mitchell, S.L., Morris, J.N., Park, P.S., *et al.* (2004) Terminal care for persons with advanced dementia in the nursing home and home care settings, *J Palliat Med*, **7**(6), pp. 808–16.

Mitchell, S.L., Teno, J., Miller, S.C., *et al.* (2005) A national study of the location of death for older persons with dementia, *J Am Geriatr Soc*, **53**(2), pp. 299–305.

Morrison R.S., and Siu, A.L. (2000) Survival in end-stage dementia following acute illness. *JAMA*, **284**(1), pp. 47–52.

Mossello, E., and Ballini, E. (2012) Management of patients with Alzheimer's disease: pharmacological treatment and quality of life, *Ther Adv Chronic Dis*, **3**(4), pp. 183–93.

National Council for Palliative Care. (2012) *National Council for Palliative Care (NCPC) Response: All-Party Parliamentary Group on Dementia 2012 Inquiry; Improving dementia diagnosis rates in the UK*. London, NCPC, available at: www.ncpc.org.uk/sites/default/files/NCPC_response_APPG_Dementia_diagnosis_inquiry.pdf

National Institute for Health and Clinical Excellence (NICE) (2005) *Pressure Ulcers: Prevention and Treatment (CG29)*, available at: www.nice.org.uk/nicemedia/pdf/cg029publicinfo.pdf

National Institute for Health and Clinical Excellence (NICE) and Social Care Institute for Excellence (2006) *CG42: Dementia. A NICE–SCIE Guideline on supporting people with dementia and their carers in health and social care*, available at: www.nice.org.uk/CG42

Richards, T. (2007) A better way to die, *BMJ*, **334**(7598), p. 830.

Roger, K.S. (2006) A literature review of palliative care, end of life, and dementia, *Palliat Support Care*, **4**(3), pp. 295–303.

Sampson, E.L., Gould, V., Lee, D., *et al.* (2006) Differences in care received by patients with and without dementia who died during acute hospital admission: a retrospective case note study, *Age Ageing*, **35**(2), pp. 187–9.

Scherder, E., Oosterman, J., Swaab, D., *et al.* (2005) Recent developments in pain in dementia, *BMJ*, **330**(7489), pp. 461–4.

Teno, J., Clarridge, B.R., Casey, V., *et al.* (2004) Family perspectives on end-of-life care at the last place of care, *JAMA*, **291**(1), pp. 88–93.

Volicer, L., Harper, D.G., Manning, B.C., *et al.* (2001) Sundowning and circadian rhythms in Alzheimer's disease, *Am J Psychiatry*, **158**(5), pp. 704–11.

CHAPTER 9

Living well with specific types of dementia: a cognitive neurology perspective

By now, almost halfway through this book, it should be evident to the reader that a genuine problem in analysing the concept of 'living well in dementia' is that, as a whole, healthcare suffers from people in different specialties working in individual 'silos'.

On top of this, dementia is a very complex construct, embracing a number of different possible diagnoses, with different time courses. There is a common perception that 'dementia' is a single disorder, further perpetuated by most of the media, but this is far from true, and indeed a critical rôle of the cognitive neurologist might be to try to identify what particular type of dementia an individual might be living with. This might best inform an approach to be taken by all specialties in helping that individual, and specific problems might be, for example, in wayfinding or social interactions at an early stage.

There are many different types of dementia, and they all tend to affect various bits of the brain as the disease progresses in a certain order. While the patterns of progression are not identical, it can be observed that certain issues are more likely to be met in some forms of dementia rather than others. For example, an individual with dementia of the Alzheimer type (DAT) is likely to have difficulty with spatial navigation or wayfinding earlier on, as the part of the brain affected in that type of dementia earlier on tends to be the areas around the hippocampus in the temporal lobe part of the human brain. Conversely, in behavioural variant frontotemporal dementia (bvFTD), individuals can be referred to health services because of a subtle change in personality and behaviour, with memory for day-to-day events relatively intact.

Any analysis of 'living well in dementia' has to acknowledge that dementia is a 'heterogeneous' condition, and a specialist view of dementia will tend to consider specific issues which may be more relevant in the activities of daily living in any individual with dementia. This focused approach is likely to be a constructive one, to help society enable individuals with dementia with their distinct issues. If these issues can be addressed in a way that appreciates the individual as a person, rather than 'medicalising' the patient, the wellbeing of immediates (e.g. family or friends) is likely to be better too.

DEMENTIA OF THE ALZHEIMER TYPE

DAT is the most common cause of dementia and a growing health problem globally, affecting 20% of the population over 80 years of age (Ferri *et al.*, 2005).

Pathology

Currently, the definite diagnosis of DAT can only be made through autopsy to find the pathological hallmarks of the disease, microscopic amyloid plaques and neurofibrillary tangles. The development of biomarkers that can reliably indicate presence of the disease at the earliest possible stage is therefore an important public health goal. Macroscopically, DAT is associated with progressive brain tissue loss (Braak and Braak, 1998), which magnetic resonance imaging (MRI) can non-invasively visualise to some extent *in vivo* (Thompson *et al.*, 2005). Unsurprisingly, MRI has attracted considerable interest as a tool to identify DAT biomarkers.

Histological studies have shown that the hippocampus is particularly vulnerable to DAT pathology and already considerably damaged at the time clinical symptoms first appear (Braak and Braak, 1998). The hippocampus has therefore become a primary target of MRI studies in DAT. In agreement with histological findings, longitudinal MRI studies have shown increased rates of hippocampal volume loss in DAT (e.g. Jack *et al.*, 2004) and mild cognitive impairment ('mild cognitive impairment' may define a window for effective therapeutic intervention) (de Pol *et al.*, 2007), in comparison with normal ageing.

Spatial cognition

The '**cognitive map theory**' proposes that the hippocampus of rats and other animals represents their environments, locations within those environments, and their contents, thus providing the basis for spatial memory and flexible navigation. When it comes to humans, the theory suggests a broader function for the hippocampus, based at least in part on lateralisation of function (Burgess, Maguire and O'Keefe, 2002). The cognitive map theory posits that the hippocampus specifically supports *allocentric* processing of space in contrast to other brain regions, such as the parietal neocortex, which support *egocentric* processing (O'Keefe and Nadel, 1978).

One of the strongest lines of evidence in support of this claim was the discovery of '**place cells**' in the rat hippocampus (O'Keefe and Dostrovsky, 1971).

Place cells are neurons that are location selective; they respond maximally when the rat's head is in a particular location in the environment. Research over the past 30 years has confirmed that the rat hippocampus has an important rôle in spatial memory and navigation; however, characterising the functions of the hippocampus is a matter of controversy.

Structural MRI scans of the brains of humans with extensive navigation experience, licensed London taxi drivers, were analysed and compared with those of control subjects who did not drive taxis (Maguire, Woollett and Spiers, 2006). The posterior hippocampi of taxi drivers were significantly larger relative to those of control subjects. A more anterior hippocampal region was larger in control subjects than in taxi drivers. Hippocampal volume correlated with the amount of time spent as a taxi driver (positively in the posterior and negatively in the anterior hippocampus). These data are in accordance with the idea that the posterior hippocampus stores a spatial representation of the environment and can expand regionally to accommodate elaboration of this representation in people with a high dependence on navigational skills. It seems that there is a capacity for local plastic change in the structure of the healthy adult human brain in response to environmental demands.

WAYFINDING

Problems in **navigation** could even be a good way to diagnose early DAT in future. Virtual reality allows naturalistic evaluation of spatial cognition disorders associated with DAT. These measures seem to be well correlated to daily difficulties of people, thus providing specific measures of cognitive deficits and their functional impact. Thus, virtual reality would be a relevant tool for the early screening of dementia and the differential diagnosis of DAT (Déjos et al., 2011).

While there is abundant evidence for spatial learning and memory decrements in patients with unilateral hippocampal lesions, remarkably little research has been done on spatial memory and learning in patients with DAT, in which relatively selective bilateral hippocampal atrophy is consistently reported in the early stages of the disease (Van de Pol, 2006). Only a few studies have examined static object-location memory tasks in DAT patients, demonstrating impaired performance compared to controls (Bucks and Willison, 1997; Kessels et al., 2010). Using a real-world wayfinding test, Monacelli and colleagues (Monacelli et al., 2003) investigated a group of DAT patients and demonstrated impaired spatial navigation and spatial orientation in the DAT group, possibly due to an underlying deficit in linking landmark information to route knowledge. Similar findings have also been reported using virtual maze-learning paradigms in Alzheimer's disease patients (Cushman, Stein and Duffy, 2008; Kalová et al., 2005).

Current pedestrian navigation systems predominantly use distance-to-turn information and directional information to enable a user to navigate. However, Cherrier and colleagues (Cherrier, Mendez and Perryman, 2001) showed that dementia patients performed better on recognition of landmarks compared with recognition and recall of spatial layout. Studies have been carried out on the quality of landmarks (May and Ross, 2005). Furthermore, relatively few studies have examined the workplaces of staff compared with those that address outcomes for patients and their families. One theme that has been receiving increasing attention over the last few years in the literature about healing environments is wayfinding. Moeser (1988) proved that mental representations of maps do not develop automatically in a complex spatial environment. The study showed that first-time visitors performed significantly better on objective measures of cognitive mapping than nurses with 2 years of experience working at the hospital.

In addition to a complex floor plan, there are other elements that contribute to poor wayfinding and inadequate or conflicting cues, such as colours and lighting (Brown, Wright and Brown, 1997). In addition to these elements, clear and understandable wayfinding and maps are fundamental to becoming oriented. However, maps should be oriented so that the top signifies the direction of movement for ease of use (Ulrich et al., 1994). Moreover, the number of signs available has a significant effect on wayfinding along many different measures including travel time, the frequencies of hesitations, the number of times directions were asked, and the reported level of stress. These results suggest that directional signs should be placed at or before every major intersection, at major destinations, and where a single environmental cue or a series of such cues (for instance, a change in flooring material) conveys the message that the individual is moving from one area into another. If there are no key decision points along a route, signs should be placed approximately every 4.6–7.6 m (Ulrich et al., 1994).

Earlier studies reviewed by Day and Calkins (2002) found that much of the orientation work revolved around '**signage**', and identified that personalised and/or unique signage assisted residents in locating desired destinations. Passini and colleagues (Passini et al., 2000) studied newly admitted residents with dementia, and noted that learning new routes was a slow process. Residents who could not identify paths to desired locations exhibited anxiety, confusion, mutism and even panic. They also noted that some residents perceived patterns on the floor as a barrier. They conclude that a 'capacity of decision-making is reduced to decisions based on immediate and visually accessible information' with such information comprising signs, landmarks, or direct visibility of the desired location. They also noted that the typical location of signs is often not seen by residents whose visual field is low to the ground.

Rule, Milke and Dobbs (1992) also found that features such as many similar doorways along corridors, lack of windows to the outside and signage resulted in poorer orientation. McGilton, Rivera and Dawson (2003) conducted a randomised control trial to ascertain the effects of using a locational map and training techniques on the ability of residents to locate distance locations (a dining room on a different floor). While residents in the treatment group showed significant effect within 1 week of starting the trial, the effect was not sustained 3 months later.

DRIVING AND DEMENTIA OF THE ALZHEIMER TYPE

Safe automobile **driving** requires a driver to perform multiple competing tasks and attend to a host of objects and ongoing events, while simultaneously monitoring traffic with central and peripheral vision to avoid roadway hazards. Impairments of visual acuity and visual fields increase crashes and traffic violations (Burg, 1971). However, drivers with certain neurological conditions may potentially fail to perceive critical roadside targets and dangers even in the absence of a measurable field defect on standard perimetry or diminished visual acuity (Owsley and McGwin, 1999).

DAT affects processing of visual sensory cues and may produce attentional decline and agnosia (for a review, *see* Hodges, 2010). These deficits can impair drivers' processing of visual information such as roadway landmarks and traffic signs that provide key information about a driver's route, upcoming road hazards, and safety regulations. Uc and colleagues (Uc *et al.*, 2005) studied 33 drivers with probable DAT of mild severity and 137 neurologically normal older adults using a battery of visual and cognitive tests and were asked to report detection of specific landmarks and traffic signs along a segment of an experimental drive. The drivers with mild DAT identified significantly fewer landmarks and traffic signs and made more at-fault safety errors during the task than control subjects.

'THE SOCIAL ANIMAL'

The Social Animal: The Hidden Sources of Love, Character, and Achievement is a highly celebrated non-fiction book by American journalist David Brooks (Brooks, 2012), who is otherwise best known for his career with the *New York Times*. The book discusses what drives individual behaviour and decision-making. Brooks asserts that people's subconscious minds largely determine who they are and how they behave. He argues that deep internal emotions, the 'mental sensations that happen to us', establish the outward mindset that makes decisions such as career choices. Brooks describes the human brain as dependent on what he calls 'scouts' running through a deeply complex neuronal network.

Ultimately, Brooks depicts human beings as driven by the universal feelings of loneliness and the need to belong – what he labels *'the urge to merge'*. He describes people going through 'the loneliness loop' of internal isolation, engagement, and then isolation again. He states that people feel the continual need to be understood by others.

We are, above all, 'social animals', and this is of fundamental importance for wellbeing. For example, Professor Mario Mendez and Professor Facundo Manes have reviewed an important collection of papers on social cognition in a number of different clinical situations, and how such neurocognitive dysfunction can give rise to problems in social interactions, immoral or even corrupt behaviour (Mendez and Manes, 2011).

> Social neuroscience has made great strides toward clarifying the neural basis of brain–behavior relationships. In the last 25 years, social neuroscience has made contributions to many fields, including cognitive neuroscience, social psychology, ethology, economics, and even philosophy. The field has spawned a highly productive collaboration between investigators in these areas, many of whom have profited from the great leap forward in functional neuroimaging. Our brains are primed for thinking about the minds of others. Making inferences about others' mental states, or theory of mind (ToM), produces increased activity in the medial prefrontal cortex (MPFC), temporoparietal junction (TPJ), and medial parietal cortex (Frith and Frith, 2006).

RESPONSE TO STRESS AND RESILIENCE

'Resilience' refers to a person's ability to adapt successfully to acute stress, trauma or more chronic forms of adversity. A resilient individual has thus been tested by adversity (Rutter, 2006) and continues to demonstrate adaptive psychological and physiological stress responses, or **'psychobiological allostasis'** (McEwen, 2003; Charney, 2004).

The study of resilience, or stress-resistance, originated in the 1970s with a group of researchers who directed their attention to the investigation of children capable of progressing through normal development despite exposure to significant adversity (Masten, 2001). For many years, research focused on identifying the psychosocial determinants of stress resistance, such as positive emotions, the capacity for self-regulation, social competence with peers and a close bond with a primary caregiver, among other factors (Masten and Coatsworth, 1998; Rutter, 1985).

The importance of resilience in policy in living well in dementia will be considered further in the final chapter, **Chapter 18**.

CONTEXTUAL LEARNING

Context-dependence effects are pervasive in everyday cognition. When we perceive objects and colours, we always perceive these among other objects and colours. We listen and speak within other word streams, and every atom of meaning emerges from a background of meanings. Acting appropriately in social interactions requires the interpretation of explicit and implicit contextual clues that orient our responses toward being polite, to make a joke or point out an irony, to say or not say something. Cognitive science and neuroscience research have evidenced context-dependence effects in similar domains of visual perception, emotion, language and social cognition in both normal and neuropsychiatric conditions.

Context is important, as shown by the **Ebbinghaus illusion**, which depicts two identical central circles, surrounded by rings of circles. Despite the fact that they are the same size, one circle is perceived as small and the other as big. The contextual information available (the surrounding circles) creates the perception that the center circles are different sizes (*see* **Figure 9.1**).

Contextual effects are present at every level, from basic perception to social interaction. This means that we do not perceive objects or process cognitive events in an abstract and universal way. The specific significance of an object, emotion, word, or social situation depends on the contextual effects. During normal cognition, our brains do not process targets and contexts separately; rather, targets are in context.

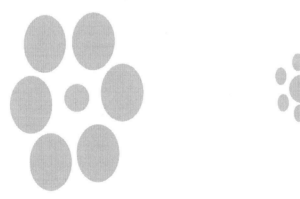

FIGURE 9.1 The Ebbinghaus illusion – in the best-known version of the illusion (the 'Titchener circles'), two circles of identical size are placed near to each other and one is surrounded by large circles while the other is surrounded by small circles; as a result of the juxtaposition of circles, the central circle surrounded by large circles appears smaller than the central circle surrounded by small circles (Roberts, Harris and Yates, 2005)

BEHAVIOURAL VARIANT FRONTOTEMPORAL DEMENTIA AND THE SOCIAL CONTEXT

The bvFTD is characterised by insidiously progressive changes in personality and social interaction that typically precede other cognitive deficits. Patients may present with compulsiveness, perseverations, or stereotyped repetitive acts, loss of self-consciousness, diminished interest for activities or hobbies, or withdrawal and apathy. Increased appetite with a tendency for sweet foods is common, and hypersexuality and hyperorality may develop, especially in the advanced stages of the disease.

Early diagnosis is difficult because behavioural problems, invariably reported by friends or family, dominate the clinical picture while cognitive functions are still relatively intact. This is why it is so important to appreciate that dementia does not equal memory problems *in every single case* (and this is discussed in **Chapter 18**). People in the early stages of bvFTD often score normally on the Mini-Mental State Examination, and conventional structural brain imaging (computed tomography and MRI) may not be sensitive to the early changes associated with bvFTD at all. Therefore, early diagnosis relies on clinical interviews and caregiver reports; it can be considerably difficult to distinguish bvFTD from primary psychiatric syndromes.

Patients with bvFTD are now reported consistently to demonstrate reliably deficits in several domains of social cognition such as recognising emotions in facial expressions, empathy processing, decision-making, figurative language, theory of mind and interpersonal norms. In the study by Rahman and colleagues (Rahman *et al.*, 1999), eight patients with relatively mild bvFTD were compared with age- and IQ-matched control volunteers on tests of executive and mnemonic function. Tests of pattern and spatial recognition memory, spatial span, spatial working memory, planning, visual discrimination learning or attentional set-shifting and decision-making were employed. Patients with bvFTD were found to have deficits in the visual discrimination learning paradigm specific to the reversal stages. Furthermore, in the decision-making paradigm, patients were found to show genuine risk-taking behaviour, with increased deliberation times rather than merely impulsive behaviour. It was especially notable that these patients demonstrated virtually no deficits in other tests that have also been shown to be sensitive to frontal lobe dysfunction, such as the spatial working memory and planning tasks.

These results were discussed at the time in relation to the possible underlying neuropathology, the anatomical connectivity and the hypothesised heterogeneous functions of areas of the prefrontal cortex. Little was known about the brains of such patients from a neuroimaging perspective. In particular, given the nature of the cognitive deficits demonstrated by these patients, the authors postulated that, relatively early in the course of the disease, the ventromedial prefrontal cortex (VMPFC) (or orbitofrontal) cortex is a major locus of dysfunction and that this may relate to the behavioural presentation of these patients clinically described in the individual case histories. A greater definition of the rôle of the ventral frontal cortex, especially given findings in the animal literature, in reversal learning and decision has been a highly influential tranche of research subsequently (Clark, Cools and Robbins, 2004).

At approximately the same time, Lough, Gregory and Hodges (2001) demonstrated relatively intact general neuropsychological and executive function, but extremely poor performance on tasks of theory of mind (ToM). This indicates a dissociation of social cognition and executive function suggesting that in psychiatric presentations of bvFTD there may be a fundamental deficit in theory of mind independent of the level of executive function. The implications of this finding for diagnostic procedures and possible behavioural management are discussed. Later, Adenzato, Cavallo and Enrici (2010) suggested a link between the progressive degeneration of the anterior regions of medial frontal structures characterising the early stages of the bvFTD, elucidated through neuroimaging data, and the ToM deficit these patients show. They also suggested the importance of using ToM tests during the diagnostic process of bvFTD.

The specificity and sensitivity of a number of tests sensitive to ventromedial prefrontal cortex functioning, in bvFTD, have latterly been investigated (Bertoux et al., 2012a). These authors found that the 'Mini-SEA' (SEA = Social cognition and Emotional Assessment), evaluating theory of mind and emotion processes, emerged as the most sensitive and specific of the VMPFC tests employed. The Mini-SEA alone successfully distinguished bvFTD and DAT in >82% of subjects at first presentation. Similarly, the Frontal Assessment Battery 'go/no-go' and reversal-learning tests also showed very good discrimination power, but to a lesser degree. The Iowa Gambling Task, one of the most common measures of VMPFC function, was found to be the least specific of these tests.

Liu and colleagues (Liu et al., 2004) later identified the behavioural features and underlying neuroanatomical correlates in clinical temporal and behavioural variants of frontotemporal dementia (tvFTD and bvFTD respectively). Volumetric measurements of the frontal, anterior temporal, ventromedial frontal cortical (VMFC), and amygdala regions were made in 51 patients with **frontotemporal dementia** (FTD) and 20 normal control subjects, as well as 22 patients with DAT who were used as dementia controls. FTD patients were classified as bvFTD or tvFTD based on the relative degree of frontal and anterior temporal volume loss compared with controls. Behavioural symptoms, cerebral volumes, and the relationship between them were examined across groups. Both variants of FTD showed significant increases in rates of elation, disinhibition and aberrant motor behaviour compared with DAT. The bvFTD group also showed more anxiety, apathy and eating disorders, and tvFTD showed a higher prevalence of sleep disturbances than DAT. The only behaviours that differed significantly between bvFTD and tvFTD were apathy, greater in bvFTD, and sleep disorders, more frequent in tvFTD. BvFTD was associated with greater frontal atrophy and tvFTD was associated with more temporal and amygdala atrophy compared with Alzheimer's disease, but both groups showed significant atrophy in the VMFC compared with DAT, which was not associated with VMFC atrophy. In FTD, the presence of many of the behavioural disorders was associated with decreased volume in right-hemispheric regions.

Using MRI, tensor-based morphometry, Lu *et al.* (Lu *et al.*, 2013) was finally used to determine distinct patterns of atrophy between these three clinical groups. The authors concluded that the bvFTD and semantic and non-fluent variants of primary progressive aphasia groups displayed distinct patterns of progressive atrophy over a 1-year period that correspond well to the behavioural disturbances characteristic of the clinical syndromes. More specifically, the bvFTD group showed significant white matter contraction and presence of behavioural symptoms at baseline predicted significant volume loss of the ventromedial prefrontal cortex. These areas of structural atrophy seem also to be correlated to functional deficits in the case of bvFTD, and now seem to suggest a dissociation in dysfunction even between reversal learning and decision learning deficits at a finer level.

Finally, to complete things, Bertoux and colleagues (Bertoux *et al.*, 2012b) reported that grey matter volume within BA 9 in the medial prefrontal was correlated with scores on the emotion recognition subtest of the social cognition and emotional assessment, and the severity of apathetic symptoms in the apathy scale covaried with grey matter volume in the lateral prefrontal cortex (BA 44/45).

THE 'SOCIAL CONTEXT NETWORK MODEL'

At a phenomenological level, **context-based predictions** make social cognition more efficient. Prototypical situations in the environment are represented in 'context frames' that integrate information about the meanings of social targets (e.g. an emotional face, a speech) that are likely to appear in a specific scene with information about their relationships.

Ibañez and Manes (2012) proposed that there exists a cortical network that mediates the processing of such contextual associations. This social context network involves regions of the frontal, insular and temporal cortices. They postulate that frontal areas (e.g. orbitofrontal cortex, lateral prefrontal cortex, superior orbital sulcus) update and associate ongoing contextual information in relation to episodic memory and target-context associations. The temporal regions (amygdala, hippocampus, perirhinal and para-hippocampal cortices) index the value learning of target-context associations. Finally, the insular cortex coordinates internal and external milieus in an internal motivational state. In this way, the insula would provide information integration from internal states and social contexts to produce a global feeling state.

Ibañez and Manes (2012) used this **social context network model** to provide an adequate model to understand bvFTD-related social impairments. Disruption of the orbitofrontal-amygdala circuit is thought to be responsible for the triad of bvFTD symptoms that includes disinhibition, stereotyped behaviours and gluttony. The mesial and orbital frontal regions atrophy first, followed by the temporal pole, hippocampal formation, dorsolateral frontal cortex and the basal ganglia. This pattern of atrophy progression has been shown to correlate with the volume of cortical and subcortical regions and with underlying neuronal loss.

A consensus has now emerged that the initial symptoms of FTD reflect the involvement of orbitofrontal cortex as well as the disruption of the rostral limbic system including the insula, the anterior cingulate cortex, the striatum, the amygdala and the medial frontal lobes. This system is involved in a number of processes, such as the evaluation of the motivational or emotional content of internal and external stimuli, error detection, response selection and decision-making, and subsequent regulation of context-dependent behaviours.

THE FOLLOWING CHAPTER

The previous chapter introduced the idea that leisure activities might be of benefit for an individual with living well, and the purpose of this chapter was to reinforce the idea that dementia is not a single medical condition (further emphasising the importance of the 'person' which was developed in **Chapter 6**). The next chapter considers other activities, which might also be enjoyed by individuals with dementa.

REFERENCES

Adenzato, M., Cavallo, M., and Enrici, I. (2010) Theory of mind ability in the behavioural variant of frontotemporal dementia: an analysis of the neural, cognitive, and social levels, *Neuropsychologia*, **48**(1), pp. 2–12.

Bertoux, M., Funkiewiez, A., O'Callaghan, C., *et al.* (2012a) Sensitivity and specificity of ventromedial prefrontal cortex tests in behavioral variant frontotemporal dementia, *Alzheimers Dement*, Epub Dec 4.

Bertoux, M., Volle, E., Funkiewiez, A., *et al.* (2012b) Social Cognition and Emotional Assessment (SEA) is a marker of medial and orbital frontal functions: a voxel-based morphometry study in behavioral variant of frontotemporal degeneration, *J Int Neuropsychol Soc*, **18**(6), pp. 972–85.

Braak, H., and Braak, E. (1998) Evolution of neuronal changes in the course of Alzheimer's disease, *J Neural Transm Suppl*, **53**, pp. 127–40.

Brooks, D. (2012) *The Social Animal: The Hidden Sources of Love, Character, and Achievement.* London: Random House.

Brown, B., Wright, H., and Brown, C. (1997) A post-occupancy evaluation of wayfinding in a pediatric hospital: research findings and implications for instruction, *J Architect Plan Res*, **14**(1), p. 35e51.

Bucks, R.S., and Willison, J.R. (1997) Development and validation of the Location Learning Test (LLT): a test of visuo-spatial learning designed for use with older adults and dementia, *Clin Neuropsychol*, **11**, pp. 273–86.

Burg, A. (1971) Vision and driving: a report on research, *Hum Factors*, **13**(1), pp. 79–87.

Burgess, N., Maguire, E.A., and O'Keefe, J. (2002) The human hippocampus and spatial and episodic memory, *Neuron*, **35**(4), pp. 625–41.

Charney, D.S. (2004) Psychobiological mechanisms of resilience and vulnerability: implications for successful adaptation to extreme stress, *Am J Psychiatry*, **161**(2), pp. 195–216.

Clark, L., Cools, R., and Robbins, T.W. (2004) The neuropsychology of the ventral prefrontal cortex: decision-making and reversal learning, *Brain Cogn*, **55**(1), 41–53.

Cherrier, M., Mendez, M., and Perryman, K. (2001) Route learning performance in Alzheimer disease patients, *Neuropsychiatry Neuropsychol Behav Neurol*, **14**(3), pp. 159–68.

Cushman, L.A., Stein, K., and Duffy C.J. (2008) Detecting navigational deficits in cognitive aging and Alzheimer disease using virtual reality, *Neurology*, **71**(12), pp. 888–95.

Day, K., and Calkins, M.P. (2002) Design and dementia. In: Churchman, R.B.A. (ed.) *Handbook of Environmental Psychology*, New York, NY: John Wiley & Sons.

De Pol, L.A., van der Flier, W.M., Korf, E.S., *et al.* (2007) Baseline predictors of rates of hippocampal atrophy in mild cognitive impairment, *Neurology*, **69**(15), pp. 1491–7.

Déjos, M., Sauzéon, H., Falière, A., *et al.* (2011) Naturalistic assessment of spatial cognition disorders in Alzheimer's disease using virtual reality: Abstracts [CO37–005–EN], *Ann Phys Rehabil Med*, **54**(Suppl.), pp. e87–94.

Ferri, C.P., Prince, M., Brayne C, *et al.* (2005) Global prevalence of dementia: a Delphi consensus study, *Lancet*, **366**(9503), pp. 2112–17.

Frith, D.C., and Frith, U. (2006) The neural basis of mentalizing, *Neuron*, **50**(4), pp. 531–4.

Hodges, J.R. (2010) Chapter 24.2.2 Dementia, in London, pp. 4795–809 In: Warrell, D.A., Cox, T.M., and Firth, J.D. (eds) *Oxford Textbook of Medicine*. Fifth edition. Oxford: Oxford University Press.

Ibañez, A., and Manes, F. (2012) Views and reviews: contextual social cognition and the behavioral variant of frontotemporal dementia, *Neurology*, **78**(17), pp. 1354–62.

Jack, C.R. Jr, Shiung, M.M., Gunter, J.L., *et al.* (2004) Comparison of different MRI brain atrophy rate measures with clinical disease progression in Alzheimer's disease, *Neurology*, **62**(4), pp. 591–600.

Kalová, E., Vlcek, K., Jarolímová, E., *et al.* (2005) Allothetic orientation and sequential ordering of places is impaired in early stages of Alzheimer's disease: corresponding results in real space tests and computer tests, *Behav Brain Res*, **159**(2), pp. 175–86.

Kessels, R.P.C., Rijken, S., Joosten-Weyn Banningh, L.W.A., *et al.* (2010) Categorical spatial memory in patients with Mild Cognitive Impairment and Alzheimer dementia: positional versus object-location recall, *J Int Neuropsychol Soc*, **16**(1), pp. 200–4.

Liu, W., Miller, B.L., Kramer, J.H., *et al.* (2004) Behavioral disorders in the frontal and temporal variants of frontotemporal dementia, *Neurology*, **62**(5), pp. 742–8.

Lough, S., Gregory, C., and Hodges, J.R. (2001) Dissociation of social cognition and executive function in frontal variant frontotemporal dementia, *Neurocase*, **7**(2), pp. 123–30.

Lu, P.H., Mendez, M.F., Lee, G.J., *et al.* (2013) Patterns of brain atrophy in clinical variants of frontotemporal lobar degeneration, *Dement Geriatr Cogn Disord*, **35**(1–2), pp. 34–50.

Maguire, E.A., Gadian, D.G., Joshnsrude, I.S., *et al.* (2000) Navigation-related structural change in the hippocampi of taxi drivers, *Procl Acad Nat Sci*, **97**(8), pp. 4398–403.

Maguire, E.A., Woollett, K., and Spiers, H.J. (2006) London taxi drivers and bus drivers: a structural MRI and neuropsychological analysis, *Hippocampus*, **16**(12), pp. 1091–101.

Masten, A.S. (2001) Ordinary magic: resilience processes in development, *Am Psychol*, **56**(3), pp. 227–38.

Masten, A.S., and Coatsworth, J.D. (1998) The development of competence in favorable and unfavorable environments: lessons from research on successful children, *Am Psychol*, **53**(2), pp. 205–20.

May, A., and Ross, T. (2005) Presence and quality of navigational landmarks: effect on driver performance and implications for design, *Human Factors*, **48**(2), pp. 346–61.

McEwen, B.S. (2003) Mood disorders and allostatic load, *Biol Psychiatry*, **54**(3), pp. 200–7.

McGilton, K.S., Rivera, T.M., and Dawson, R. (2003) Can we help persons with dementia find their way in a new environment? *Aging Ment Health*, **7**(5), pp. 363–71.

Mendez, M.F., and Manes, F. (2011) The emerging impact of social neuroscience on neuropsychiatry and clinical neuroscience, *Soc Neurosci*, **6**(5–6), pp. 415–19.

Moeser, S.D. (1988) Cognitive mapping in a complex building, *Environ Behav*, **20**(1), p. 21e49.

Monacelli, A.M., Cushman, L.A., Kavcic, V., *et al.* (2003) Spatial disorientation in Alzheimer's disease: the remembrance of things passed, *Neurology*, **61**(11), pp. 1491–7.

O'Keefe, J., and Dostrovsky, J. (1971) The hippocampus as a spatial map, *Behav Brain Res*, **34**(1), pp. 171–5.

O'Keefe, J., and Nadel, L. (1978) *The Hippocampus as a Cognitive Map*. Oxford: Oxford University Press.

Owsley, C., and McGwin, G. (1999) Vision impairment and driving, *Surv Ophthalmol*, **43**, pp. 535–50.

Passini, R., Pigot, H., Rainville, C., *et al.* (2000) Wayfinding in a nursing home for advanced dementia of the Alzheimer's type, *Environ Behav*, **32**(5), pp. 684–710.

Rahman, S., Sahakian, B.J., Hodges, J.R., *et al.* (1999) Specific cognitive deficits in early frontal variant frontotemporal dementia, *Brain*, **122**(Pt. 8), pp. 1469–93.

Roberts, B., Harris, M.G., and Yates, T.A. (2005) The roles of inducer size and distance in the Ebbinghaus illusion (Titchener circles), *Perception*, **34**(7), pp. 847–56.

Rule, B.G., Milke, D.L., Dobbs, A.R. (1992) Design of institutions: cognitive functioning and social interactions of the aged resident, *J Appl Gerontol*, **11**(4), pp. 475–88.

Rutter, M. (1985) Resilience in the face of adversity: protective factors and resistance to psychiatric disorder, *Br J Psychiatry*, **147**, pp. 598–611.

Rutter, M. (2006) Implications of resilience concepts for scientific understanding, *Ann NY Acad Sci*, **1094**, pp. 1–12.

Thompson, P.M., Hayashi, K.M., Dutton, R.A., *et al.* (2005) Driver landmark and traffic sign identification in early Alzheimer's disease, *J Neurol Neurosurg Psychiatry*, **76**(6), pp. 764–8.

Uc, E.Y., Rizzo, M., Anderson, S.W., *et al.* (2005) Driver landmark and traffic sign identification in early Alzheimer's disease. *J Neurol Neurosurg Psychiatry*, **76**(6), pp. 764–8.

Ulrich, R.S., Quan, X., Zimring, C., *et al.* (2004) *The Role of the Physical Environment in the Hospital of 21st Century: A Once-in-a-lifetime Opportunity*. Concord, CA: Center for Health Design.

Van de Pol, L.A., Hensel, A., van der Flier, *et al.* (2006) Hippocampal atrophy on MRI in frontotemporal lobar degeneration and Alzheimer's disease, *J Neurol Neurosurg Psychiatry*, **77**(4), pp. 439–42.

Zubicaray, G., Becker, J.T., Lopez, O.L., *et al.* (2007) Tracking Alzheimer's disease, *Ann N Y Acad Sci*, **1097**, pp. 183–214.

CHAPTER 10

General activities that encourage wellbeing

There are a number of activities that encourage wellbeing. The focus of this chapter, however, will be '**reminiscence therapy**'. This is particularly relevant to where memory problems constitute the prominent presenting feature of dementia, and therefore will be especially important in the dementia of the Alzheimer type (DAT).

REMINISCENCE THERAPY

Reminiscence therapy is a biographical intervention that involves either group reminiscence work, where the past is discussed generally, or the use of stimuli such as music or pictures. Although closely related to reminiscence therapy, '**life story work**' tends to focus on putting together a life story album for an individual (Moos and Bjorn, 2006).

Reminiscence work was introduced to dementia care over 20 years ago (Norris, 1986) and has taken a variety of forms. At its most basic, it involves the discussion of past activities, events and experiences, usually with the aid of tangible prompts (e.g. photographs, household and other familiar items from the past, music and archive sound recordings).

Reed, who has helped to popularise reminiscence approaches through various approaches (one of which (**the 'Many Happy Returns' innovation**) (Reed, 2012) is described later in this chapter), describes here the essence of reminiscence therapy:

Reminiscence can be very beneficial. What a person with dementia has to say about their life experiences is a great way of demonstrating their value as a person – both to them and you, and even when their memory storage system is inconsistent, to really engage with them while they remember happy times is therapeutic and valuable to you both. Old photographs are a great way to get going and since home and family (assuming it was relatively happy) is so central to all our lives, this may be a good place to start.

People with dementia can access a wealth of long-term memories although it works better if you can avoid direct questions. To help them, you can slip some facts into a comment while looking at (say) an old photograph, for example – '… oh look, there's your brother Peter – he looks nice in that jacket doesn't he, and there's Freddie the dog, he's looking very alert!'; now the person won't have the embarrassment of having forgotten the person's – or the dog's name, and the comment might lead to other memories.

The development of reminiscence work is usually traced to Butler's early work (Butler, 1963) on **'life review'**. Butler described life review as a naturally occurring process where the person looks back on his or her life and reflects on past experiences, including unresolved difficulties and conflicts. This concept was incorporated into psychotherapy for older people, which emphasises that life review can be helpful in promoting a sense of integrity and adjustment. Butler's seminal work contributed critically to the change in professional perspectives on reminiscence. Rather than being viewed as a problem, with the older person 'living in the past', reminiscence is now seen as a **'dynamic process of adjustment'**.

Reminiscence work also has a cognitive rationale. People with dementia often appear able to recall events from their childhood, but not from earlier the same day. Accordingly, a promising strategy appeared to be able to tap into the apparently preserved store of remote memories. By linking with the person's cognitive strengths in this way, it was thought that the person's level of communication might be enhanced, allowing the person to talk confidently of his or her earlier life and experiences. In fact, studies of remote memory suggest that recall for specific events is not relatively preserved; performance across the lifespan is impaired but people with dementia, like all older people, recall more memories from earlier life (Morris, 1994). Some of the memories represent well-rehearsed, much-practised items or anecdotes. The almost complete absence of autobiographical memories from the person's middle years could lead to a disconnection of past and present, which could contribute to the person's difficulty in retaining a clear sense of personal identity. From a cognitive standpoint, autobiographical memory and level of communication appear key outcomes.

Evidence suggests that reminiscence therapy can lead to overall improvements in depression and loneliness and promote psychological wellbeing (Chiang *et al.*, 2010). Research also supports the view that reminiscence therapy, including life story work, can improve relationships between people with dementia and their carers, and thereby 'benefits both' (Woods *et al.*, 2009;

Clarke *et al.*, 2003; McKeown, Clarke and Repper,2006). Other reported benefits include enhancing the opportunity to provide personal and individualised care and assisting the individual move between different care environments such as home to care home, or between care homes (Murphy, 2000).

However, Clarke and colleagues (Clarke, Hanson and Ross, 2003) revealed an expressed concern of care staff that psychological types of therapy involving discussion and personal interaction are often not viewed as 'real work'. Another view explored by Kerr and colleagues (Kerr *et al.*, 2005) suggests that depression in older people is viewed as somehow natural, even when evidence indicates that a range of interventions, many of them psychotherapeutic, can be effective. If reminiscence therapy and life story work are to be used as effective treatments for those with mild to medium cognitive impairment, it is important that the potential value of these psychotherapeutic approaches is understood by care staff and endorsed by those in managerial positions.

The research evidence on reminiscence therapy has examined its impact on older people with dementia and those without dementia. Research by Chiang and colleagues (Chiang *et al.*, 2010) among older people without dementia in institutions in Taiwan, found that there was a positive effect among research subjects involved in reminiscence therapy that was not found in the control group. This study found that those participants involved in reminiscence therapy were more sociable, were less depressed and showed stronger signs of wellbeing than control group members. The relatively small sample size, its composition (all male) and short-term nature of the study (3 months) mean that the results, although favourable, cannot be generalised to the whole population necessarily.

Other studies conducted among individuals with dementia have delivered very encouraging findings on the effect of reminiscence therapy. The first study to be done with a group of older people with dementia was reported by Kiernat (1979). Although this was an uncontrolled study using subjective assessment, Kiernat (1979) concluded that, *'Conversation can be stimulated, interest can be sparked and attention span can be increased'*. Since 1979, there have been various studies using reminiscence approaches with dementia populations, usually in a group context (including Cook, 1984; Lesser *et al.*, 1981). However, very few randomised controlled trials have been conducted (Baines *et al.*, 1987; Goldwasser, Auerbach and Harkins 1987; Orten, Allen and Cook, 1989). More recently, there have been yet further developments in reminiscence therapy research; for example, there has been much interest in conducting reminiscence sessions jointly with people with dementia and their family caregivers (Bruce and Gibson, 1998), and an increasing interest in psychotherapeutic work with people with dementia has led to some attempts to utilise life review with people with dementia (Lai, Chi and Kayser-Jones, 2004) and life review with the person with dementia and family caregiver together (Haight *et al.*, 2003).

Although the Cochrane review (Woods *et al.*, 2009) found that evidence in support of reminiscence therapy for those with dementia was inconclusive, they indicated that at a meta-analytical level the combined results of the studies suggest that reminiscence therapy has the following positive effects:

- improvements in cognition and mood of those with dementia
- reductions in the strain experienced by care-givers and relatives
- improvements in functional ability of dementia participants
- reductions in the symptoms of depression.

Of particular significance perhaps is the finding that, *'no harmful effects were identified on the outcomes measures reported'*.

The study by McKee and colleagues (McKee *et al.*, 2003) identified several positive effects of reminiscence therapy and emphasised the enjoyment of those involved. The main benefits to the individual are cited as follows:

- empowerment
- raised self-esteem
- improved communication
- stimulation and fun
- enhanced mood.

While current research findings might be encouraging and supportive of the use of reminiscence therapy, there is still a need for thorough, rigorous research on the therapy further to substantiate the effectiveness of the approach. Furthermore, reminiscence therapy and life story work can be utilised in a number of important ways.

The aims of reminiscence therapy and life story work appear to be quite varied:

- uncover or preserve the identify of older people (Murphy, 2000; Clarke, Hanson and Ross, 2003)
- improve the quality of life through the impact of 'being listened to' (McKee *et al.*, 2003)
- allow staff to see beyond the diagnosis (Murphy 2000; Clarke, Hanson and Ross, 2003)
- facilitate communication between the person with dementia and their families (Batson, Thorne and Peak, 2002)
- provide enjoyment for the recipient of therapy (Murphy, 2000).

Reminiscence therapy and life story work therapy can range from one-to-one delivery to group work. It may involve the development of a life story album for a person (care home staff and relatives can assist with its formation), or it may involve group reminiscence work where memory prompts such as photographs are shown. The life story approach allows the individual to map where he or she has been, his or her jobs, the food he or she enjoys and other information specific to his or her life. It provides a context and focus for engagement with care home staff and family members.

STORYTELLING

While individuals with dementia have difficulty recalling and discussing recent events, they find it easier to speak about memories from earlier in their lives. The benefits of reminiscing for people with a dementia diagnosis are clearly outlined in existing research (e.g. Astell *et al.*, 2010a, 2010b; Basting, 2003; Bender, Bauckham and Norris, 1998; Brooker and Duce, 2000). For example, Astell and colleagues (2010a) identified three specific functions for people with dementia provided by engaging in reminiscing: **Social**, **Skills** and **Self**, where 'social' refers to the social benefits of engaging and sharing stories with other people, 'skills' alludes to the benefits for people with dementia of keeping using their social and cognitive skills, and 'self' applies to the opportunity afforded to people with dementia to participate as equals in a social situation and feel positive about themselves.

Studies of **storytelling** with people with dementia have included one-to-one (e.g. Astell *et al.*, 2010b) and group settings (e.g. Lepp *et al.*, 2003). To facilitate storytelling, Lepp and colleagues (Lepp *et al.*, 2003) used a formalised story-telling and dramatic workshop process to involve people with dementia and caregivers together in conversational activities. They used generic prompts relat-ing to (a) everyday life, such as the seasons, nature and love, and (b) categories fitting Erikson's model of the **'lifecycle'**, such as childhood, adulthood and mar-riage (Lepp *et al.*, 2003). The dramatic workshops involved formal elements of performance in that people could sing and dance as well as narrate their stories. They found that people with dementia were stimulated to tell personal stories that were engaging and encouraged greater interaction and understanding bet-ween people with dementia and their caregivers (Lepp *et al.*, 2003).

Group processes in storytelling were explored further in the TimeSlip project (Basting, 2003). This used a formal, structured process to support and enable a group of people with DAT to produce one common story based on a series of prompts (e.g. newspaper articles or headlines, images, greeting cards) and questions asked by a facilitator (e.g. What should we name this character?). In this study the stories that emerged tended to be non-linear and did not neces-sarily follow the traditional beginning, middle and end structure. This may be due to the group process or it may reflect changes in the storytelling abilities of people with dementia.

In their comparison of personal and generic photographs as prompts for reminiscing, Astell and colleagues (Astell *et al.*, 2010a) found that, while older people with dementia produced fewer stories than their relatives about fam-ily photographs, they generated as many personal autobiographical stories in response to generic photographs as a matched group of older people. In their study, stories were loosely defined and analysed as the total number of words and turns taken, providing an overview of storytelling (Astell *et al.* 2010a).

'MANY HAPPY RETURNS'

Sarah Reed is the remarkable founder and creator of reminiscence activity **'Many Happy Returns'** (www.manyhappyreturns.org). This activity is a set of cards for younger and older people to share, with pictures and words that are reminders of people's everyday memories where most of their experiences reside, making conversation easier and more fun and helping to capture family memories that would otherwise be lost (Reed, 2012). She has 15 years' volunteering experience with two national elderly people's charities, and her mother has had dementia for ten years.

THE CIRCA PROJECT

The **Computer Interactive Reminiscence and Conversation Aid** (CIRCA), supported by the Engineering and Physical Sciences Research Council (EPSRC, a major research council), project aims to develop an innovatively designed reminiscence experience based on a computer, using multimedia techniques, that could provide the user with a livelier and more engaging form of reminiscence activity than, for instance, a paper scrapbook. The main objective of using a computer-based system over traditional materials is the bringing together of the various media into one easily accessible system.

CIRCA is the first dedicated computer-based system to support reminiscence and conversation. It is an easy-to-use computer program that helps support conversation between people with dementia, and their caregivers and relatives. The system contains an extensive collection of archive photographs, video clips and popular music, which can be easily accessed by simply touching the screen. The system involves the user by stimulating thoughts and memories and well-rehearsed scripts. Contemporary footage of city life, local beauty spots, and festive and traditional events are juxtaposed with archive material to bridge the old and new.

'Hypermedia' provides abundant opportunities for users to make decisions as they explore the system. Random scripting in the programming ensures that the process of involvement need not be repetitive – each use of the material will be a different experience if desired, while an index or search facility allows for more predictable options. The person with dementia can use CIRCA in different ways. He or she may wish to tell a story or to simply enjoy the experience of exploring the presentations with another person. By 'filling in the gaps' of a typical conversation, CIRCA encourages a failure-free social interaction.

Early prototypes taken into the field have met with a great deal of interest from potential users, carers and professionals. The system was evaluated by comparing it with traditional reminiscence and CIRCA-facilitated interactions between people with dementia and caregivers gave those with dementia a more equal partner in social situations. Users operated the touch screen and made choices about what they wanted to see or hear. Caregivers found it easy to give the people with dementia freedom of choice and were surprised at the quick adaptation to using the computer. Both conversation partners enjoyed the using the multimedia system as it provided a shared experience rather than a one-way series of questions with one partner passive. The developers are currently exploring the commercial development of CIRCA with a European and North American company.

OTHER TYPES OF ACTIVITIES THAT PROMOTE WELLBEING

Dancing

Research has elicited many positive results in terms of the impact which dance can have on depression on older people. Much of the research so far has focused on populations within residential care, or those with cognitive impairment including the dementias. A focus group (Harmer and Orrell, 2008), around the topic of 'what constitutes meaningful activity for people with dementia living in care homes', found that various themes emerged among older people with dementia, care home staff and family carers: (1) reminiscence, (2) family, (3) social, (4) musical and (5) individual. Listening to music, singing and dancing were all highlighted as being important aspects of care-home residents' lives. The main factors identified that made activities meaningful for the residents were ones that were *based on values and beliefs related to their past roles, interests and routines*.

Further research has focused on social dancing as a means to support intellectual, emotional and motor function in persons with dementia, and has demonstrated positive responses among participants of social dancing (Palo-Bengsston, Winblad and Ekman, 1998). The **2009 Dance 4 Health study** (Nordin and Hardy, 2009), found that the participants among its frail elderly people group who had DAT generally remained 'actively engaged' in the dance sessions, and demonstrated a strong level of commitment towards the dance sessions. This study, while small in number of participants demonstrated that dance can be an appropriate and engaging activity for those with DAT as well as for healthy older people.

However, a study that researched emotional responses to social dancing and walking among individuals with dementia found that none of the participants had difficulty understanding how to execute movements in dance. The study also highlighted music as a key element in creating a positive atmosphere, and therefore eliciting positive emotional responses among the participants during the activity (Palo-Bengsston and Ekman, 2002).

A pilot study of waltz lessons with patients with moderate DAT also demonstrated a significant effect in procedural learning among participants, suggesting potential implications for dance to serve as a therapeutic intervention for patients with moderate Alzheimer's disease (Rösler *et al.*, 2002). Patients with DAT were compared to patients with major depresssion, in relation to an intervention that involved a 12-day series of half-hour waltz lessons. In comparison with the depressed patients, the participants with DAT showed significant improvements in procedural learning in the dance classes. While this study was a trial, with a small sample group, it nonetheless produced positive results for individuals with DAT, and it suggested further studies with a larger sample group be conducted to validate its findings.

A more recent study (Hackney and Earhart, 2010), which explored the effects of social partnered dance for patients with '*serious and persistent mental illness*', found trends towards improvement in anxiety and depression (measured by Beck Depression II and Beck Anxiety inventories).

Whatever the exact research, and all the methodological considerations, a steady flurry of reports has now emerged concerning the potential beneficial effects of dance in the popular press (the Case Study by Sue Learner is an interesting example).

Case Study: Care homes urged to run dance classes after they were found to calm dementia patients

ADAPTED FROM AN ARTICLE BY SUE LEARNER, 2 APRIL 2013

www.carehome.co.uk/news/article.cfm/id/1559589/call-for-all-care-homes-to-run-dance-classes-after-they-were-found-to-calm-dementia-patients

An academic is calling for all care homes to run structured and regular dance sessions after she found a popular dance from the streets of Mexico helped to calm dementia patients when they were agitated.

Dr Azucena Guzmán García's research has revealed dancing improves mood, is good for physical wellbeing and also helps to strengthen the bond of trust between staff and residents.

Care homes are increasingly being encouraged to use therapies such as psychomotor intervention (using activities requiring physical and mental skills) and cognitive stimulation to reduce the use of antipsychotic medication.

Dr Azucena Guzmán García used a simple-to-follow Latin ballroom style dance called Danzón, in care homes in Tyneside as part of her PhD research at Newcastle University.

Residents were introduced to some simple steps allowing them to dance together to uplifting Danzón music. The lessons brought together cognitive, behavioural and emotional functions and also enabled residents to enjoy the music and the social interaction.

Dr Guzmán García, who now works at the Dementia Research Centre, North East London NHS Foundation Trust, said: 'While dancing is often considered entertainment in care homes, I believe that it can be useful practice. I found that these dance classes helped calm agitation and improved mood and quality of life for people with dementia. There are also obvious advantages in terms of physical fitness.'

Reproduced by kind permission of Sue Learner at www.carehome.co.uk

Exercise

Daily walks can be beneficial, but so can a whole manner of exercises. It will be worth seeing what others recommend, particularly the GP in light of the individual's general health.

Animal therapy

If an individual particularly likes animals, 'animal therapy' might be beneficially considered. Visits from calm animals are a great way to introduce something new and interesting to an individual's environment, and the interaction between humans and animals may be of therapeutic benefit.

Socialising

Every person has different social needs. Some people prefer to be left alone for long periods of time, while others enjoy companionship. Often volunteers can be integrated into a schedule so as to provide companionship and allow you

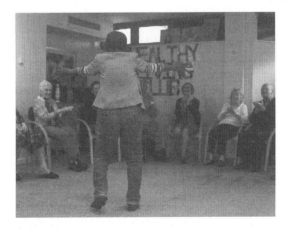

FIGURE 10.1 This picture shows members of 'Healthy Living Club' (described in Chapter 7) participating in a pleasant socialising activity. Individuals report enjoying companionship of their peers in such semi-structured events. (Photograph by kind permission of the 'Healthy Living Club'.)

a chance for your own personal time. Adult day care and adult day healthcare programmes often allow older adults the opportunity to socialise with a group of peers.

Music

Music appears to have significant effects for people with cognitive impairments. Many of those with DAT, despite aphasia and memory loss, continue to remember and sing old songs, and dance to old tunes (Braben, 1992; Brotons, 2000). Furthermore, musical abilities appear to be retained among those who could play instruments prior to the onset of dementia, indicating that musical abilities may be spared in the progression of the disease (Crystal, Grober and Masur, 1989; Cuddy and Duffin, 2005).

Such research has also indicated that musical abilities and memories may not be connected to deterioration in the brain relating to speech and language, raising the possibility of music as a valid non-verbal form of communication for people with dementia (Aldridge, 2000; Brotons, 2000; Hubbard *et al.*, 2002).

Several literature reviews have illustrated the potential of music therapy for people with dementia, although the underlying cognitive and behavioural processes are still somewhat presently uncertain (Brotons, Koger and Pickett-Cooper, 1997; Brotons, 2000; Vink *et al.*, 2003; Kneafsey, 1997; Sherratt, Thornton and Hatton, 2004). Music therapies have been shown to have many beneficial outcomes, including providing frameworks for meaningful activity and stimulation, the management of problematic behaviour such as agitation, improved activity participation, social interaction and social, emotional and cognitive skills, and improved eating at mealtimes (Pulsford, 1997; Ragneskog *et al.*, 1996; Ragneskog and Kihlgren, 1997; Denney, 1997; Biley, 2000; Gotell, Brown and Ekman, 2000).

While therapeutic interventions involving music have been shown to have benefits for people with dementia, little research has examined the rôle of music and music-related activities in their everyday lives. Sixsmith and Gibson (2007) have presented the results of qualitative research that explored this rôle in terms of the meaning and importance of music in everyday life; the benefits derived from participation in music-related activities; and the problems of engaging with music. Data were collected during in-depth interviews with 26 people with dementia and their carers, with the 26 people living either in their own homes or in residential care in different parts of England.

The paper illustrates the many different ways in which people with dementia experience music. As well as being enjoyed in its own right, music can enable people to participate in activities that are enjoyable and personally meaningful. It is an important source of social cohesion and social contact, supports participation in various activities within and outside the household, and provides a degree of empowerment and control over their everyday situations.

Gardening

In **Chapter 13**, I will introduce the idea of the importance of the design of gardens for promoting wellbeing in dementia.

Rachel Pugh's (2013) recent article in the *Guardian*, 'How gardening is helping people with dementia', discusses the therapeutic impact of gardens themselves. The therapeutic qualities of gardens are increasingly being recognised as a way to improve the health of care home residents. The article also mentions the therapeutic effect of the activity of gardening itself.

> The charity Thrive uses gardening to help people with a range of mental health problems, including soldiers experiencing post-traumatic stress. Its recent research with early-onset dementia patients showed that, over a year, participants' memory and concentration remained unchanged, but that mood and sociability improved. (Pugh, R., 2013)

WEBSITES

- **CIRCA (Computer Interactive Reminiscence and Conversation Aid):**
  - **background:** www.computing.dundee.ac.uk/projects/circa/
  - **more detailed document:** www.computing.dundee.ac.uk/projects/circa/5EAD.pdf

REFERENCES

Aldridge, D. (2000) Overture: it's not what you do but the way that you do it. In: Aldridge, D. (ed.) *Music Therapy in Dementia Care*, London: Jessica Kingsley, pp. 9–32.

Astell, A.J., Ellis, M.P., Alm, N., *et al.* (2010a) Stimulating people with dementia to reminisce using personal and generic photographs, *Int J Comput Healthc*, 1(2), pp. 177–98.

Astell, A.J., Ellis, M.P., Bernardi, L., *et al.* (2010b) Using a touch screen computer to support relationships between people with dementia and caregivers, *Interact Comput*, 22(4), pp. 267–75.

Baines S., Saxby P., and Ehlert K. (1987) Reality orientation and reminiscence therapy: a controlled cross-over study of elderly confused people, *Br J Psychiatry*, 151, pp. 222–31.

Basting, A.D. (2003) Reading the story behind the story: context and content in stories by people with dementia, *Generations*, 27(3), pp. 25–9.

Batson, P., Thorne, K., and Peak, J. (2002) Life story work sees the person beyond the dementia, *J Dement Care*, 10(3), pp. 15–17.

Bender, M., Bauckham, P., and Norris, A. (1998) *The Therapeutic Purposes of Reminiscence*. London: Sage.

Biley, F. C. (2000) The effects on patient wellbeing of music listening as a nursing intervention: a review of the literature, *J Clin Nurs*, 9(5), pp. 668–77.

Braben, L. (1992) A song for Mrs Smith, *Nurs Times*, 88(41), p. 54.

Brooker, D., and Duce, L. (2000) Wellbeing and activity in dementia: a comparison of group reminiscence therapy, structured goal-directed group activity and unstructured time, *Aging Ment Health*, **4**(4), pp. 354–8.

Brotons, M. (2000) Overview of the music therapy literature relating to elderly people. In: Aldridge, D. (ed.) *Music Therapy in Dementia Care*, London: Jessica Kingsley, pp. 33–62.

Brotons, M., Koger, S. M., and Pickett-Cooper, P. (1997) Music and dementias: a review of literature, *J Music Ther*, **34**(4), pp. 204–45.

Bruce, E., and Gibson, F. (1988) *Remembering Yesterday, Caring Today: Evaluators' Report*. London: Age Exchange.

Butler, R.N. (1963) The life review: an interpretation of reminiscence in the aged, *Psychiatry*, **26**(1), pp. 65–76.

Chiang, K.J., Chu, H., Chang, H.J., *et al.* (2010) The effects of reminiscence therapy on psychological wellbeing, depression, and loneliness among the institutionalized aged, *Int J Geriatr Psychiatry*, **25**(4), pp. 380–8.

Clarke, A., Hanson, E.J., and Ross, H. (2003) Seeing the person behind the patient: enhancing the care of older people using a biographical approach, *J Clin Nurs*, **12**(5), pp. 697–706.

Cook, J.B. (1984) Reminiscing: how it can help confused nursing home residents, *Soc Casework*, **65**(2), pp. 90–3.

Crystal, H.A., Grober, E., and Masur, D. (1989) Preservation of musical memory in Alzheimer's disease, *J Neurol Neurosurg Psychiatry*, **52**(12), pp. 1415–16.

Cuddy, L.L., and Duffin, J. (2005) Music, memory, and Alzheimer's disease: is music recognition spared in dementia, and how can it be assessed? *Med Hypotheses*, **64**(2), pp. 229–35.

Denney, A. (1997) Quiet music: an intervention for mealtime agitation, *J Gerontol Nurs*, **23**(1), pp. 16–23.

Goldwasser, A.N., Auerbach, S.M., and Harkins, S.W. (1987) Cognitive, affective and behavioural effects of reminiscence group therapy on demented elderly, *Int J Aging Hum Dev*, **25**(3), pp. 209–22.

Gotell, E., Brown, S., and Ekman, S.L. (2000) Caregiver-assisted music events in psychogeriatric care, *J Psychiatr Ment Health Nurs*, **7**(2), pp. 119–25.

Hackney, M.E., and Earhart, G.M. (2010) Effects of dance on gait and balance in Parkinson's disease: a comparison of partnered and nonpartnered dance movement, *Neurorehabil Neural Repair*, **24**(4), pp. 384–92.

Haight, B.K., Bachman, D.L., Hendrix, S., *et al.* (2003) Life review: treating the dyadic family unit with dementia, *Clin Psychol Psychother*, **10**(3), pp. 165–74.

Harmer, B.J., and Orrell, M. (2008) What is meaningful activity for people with dementia living in care homes? A comparison of the views of older people with dementia, staff and family carers, *Aging Ment Health*, **12**(5), pp. 548–58.

Hubbard, G., Cook, A., Tester, S., *et al.* (2002) Beyond words: older people with dementia using and interpreting nonverbal behavior, *J Aging Stud*, **16**(2), pp. 155–67.

Kerr, B., MacDonald, C., Gordon, J., *et al.* (2005) *Effective Social Work with Older People*. Edinburgh: Scottish Executive Social Research.

Kiernat, J.M. (1979) The use of life review activity with confused nursing home residents, *Am J Occup Ther*, **33**(5), pp. 306–10.

Kneafsey, R. (1997) The therapeutic use of music in a care of the elderly setting: a literature review, *J Clin Nurs*, **6**(5), pp. 341–6.

Lai, C.K.Y, Chi, I, Kayser-Jones, J. (2004) A randomized controlled trial of a specific remin-iscence approach to promote the well-being of nursing home residents with dementia, *Int Psychogeriatr*, **16**(1), pp. 33–49.

Lepp, M., Ringsberg, K.C., Holm, A., *et al.* (2003) Dementia: involving patients and their caregivers in a drama programme; the caregivers' experience, *J Clin Nurs*, **12**(6), pp. 873–81.

Lesser, J., Lazarus, L.W., Frankel, R., *et al.* (1981) Reminiscence group therapy with psych-otic geriatric inpatients, *Gerontologist*, **21**(3), pp. 291–6.

McKee, K., Wilson, F., Elford, H., *et al.* (2003) Reminiscence: is living in the past good for wellbeing? *Nurs Residential Care*, **5**(10), pp. 489–91.

McKeown, J., Clarke, A., and Repper, J. (2006) Life story work in health and social care: systematic literature review, *J Adv Nurs*, **55**(2), pp. 237–47.

Moos, I., and Bjorn, A. (2006) Use of life story in the institutional care of people with dementia: a review of intervention studies, *Ageing Soc*, **26**(3), pp. 431–54.

Morris, R.G. (1994) Recent developments in the neuropsychology of dementia, *Int Rev Psychiatry*, **6**(1), pp. 85–107.

Murphy, C. (2000) *Crackin' Lives: An Evaluation of a Life Story Book Project to Assist Patients from a Long Stay Psychiatric Hospital in their Move to Community Care Situations*. Stirling: Dementia Services Development Centre.

National Institute for Health and Care Excellence (NICE) (2013) *Supporting people to live well with dementia (Quality Standard 30)*, statement 2, available at: http://publications. nice.org.uk/quality-standard-for-supporting-people-to-live-well-with-dementia-qs30/ quality-statement-2-choice-and-control-in-decisions

National Institute for Health and Care Excellence (NICE) (2013) *Supporting people to live well with dementia (Quality Standard 30)*, statement 3, available at: http://publications. nice.org.uk/quality-standard-for-supporting-people-to-live-well-with-dementia-qs30/ quality-statement-3-reviewing-needs-and-preferences

Nordin, S., and Hardy, C. (2009) *Assessing the Impact of Community Dance on Physical Health, Psychological Wellbeing and Aspects of Social Inclusion: Evaluation Report*, quoted in 'dance 4 your life': a dance and health report] (Report by NKLA Art Partnership and LABAN), available at: www.trinitylaban.ac.uk/media/55963/dance%20for%20life.pdf

Norris, A.D. (1986) *Reminiscence with Elderly People*. London: Winslow.

Orten, J.D., Allen, M., and Cook, J. (1989) Reminiscence groups with confused nursing centre residents: an experimental study, *Soc Work Health Care*, **14**(1), pp. 73–86.

Palo-Bengtsson, L., and Ekman, S.L. (2002) Emotional response to social dancing and walks in persons with dementia, *Am J Alzheimers Dis Other Dement*, **17**(3), pp. 149–53.

Palo-Bengtsson, L., Winblad, B., and Ekman, S.L. (1998) Social dancing: a way to support intellectual, emotional, and motor functions in persons with dementia, *J Psychiatr Ment Health Nurs*, **5**(6), pp. 545–54.

Pugh, R. (2013) How gardening is helping people with dementia, *Guardian*, Tuesday 30 July, available at www.theguardian.com/society/2013/jul/30/dementia-gardening-helping-people

Pulsford, D. (1997) Therapeutic activities for people with dementia: what, why ... and why not? *J Adv Nurs*, **26**(4), pp. 704–9.

Ragneskog, H., and Kihlgren, M. (1997) Music and other strategies to improve the care of agitated patients with dementia: interviews with experienced staff, *Scand J Caring Sci*, **11**(3), pp. 176–82.

Ragneskog, H., Kihlgren, M., Karlsson, I., *et al.* (1996) Dinner music for demented patients; analysis of video-recorded observations, *Clin Nurs Res*, **5**(3), pp. 262–77.

Reed, S. (2012) *Ten Tips for Better Dementia Caring* available at: www.saga.co.uk/care/carers-tips/ten-tips-for-better-dementia-caring.aspx

Rösler, A., Seifritz, E., Kräuchi, K., *et al.* (2002) Skill learning in patients with moderate Alzheimer's disease: A prospective pilot-study of waltz-lessons, *Int J Geriatr Psychiatry*, **17**(12), pp. 1155–6.

Sherratt, K., Thornton, A., and Hatton, C. (2004) Music intervention for people with dementia: a review of the literature, *Aging Ment Health*, **8**(1), pp. 3–12.

Sixsmith, A., and Gibson, G. (2006) Music and the wellbeing of people with dementia, *Ageing Soc*, **27**(1), pp. 127–45.

Vink, A.C., Birks, J.S., Bruinsma, M.S., *et al.* (2003) Music therapy for people with dementia, *Cochrane Database Syst Rev*, **4**, pp. 1–19.

Woods, B., Spector, A.E., Jones, C.A., *et al.* (2005) Reminiscence therapy for dementia, *Cochrane Database Syst Rev*, (2), CD001120, available at: www.ncbi.nlm.nih.gov/pubmedhealth/PMH0010870/

CHAPTER 11

Decision-making, capacity and advocacy in living well with dementia

Statement 2. People with dementia, with the involvement of their carers, have choice and control in decisions affecting their care and support.

Statement 3. People with dementia participate, with the involvement of their carers, in a review of their needs and preferences when their circumstances change.

Statement 9. People with dementia are enabled, with the involvement of their carers, to access independent advocacy services.

Statement 10. People with dementia are enabled, with the involvement of their carers, to maintain and develop their involvement in and contribution to their community.

There is currently debate – yet to reach proper fruition – on the extent to which individuals can 'maintain and manage their own health', and that healthy living is not always an individualised, purely rational process of information-seeking and correct choices that result in improved health and independence (Henwood, Harris and Spoel, 2011).

Living well with dementia nonetheless appears to involve supporting individuals in making decisions appropriate for them, and these are decisions that directly affect their care and support. However, as a result of the dementia itself, a person's mental capacity can change, and the nature of this decision-making process will change, with carers involved in reviewing the needs and preferences of individuals with dementia as their circumstances change. While the focus of this book is not legal, and certainly an intention of this book is not to give any medical or legal advice, this chapter introduces the very important issue of independent advocacy services, as access-to-justice is an important feature of all civilised societies.

INFORMATION

A key to making informed decisions is having **full, accurate information**. However, the information can be incredibly overwhelming. Lee (@dragon misery) decided to organise this information for carers in an organised way. Her impressive website, **Dementia Challengers: Signposting Carers to Online Resources** (www.dementiachallengers.com), is a great place for information about dementia, and this website contains information specifically for carers. Clearly, accurate and complete information such as on this website is essential for individuals with dementia and their immediates to be able to exercise control and choice properly in negotiating access to resources.

A previous policy document, *Putting People First: A Shared Vision and Commitment to the Transformation of Adult Social Care* (UK Government/LGA/ADASS/NHS, 2007), among others, had made a close link between person-centred care and 'choice and control'.

> Ensuring older people, people with chronic conditions, disabled people and people with mental health problems have the best possible quality of life and the equality of independent living is fundamental to a socially just society. For many, social care is the support which helps to make this a reality and may either be the only non-family intervention or one element of a wider support package. The time has now come to build on best practice and replace paternalistic, reactive care of variable quality with a mainstream system focussed on prevention, early intervention, enablement, and high quality personally tailored services. In the future, we want people to have maximum choice, control and power over the support services they receive.

Lee is specifically mentioned by Anna Hepburn (2013), Digital Communications Manager for Social Care, in an article entitled 'Digital engagement on dementia' on the Department of Health website.

> One of the #dementiachallengers, Lee (@dragonmisery) has set up the Dementia Challengers site to signpost online resources for people caring for someone with dementia. Nothing demonstrates better how the Dementia Challenge is more than a government initiative – and how it has its own digital life – than people who care about dementia creating their own digital community and helping others.

Anna Hepburn in her online article from 16 April 2013 then explains how this is consistent with the wider 'digital strategy' from the Department of Health (and other government departments):

> Digital isn't just about publishing anymore. The Department of Health (DH) digital team certainly knows that, but there are plenty of people within the department – and across government – still to be convinced of the wider benefits of digital, or uneasy about new ways of working.
>
> …
>
> Tapping into this community provides a great opportunity for policy colleagues to engage with people with day-to-day experience of living, caring or working with dementia. I've learnt a great deal from them myself and now I want to find ways of extending those benefits to the dementia policy team. So this is the next step, to fulfil some of the central aims of the DH digital strategy – embedding digital processes in the way we work, giving policy colleagues the tools and confidence to engage digitally, and helping them identify the most appropriate digital tools and techniques for each stage of the policy cycle, and I'll continue to try out new digital ways of opening up our work, such as the live blog from the Dementia Village, which helped extend the reach of the event.

Stephen Hale is the Head of Digital for the UK Department of Health. The emphasis on open policymaking by the Department of Health is a welcome aspect of its digital strategy (Strategy). It is through this Strategy that the Department of Health has committed to using digital tools and techniques to improve upon an open policymaking process. The four stages are as follows:
- Stage 1: Shaping the policy product
- Stage 2: Engaging stakeholders
- Stage 3: Building robust analysis and evaluation
- Stage 4: Finding practical solutions and enabling delivery.

In the business sector, Gomes-Casseres (1996), in a very famous work called, *The Alliance Revolution: The New Shape of Business Rivalry*, has advanced the thesis of constructing networks actively to seek out and incorporate external knowledge into the innovative processes of businesses. Social networks play an important rôle in the sourcing and sharing of information, ideas and knowledge, particularly where they span functional, divisional and organisational boundaries. However, social networks are dynamic, personal and unrecorded, and, as a result, they are difficult to manage and direct. Organisational networks also play an important rôle in the innovation process; they are flexible, enabling network members to reposition themselves more speedily in response to changes in technology and market. They also bring together distributed resources, knowledge and competences.

The **open innovation paradigm** for firms, pioneered by Henry Chesbrough (2003), can be interpreted going beyond just using external sources of innovation such as customers, rival companies and academic institutions, and can be as much a change in the use, management and employment of intellectual property as it is in the technical and research driven generation of intellectual property. There are clear lessons to be learned in the development of policy about dementia in a way that includes opinions of all stakeholders, not just the usual ones.

THE PURPOSE OF ADVOCACY

As reviewed in the Social Care Institute for Excellence (SCIE) **guidance 15** on 'Choice and Control', the three key principles of advocacy are: independence, inclusion and empowerment. Advocacy services form an essential part of the inter-agency framework for the protection of vulnerable adults (Department of Health, 2000)

Wright (2006) defines '**advocacy**' as:

> A one-to-one partnership between a trained, independent advocate and an older person who needs support in order to secure or exercise their rights, choices and interests. (Wright, 2006)

The study found the following.
- Older people thought awareness should be raised about advocacy.
- Advocacy had been used for a number of reasons: protection from abuse; combating discrimination; obtaining and changing services; securing and exercising rights; being involved in decision-making and being heard.
- Participants identified two sets of successful outcomes – those relating to tangible or material gains (e.g. obtaining a service) and those bound up in feelings of greater confidence and self-esteem and of being better equipped to deal with life situations themselves.

QUALITY STATEMENT ON THE NEED FOR INDEPENDENT DEMENTIA ADVOCACY

Having reached a view about what the person with dementia wants, the advocate's task is to represent that view to others and to assist the person with dementia to achieve their wishes. The way that the advocate pursues this will depend upon the retained skills and abilities of the person with dementia. When people have less advanced dementia the advocate's task may be to support them in self-advocacy. More often, however, advocates are working with people with dementia who are unable to effectively voice their wishes.

Dementia advocates may have to represent the views of people with dementia to a range of **'audiences'** (e.g. relatives, doctors, or care managers). These audiences inevitably vary in the extent to which they are open to hearing and acting on what the advocate has to say. Whether or not the advocate expects the reaction from others to be sympathetic or resistant, it is important for advocates to maintain a consistent, professional approach.

Advocacy has for some time been recognised as having the potential to make a valuable contribution to achieving greater empowerment of vulnerable older people, particularly those with mental health needs:

> [Advocacy] can be invaluable in helping a patient to express his or her views if there are difficulties in communication. As the advocates are neither a relative nor associated with the health care facility, they can offer assistance without being influenced by conflicting interests. (BMA and RCN, 1995)

The **ninth NICE Quality Statement 30** provides that

> People with dementia are enabled, with the involvement of their carers, to access independent advocacy services.

The importance of advocacy services is enshrined in **1.1.4.2 of CG42**, the **National Institute for Health and Clinical Excellence (NICE) guidance** on dementia:

> Health and social care professionals should inform people with dementia and their carers about advocacy services and voluntary support, and should encourage their use. If required, such services should be available for both people with dementia and their carers independently of each other.

When significant decisions are being made concerning the current and future care of someone with dementia, it is important that they can access independent advocacy services, if they are not fully able to present their own views. Indeed, a guiding measure is the proportion of people with dementia accessing independent advocacy services.

The group **Action for Advocacy** defines 'independent advocacy' as:

'Advocacy is taking action to help people say what they want, secure their rights, represent their interests and obtain services they need. Advocates and advocacy schemes work in partnership with the people they support and represent their views. Advocacy promotes social inclusion, equality and social justice.' This includes instructed advocacy and non-instructed advocacy for people who do not have capacity to instruct advocacy services on their own behalf. A non-instructed advocate seeks to uphold the person's rights; ensure fair and equal treatment and access to services; and make certain that decisions are taken with due consideration for all relevant factors, which must include the person's unique preferences and perspectives.

ADVOCACY STANDARDS

The '**advocacy standards**' (Action for Advocacy, 2006) are designed to ensure that advocacy is free, confidential and independent to those who require its services. They also give guidelines on providing clear aims and objectives, supporting advocates through training and supervision and clear boundaries to their rôle. Advocacy standards also ensure that the wishes and views of the person being advocated for direct the advocate's work and wherever possible they are involved. Many schemes follow the standards set in the **Advocacy Charter** (Action for Advocacy, 2002) **and Code of Practice** (Action for Advocacy, 2006) developed by Action for Advocacy or similar guidelines.

PERSON-CENTRED ADVOCACY

Advocacy is '**person-centred**' by definition. This is particularly relevant to the dementia advocacy and dementia care process, which puts the individual and their needs foremost, recognising and supporting their unique personal history and personality

SCIE guidance 47 discusses 'personalisation'. **Personalisation means recognising people as individuals who have strengths and preferences and putting them at the centre of their own care and support.** The traditional service-led approach has often meant that people have not been able to shape the kind of support they need, or receive the right kind of help.

According to this guidance, the essence of personalisation means tailoring support to individual needs of people. This means ensuring that people have access to information, advocacy and advice, including peer support and mentoring, to make informed decisions about their care and support, or personal budget management.

Principles of advocacy

There are **two** sides to advocacy that are particularly relevant to those with dementia.

First, advocacy is supposed to provide the individual with a **'voice'**, including them in all decisions that affect their lives, enabling them to make decisions, express their views, wishes and choices.

Second, in particular when the individual may no longer be able to express themselves and make choices, the advocate takes on a **'safeguarding rôle'**, protecting them from abuse, discrimination and neglect, ensuring that their rights are respected and upheld, and determining that all decisions are made, taking into account any expressed wishes and known aspects of their life that may enhance their general wellbeing.

Impact of dementia on the individual

To be an effective advocate for someone with dementia, an advocate needs to have an understanding of dementia and its impact on each individual, adapting their approach to the needs of that individual.

Communication and interpersonal skills

The advocate will have developed communication skills that are flexible and innovative, responding to the assessed communication skills of the person with dementia and enabling engagement and meaningful interaction.

HOW ADVOCACY AFFECTS DIFFERENT POPULATIONS

- **Individuals themselves with dementia** can have help from independent advocacy.
- **Carers of people with dementia** are involved in helping the person they support to access independent advocacy services to present their views.
- **Local authorities and others commissioning services** work with providers to ensure the services they commission enable people with dementia, with the involvement of their carers, to access independent advocacy services.
- **Organisations** providing care and support ensure people with dementia are enabled, with the involvement of their carers, to access independent advocacy services.
- **Social care and healthcare staff** ensure they enable people with dementia, with the involvement of their carers, to access independent advocacy services.

MENTAL CAPACITY ACT 2005

Mental capacity describes the ability to make decisions about some or all aspects of your life. The English law assumes that every adult has the mental capacity (or is competent) to make their own decisions if he or she is given sufficient information, support and time to do so.

Capacity is an issue that can affect us all at any stage. Sudden illness (e.g. stroke) or an accident (e.g. severe head injury) could temporarily or permanently affect one's ability to make decisions. Other groups of people may also be affected – people with dementia, people with a learning disability, autism, or severe mental health problems.

Sadly, some individuals will permanently lack capacity, and for others it will fluctuate.

The **Mental Capacity Act** 2005 (MCA) is a law that fundamentally protects and supports people who do not have the ability to make decisions for themselves. This could be due to a condition such as dementia. The Act applies to people aged 16 and over in England and Wales. It also provides guidance to support people who need to make decisions on behalf of someone else.

The key principles state clearly that everyone has capacity until proved otherwise and that every practicable effort should be made to help that person reach a decision for themselves. Even if they are unable to make a decision their views, wishes and preferences are to be taken into account when others make a decision on their behalf and in their best interests. Mental capacity is the ability to make decisions for yourself. People who cannot do this are said to 'lack capacity'.

To have capacity a person must be able to:
- understand the information that is relevant to the decision he or she wants to make
- retain the information long enough to be able to make the decision
- weigh up the information available to make the decision
- communicate his or her decision by any possible means, including talking, using sign language, or through simple muscle movements such as blinking an eye or squeezing a hand.

The **key principles** of the MCA are as follows.
- Every adult has the right to make decisions for him- or herself. It must be assumed that the adult is able to make his or her own decisions, unless it has been shown otherwise.
- Every adult has the right to be supported to make his or her own decisions – all reasonable help and support should be provided to assist a person to make his or her own decisions and to communicate those decisions, before it can be assumed that he or she has lost capacity.
- Every adult has the right to make decisions that may appear to be unwise or strange to others.
- If a person lacks capacity, any decisions taken on his or her behalf must be in his or her best interests. (The Act provides a checklist that all decision-makers must work through when deciding what is in the best interests of

the person who lacks capacity – *see* later in this chapter.)
- If a person lacks capacity, any decisions taken on his or her behalf must be the option least restrictive to the person's rights and freedoms.

There is currently a consultation in progress about the future of this statutory instrument.

A 'two stage test of mental capacity'

A guide to mental capacity and the MCA, by the Mental Health Foundation and Foundation for People with Learning Disabilities (2005), helpfully sets out the **two stage test** for assessing capacity, stipulated by the Act.

> The MCA and Code of Practice explain how and when capacity is to be assessed, which is through a two-stage process. Firstly, the cause of the inability to make the decision must be established as being due to a disturbance of the mind or brain, regardless of whether it is permanent or temporary. Secondly, in establishing an individual's capacity, their ability to understand, retain, use and weigh up the relevant information presented to them should be assessed. Incapacity to make a decision can only be established if all practicable steps to help the individual to make the decision autonomously have been attempted without success. The individual must be unable to make the decision at the time the decision is required. A medical or psychological professional is not required to ascertain capacity but they are often involved in the assessment process. An assessment of capacity must not be done solely on the basis of a person's age, appearance, condition or behaviour.

Key questions for determining whether someone can make a decision

- Does the person have a general understanding of what the decision is and why s/he is being asked to make it?
- Does the person have a general understanding of the consequences of making, or not making, this decision?
- Is the person able to understand, retain, use and weigh up the information relevant to this decision as part of the process of making a decision?
- Can the person communicate his or her decision (whether by talking, using sign language or any other means)?

The English law currently provides that every effort should be made to provide information in a way that is the easiest and most appropriate to help the person to understand; this can be a key rôle for an advocate who takes the time to ensure this happens. A person may only be able to retain the information for a short time – for example, because of memory problems, but this may still be long enough to make a decision. An advocate may identify that the person could benefit from another professional – for example, a speech and language therapist or an interpreter. Advocates are often experienced at putting people at ease to enable communication. It is also worth asking whether there are times of the day when a person's understanding is better or a place where they feel more at ease. To claim that an individual lacks capacity requires evidence.

An **independent advocate** can support or represent someone with dementia by:

- listening to his or her views and wishes
- ensuring his or her voice is heard
- helping the person to be involved in decisions about his or her life
- supporting the person to get the rights he or she is entitled to, enabling the person to obtain the services he or she needs.

INDEPENDENT MENTAL CAPACITY ADVOCACY

The MCA covers England and Wales, and was developed after many years of campaigning and consultations. It finally came into force in 2005 and has brought much clarity to the issue of mental capacity, and who determines it.

The MCA has created a legal right for **Independent Mental Capacity Advocacy** (IMCA) in certain very specific situations for those who lack mental capacity to make their own decisions and have no one else to represent them (i.e. family or friends). Changes to the **Mental Health Act** 1983 in 2007 (under section 30) introduced Independent Mental Health Advocacy for those detained under that Act.

For decisions or support outside of those situations there is no legal right to an advocate. However, the MCA outlines good practice that advocates should follow when supporting people with dementia who may have fluctuating or deteriorating mental capacity.

Advocates should know the key principles of the MCA. Advocates should be aware of the guidance on determining someone's best interests and always look for the least restrictive option. The **Code of Practice** also gives guidance on the kind of help that can be given to enable someone to understand issues, or to enable people properly to express themselves.

Situations requiring IMCA services include decisions about change of accommodation and serious medical decisions. The IMCA's rôle is to find out and represent the views of the individual who lacks capacity. The MCA also established a Court of Protection, which can deal with complex or disputed cases involving mental capacity. It has the power to appoint a 'deputy' who can be authorised to make decisions on behalf of someone who lacks mental capacity but they must do these in accordance with the best interests principle and procedures.

BEST INTERESTS

As reviewed by Hope, Slowther and Eccles (2009), with regard to adults who lack capacity the MCA makes explicit **a three-step approach to decision-making**.

- Step 1: Enable the patient to make a valid choice at the time the decision needs to be taken if at all possible, and respect that choice.
- Step 2: If the patient lacks capacity and cannot be enabled to gain capacity then follow the choice that the patient has expressed in a valid and applicable advance decision, if one exists.
- Step 3: If the patient lacks capacity, and he or she cannot be enabled to gain capacity, and no valid and applicable advance decision exists (or can be found), then the patient should be treated in his or her best interests.

The MCA, in keeping with most ethical and conceptual constructs, does not view a person's valid choice as necessarily the same as his or her best interests. A person can be mistaken, for example, about what is best for him or her; or can make a valid decision knowing that it is unlikely to be in his or her best interests. Neither does the MCA see a valid and applicable advance decision as a component of best interests but instead as separate from and as trumping best interests (**Step 2**).

Everything that is done for or on behalf of a person who lacks capacity must be in that person's best interests. The Act does not define what 'best interests' means because every case and every decision is different.

It does, however, provide a checklist of factors that decision-makers must work through in deciding what is in a person's best interests.

- Every effort should be made to encourage and enable the person to take part in making the decision.
- The person's past and present wishes and feelings, beliefs and values should be taken into account.
- There should be no discrimination based on age, appearance, condition or behaviour.
- If there is a possibility that the person might regain capacity and the issue is not urgent then the decision might be delayed.
- The views of other people who are close to the person should be considered, as well as the views of an attorney or deputy.
- Any advance decisions or statements made by the person who lacks capacity should be considered.

Hope, Slowther and Eccles (2009) have produced a classification of approaches to decision-making (*see* Table 11.1).

TABLE 11.1 A classification of approaches to decision-making: three approaches to decision-making together with some distinctions relevant to each

A classification of approaches to decision-making

1. Valid choice

    (a) Contemporaneous valid choice. A choice (e.g. refusal of treatment) made about a current situation is valid if the person has capacity, is properly consulted and can make the choice voluntarily and without coercion.

    (b) Prior (advance) valid and applicable choice. The person now lacks the capacity to make the choice but had previously, when he or she had capacity, made a choice that was valid (see (a) above) and that is applicable to the current circumstances.

2. Hypothetical choice (substituted judgements)

    (a) External sense. The choice that the person would have made at a time shortly before losing capacity, had he or she considered the current situation. In other words, what the person would have written or said in a valid and applicable advance directive had he or she made one shortly before losing capacity.

    (b) Internal sense. What the person would now choose were he or she (magically) to regain capacity for long enough to make a valid choice.

2. Best interests

The decision that would maximise the person's wellbeing. Wellbeing is not necessarily the same as what a person validly chooses; people may make valid choices that do not maximise their own wellbeing; for example a choice may be foolish, or it may be made for the benefit of another. Various accounts of wellbeing have been proposed and these have been usually classified into three types (although the classification is not entirely satisfactory.)

(a) Mental state themes. Wellbeing is defined in terms of mental states. At its simplest (hedonism) it is the view that happiness or pleasure is the only intrinsic good and unhappiness or pain the only intrinsic bad. The theory can be enriched (and complicated) by allowing a greater plurality of states of mind as contributing to wellbeing, although this raises the problem of which mental states these should be.

(b) Disease-fulfilment theories. Wellbeing consists in having one's desires fulfilled. It is plausible that to maximise a person's wellbeing we ought to give him or her what he or she wants. If desire-fulfilment theories are to provide a reasonable account of wellbeing, it is necessary to restrict the relevant set of desires. On one view only those desires pertaining to life as a whole count as relevant on the analysis of wellbeing. These are desires that relate to a person's life plan.

(c) Objective list theories. According to these theories certain things can be good or bad for a person and can contribute to his or her wellbeing, whether or not they are desired or whether or not they lead to a 'pleasurable' mental state. Examples of this kind of thing that have been given as intrinsically good in this way are engaging in deep personal relationships, rational activity and the development of one's abilities. Examples of things that are bad might include being betrayed or deserted, or gaining pleasure from cruelty.

Source: Hope, Slowther and Eccles (2009).

COMMUNICATION DIFFICULTIES AND ADVOCACY

Some people with **social or communication difficulties** may appear to be incapable of making choices. They may, however, be fully able to make decisions, if given the means to express themselves. Others may appear to have very good communication skills but this may hide their impaired capacity to make decisions.

Many communication difficulties can be overcome with time, patience and skill – by building trusting relationships which are sensitive to an individual's needs and circumstances, and by using tailored communications systems and equipment. People unable to speak, for example, can use pictures or photographs to communicate.

Communication is considered in detail on its own, in the next chapter (**Chapter 12**).

PROVISION OF ADVOCACY

Advocacy schemes can vary according to:

- ages of clients: children, adults, older people
- client groups supported (e.g. people with mental health needs or learning disabilities)
- type of advocacy provided (e.g. self-advocacy, group advocacy, one-to-one advocacy)
- type of advocate (e.g. paid or volunteer)
- the setting they work in (e.g. in the community, on a hospital ward, in a care home)
- instructed or non-instructed (e.g. where someone no longer has the mental capacity to consent or give instruction)
- statutory or voluntary – IMCAs and IMHAs (Independent Mental Health Advocates) provide statutory advocacy for specific client groups.
  1. *Non-instructed advocacy.* Some people may be unable to communicate their wishes or views or have the mental capacity to make decisions, consent or instruct advocates. In these situations advocates work **on a non-instructed basis**.
  2. *Person-centred advocacy.* This involves taking time to build a picture of the **person's life history, lifestyle and preferences including their cultural background**. It requires time to talk to the individual, learning how they communicate best, talking to others that know them well.
  3. *Rights-based advocacy.* Sometimes people forget or overlook the fact that the person with dementia's **rights** are no different to any other citizen. He or she has entitlements and rights as other users of health and social services.
  4. *Observation/witness.* This is about acting as a witness or observer in the settings in which the individual spends time, seeing how the individual

responds to his or her environment, the routine, the people around the individual, how others treat and relate to him or her.

5. *Questioning/watching brief.* This approach requires the advocate to question and challenge those making decisions about the individual's life. The questions will be based around what constitutes quality of life, looking at eight specific domains or indicators and how they will be affected by any decisions.

6. *Holistic approach.* The skilled advocate will use these approaches in a flexible, holistic way.

FUNDAMENTAL PRINCIPLES OF ADVOCACY

The processes of dementia advocacy typically involve some or all of the following:

- building a relationship with the person with dementia
- ascertaining their views and wishes
- enabling them to exercise choice
- supporting them in having their views heard
- representing their interests
- influencing, often powerful, others
- resolving conflicts.

Key elements are communication, capacity, consent and changes.

Communication

Communication is considered the key to a good advocacy relationship, the building of trust and rapport that gives the person confidence that their advocate will speak on their behalf accurately and represent them well.

Capacity

The nature of dementia as a progressive illness means that the mental capacity of someone with dementia is likely to change over time. As a person progresses through their dementia, their capacity to understand the issue and to make a decision based on their ability to reason lessens.

Following the principles of the **Mental Capacity Act** 2005 advocates start working with a person with dementia with the assumption that they **do** have mental capacity. People with dementia especially in the early stages are often able to understand the issues and retain relevant information if they are given time and information in a manageable and appropriate format – that is, using simple language to explain something more complex or presenting it in a visual format.

Mental capacity in someone with dementia may also fluctuate from day-to-day and visit-to-visit. The advocate therefore needs to be flexible and innovative in their approach. In these situations the advocate cannot always take the first response to a question.

Dementia advocacy services, like advocacy services more generally, operate on the basis that they represent the person's case to decision-makers but do not make decisions on behalf of the person with dementia.

The level of insight the person has into their own situation and abilities is also likely to be affected and will diminish with time. This can often present a challenge for the advocate – representing the wishes of a client who has no insight into their needs, is living in a different reality and is unable to understand the risks of some decisions. The Mental Capacity Act provides clear guidelines as to what needs to be considered when assessing mental capacity; all professionals, including advocates should be using these as the benchmark.

Consent

Gaining a client's consent to work with and on behalf of them is an essential principle for an advocate. However, because of the nature of dementia, it is not always possible to gain consent from a client or in fact be sure that the consent you gained previously is still relevant. Therefore, the client's consent needs to

TABLE 11.2 Suggestions about dealing with consent and other ethical issues (advocates need to be constantly mindful of issues of confidentiality and to ensure that they have consent before they share information that may have been given in confidence; this table provides some ideas about how dementia advocates and their services can deal with ethical issues)

Suggestions about dealing with consent and other ethical issues
Treat consent as an ongoing process not a one-off decision.
Record how consent is obtained at the beginning and throughout the advocacy process.
Record the basis on which you form your views about what the person with dementia wants.
Explain to the person with dementia what you are recording, and how the information will be used.
Try to establish the issue(s) that are important to the person with dementia and agree which to prioritise.
Continually reflect on what you are doing, why and in whose interests.
Ensure that confidentiality is maintained and that you have consent to share information with others in the family or the service system.
Ensure that you receive regular supervision in which potential and actual ethical issues are identified and discussed with clear recording of agreed action and the reasoning underpinning those actions.
Ensure you have received appropriate training/education on issues of capacity, human rights, and other ethical issues.

Source: '"Hear what I say" Developing dementia advocacy services', by Cantley, C., Steven, K., Smith, M. (2003), available at: www.bjf.org.uk/web/documents/resources/HearWhatISay.pdf.

be reviewed regularly – in fact at every visit. This will allow the advocate to be confident that the client is still comfortable with their presence. The impact of memory loss and lack of mental capacity may mean that the advocate will continually need to review consent, even during a visit.

Table 11.2 provides some ideas about how dementia advocates and their services can deal with ethical issues.

Changes

The progression of dementia means that there may be changes all along the development of the advocacy relationship; changes in the ability of the person with dementia to express themselves or understand what is said to them, changes in the ability to make decisions, changes in the ability to consent to an advocate's support, changes in behaviour and other symptoms of dementia.

More often, advocates are working with people with dementia who are unable to effectively voice their wishes: the rôle of the independent advocate is to ensure that people with dementia are treated with respect, their wishes and concerns listened to and addressed and to redress any disadvantage or discrimination they experience because of their dementia.

AUTONOMY, CONTROL AND CHOICE

Autonomy is a key factor relating to the dignity of older people and is set within the context of human rights and equality. Dictionary definitions of autonomy include: 'the power of self direction' and 'the ability to make independent choices'. Autonomy is about a freedom to act, for example to be independent and mobile, as well as freedom to decide.

Control and choice over one's life and involvement – in day-to-day living and the wider community – support autonomy and self-esteem. For example, being given support to cook a meal will help the person to remain in control and be far more rewarding and meaningful than passively waiting for staff to cook the meal. In terms of involvement in the wider community, being supported to continue with routine daily tasks such as shopping, walking a dog or going to a place of worship, as well as involvement in community activities such as social clubs, can be instrumental in maintaining a person's autonomy.

The issues of choice, control, involvement and self-determination are at the forefront of current government policy. Department of Health research (Department of Health, 2005) found that health and social care recipients value having information to make choices and decisions for themselves, and that feeling confident and maintaining control is important. The need to know about, and access, advocacy services was also raised. Information, advice, advocacy and support with decision-making, are all key to ensuring that older people can exercise autonomy.

A key observation was that the national minimum standards for domiciliary care require that: *'Managers and care and support workers enable service users to make decisions in relation to their own lives, providing information, assistance, and support where needed'* (Department of Health, 2003). This includes ensuring that service users and their carers are informed about local advocacy and self-advocacy schemes.

Case Study: A blogpost by Andrea Sutcliffe, previously CEO of Social Care Institute for Excellence (but recently appointed as the Chief Inspector of Social Care for England)

(This was first published on 'Whose Shoes' blog, created by Gill Phillips: http://whoseshoes. wordpress.com/2013/03/04/in-the-shoes-of-andrea-sutcliffe-ceo-of-the-social-care-institute-for-excellence-find-me-good-care/)

The majority of adults unaware of what care is available (59%) and have no idea how much it costs (66%). More than two-thirds of people say that they are not likely to consider care decisions until they become urgent, increasing the risk of not choosing the best provision A quarter of adults who already use care provision say they struggled to find appropriate care and now feel they ended up with the wrong type of support. SCIE [Social Care Institute for Excellence] launches online service Find Me Good Care to help public navigate complex world of care and support; including a range of services on Find Me Good Care, for adults of all ages, shows just how much support is available if you know where to look.

www.scie.org.uk/news/mediareleases/2012/221012.asp

As we, or our loved ones, get older the reality that we may have to think about needing a little bit of extra care and support (or maybe a lot more care and support) gradually dawns on us. Lots of us leave it to the last minute when a crisis intervenes and rapid decisions have to be made, and sadly research suggests that those decisions may not end up being the right ones. At SCIE, we firmly believe that people should have access to enough information to enable them to take control and make informed choices about the support they need to live their lives in the way they want. This is true for everyone but how much more important for someone living with dementia or their family?

To help anyone choose the right kind of care, we need to know what our options are and to be well armed with that knowledge. That is why we set up 'Find me good care' – to help people taking their first steps in navigating the care system, offering advice and guidance on care and support options, whether that is to do with paying for care, getting to know the different types of care available, finding out what to ask and look for, or being aware of your rights. We have included a searchable directory with the option of leaving feedback – you can search by location, type of care, lifestyle preferences e.g. hobbies, pets or holidays, faith, sexuality and so on.'

Reference
'Find me good care': www.findmegoodcare.co.uk set up by Andrea Sutcliffe/SCIE.

Reproduced by kind permission of Gill Phillips, author of the 'Whose Shoes' blog.

'ADVOCACY MANIFESTO'

In 2010, several national organisations worked with over 150 advocates to develop an '**Advocacy Manifesto**' for independent advocacy services in England and Wales. The manifesto sets out a series of core beliefs relating to advocacy services and a number of expectations in respect to our sector's relationship with government at all levels (local, regional and national). Much work has gone into ensuring these expectations are realistic and achievable. It covers what independent advocacy is; access and diversity; funding; advocacy and safeguarding; volunteering; training and support and also personalisation (*A Manifesto for Independent Advocacy Services in England and Wales*, 2010).

DIVERSITY AND EQUALITY

Individuals with dementia vary enormously according to age, gender, social and ethnic backgrounds, education, type of dementia, degree of dementia and so on. Responding to their diverse needs and circumstances requires a range of advocacy approaches and skills.

NICE CG42 recommendation 1.1.1.7 lists alternative and additional support that may be needed if language or acquired language impairment is a barrier to accessing or understanding support. Social care and healthcare staff should identify the specific needs of people with dementia and their carers arising from diversity, including gender, sexuality, ethnicity, age and religion. These needs should be recorded in care plans and addressed (**NICE CG42 recommendations 1.1.1.3 and 1.1.1.5**).

FINANCIAL ABUSE

Action for Advocacy and Action on Elder Abuse are collaborating in a noteworthy project to explore what is happening in advocacy services working with people who are **at risk of of experiencing financial abuse**. The project focuses on older people who lack capacity to manage their finances but will include younger adults in the same circumstances. It is funded by the Department of Health, and covers England only. The aim of the project is to ascertain the most appropriate methods of advocating for people in financial abuse situations and to develop a toolkit and good practice guidance for advocacy services working in this area.

DECISION-MAKING FOR PEOPLE WITH DEMENTIA WHO LACK CAPACITY

Decisions often have to be made on behalf of people without capacity, which includes many people with dementia, and relatives often do this, either by themselves or by acting as an advocate and giving advice to professionals for the person for whom they care. They report major barriers to doing so, including difficulties in deciding what to do and the family member experiencing distress in making a decision (Hirschman, Kapo and Karlawish, 2006).

In addition, lack of emotional support for families of people with early dementia who still have capacity acts as a barrier to the difficult discussion of future care options, including placement in residential institutions with 24-hour care (care homes), and makes reaching a decision more difficult (Davies and Nolan, 2003). Decision-making will differ according to previous experiences, education, and social and cultural background. Some people seek information, whereas others do not (Wackerbarth, 2002). All are facilitated in making decisions if they have access to good information and support (Hansen, Archbold and Stewart, 2004). A discussion about the English law relating to the 'lasting power of attorney' is beyond the scope of this chapter. You are advised to reputable sources such as 'NHS Choices' for an introduction to this important topic.

A discussion about the English law relating to the 'lasting power of attorney' is beyond the scope of this chapter. You are advised to refer to reputable sources such as 'NHS Choices' for an introduction to this important topic.

CONCLUSION

It is therefore increasingly clear that the medical and legal professions have converged on a sense of agreement that a law of 'mental capacity' should guide our perception of what individuals with dementia are capable of doing and not capable of doing. The aim of this approach is to give a genuine sense of empowerment for individuals with dementia to make decisions where they can.

The next chapter considers another critical plank of the philosophy of individuals 'living well with dementia' – that of effective communication.

WEBSITE

- **Dementia Advocacy Network ('The Advocacy Manifesto'):** http://dan.advocacyplus.org.uk/data/files/publications/ADVOCACY_MANIFESTO_pdf.pdf

- **Dementia Challengers: Signposting Carers to Online Resources** (www.dementia challengers.com)

REFERENCES

Action for Advocacy (2002) *Advocacy Charter: Defining and Promoting Key Advocacy Principles.* London: A4A.

Action for Advocacy (2006) *Quality Standards for Advocacy Schemes.* London: A4A.

Action for Advocacy (2006) *A Code of Practice for Advocates: Based on the Advocacy Charter.* London: A4A.

British Medical Association and Royal College of Nursing (BMA and RCN) (1995) *The Older Person: Consent and Care.* London: British Medical Association.

Chesbrough, H.W. (2003) *Open Innovation: The New Imperative for Creating and Profiting from Technology.* Boston, MA: Harvard Business School Press.

Davies, S., and Nolan, M.R. (2003) 'Making the best of things': relatives' experiences of decisions about care-home entry, *Ageing Soc*, **23**(4), pp. 429–50.

Department of Health (2000) *No Secrets: Guidance on Developing and Implementing Multi-agency Policies and Procedures to Protect Vulnerable Adults from Abuse.* London: The Stationery Office, available at: www.elderabuse.org.uk/Documents/Other%20Orgs/No%20Secrets.pdf

Department of Health (2003) *Domiciliary Care: Minimum Care Standards (regulations),* available at: www.age-platform.eu/images/stories/uk_minimumcarestandarts_athome.pdf

Department of Health (2005) *Now I Feel Tall: What a Patient-led NHS feels like.* London: The Stationery Office, available at: www.scie.org.uk/publications/guides/guide15/files/nowifeeltall.pdf

Department of Health (2012) *The DH Digital Strategy, 20 December,* available at: http://hale.dh.gov.uk/2012/12/20/the-dh-digital-strategy/

Gomes-Casseres, B. (1996) *The Alliance Revolution: The New Shape of Business Rivalry,* Cambridge, MA: Harvard University Press.

Hansen, L., Archbold, P.G., Stewart, B.J. (2004) Role strain and ease in decision-making to withdraw or withhold life support for elderly relatives, *J Nurs Scholarsh*, **36**(3), pp. 233–8.

Henwood, F., Harris, R., and Spoel, P. (2011) Informing health? Negotiating the logics of choice and care in everyday practices of 'healthy living', *Soc Health Med*, **72**(12), 2026–32.

Hepburn, A. (2013) *Digital Engagement on Dementia,* 16 April, available at: http://digital health.dh.gov.uk/digital-engagement-on-dementia/

Hirschman, K., Kapo J., and Karlawish, J. (2006) Why doesn't a family member of a person with advanced dementia use a substituted judgment when making a decision for that person? *Am J Geriatr Psychiatry*, **14**(8), pp. 659–67.

Hope, T., Slowther, A., and Eccles, J. (2009) Best interests, dementia and the Mental Capacity Act (2005), *J Med Ethics*, **35**(12), pp. 733–8.

Joseph Rowntree Foundation/'Dementia North' and Northumbria University/Cantley, C., Steven, K., and Smith, M. (2003) *Hear what I say: Developing dementia advocacy services,* available at: www.bjf.org.uk/web/documents/resources/HearWhatISay.pdf

A Manifesto for Independent Advocacy Services in England and Wales (2010) London: Action for Advocacy; Leeds: Advocacy Consortium UK.

Mental Health Foundation and Foundation for People with Learning Disabilities (2005) *Mental Capacity and the Mental Capacity Act 2005: A Literature Review.* London: Mental Health Foundation.

National Institute for Health and Care Excellence (NICE) (2013) *Supporting people to live well with dementia (Quality Standard 30)*, statement 9, available at: http://publications. nice.org.uk/quality-standard-for-supporting-people-to-live-well-with-dementia-qs30/quality-statement-9-independent-advocacy

National Institute for Health and Care Excellence (NICE) (2013) *Supporting people to live well with dementia (Quality Standard 30)*, statement 10, available at: http://publications. nice.org.uk/quality-standard-for-supporting-people-to-live-well-with-dementia-qs30/quality-statement-10-involvement-and-contribution-to-the-community

National Institute for Health and Clinical Excellence (NICE) and Social Care Institute for Excellence (2006) *CG42: Dementia.* A NICE–SCIE Guideline on supporting people with dementia and their carers in health and social care, available at: www.nice.org.uk/CG42

Social Care Institute for Excellence (SCIE). *Choice and Control. Adults' Services Practice Guide 15*, London: Social Care Institute for Excellence, available at: www.scie.org.uk/publications/guides/guide15/files/guide15.pdf

Social Care Institute for Excellence (SCIE). *Personalisation. Adults' Services Practice Guide 47*, London: Social Care Institute for Excellence, available at: www.scie.org.uk/publications/guides/guide47/files/guide47.pdf

UK Government. *Mental Capacity Act 2005*, available at: www.legislation.gov.uk/ukpga/2005/9/contents

UK Government/LGA/ADASS/NHS (2007) *Putting People First: A Shared Vision and Commitment to the Transformation of Adult Social Care.* London: The Stationery Office, available at: www.cpa.org.uk/cpa/putting_people_first.pdf

Wackerbarth, S. (2002) The Alzheimer's family caregiver as decision maker: a typology of decision styles, *Gerontologist*, **42**, pp. 340.

Wright, M. (2006) *A Voice that Wasn't Speaking: Older People Using Advocacy and Shaping Its Development.* Stoke-on-Trent: Older People's Advocacy Alliance (OPAAL) UK, available at: www.opaal.org.uk/Libraries/Local/1013/Docs/Resources/A%20Voice%20that%20Wasn't%20Speaking.pdf

CHAPTER 12

Communication and living well with dementia

Statement 1. People worried about possible dementia in themselves or someone they know can discuss their concerns, and the options of seeking a diagnosis, with someone with knowledge and expertise.

A recent YouGov survey – released to mark Dementia Awareness Week for May 2013 – found that 45% of people agreed that they would find it difficult to tell their families if they thought they had dementia (quoted on the Department of Health 'Dementia Challenge' webpage, 'About dementia') Those aged 55 and over are more likely to find this difficult (50%). Fifty-six per cent of people agreed they would find it difficult to broach the subject of dementia with someone they knew if they were worried they were developing the condition. Those aged between 18 and 24 were most likely to agree they would find this difficult (64%) followed closely by those aged 55 and over (60%).

Communication is extremely important in living well with dementia.

Any 'strategy' for effective communication with a person with dementia must, above all, take into account that person's 'uniqueness' (as indeed reflected in the SCIE research briefing 3: *Aiding Communication with People with Dementia*, originally published in 2004 and updated in 2005).

Individuals worried about dementia for themselves and other people need to be able to communicate with individuals who not only know what they are talking about, but also can communicate issues carefully.

The National Dementia Strategy (Department of Health, 2009) itself has given much attention to the nature of information provision in dementia, and recent years have seen scrutiny on the communication process itself. It is widely felt that understanding barriers to communication is critical for facilitating wellbeing in individuals with dementia, and their carers.

THE NATIONAL DEMENTIA STRATEGY AND COMMUNICATION

The National Dementia Strategy in 2009 emphasised that 'good quality information for people with dementia and carers' is essential:

> Good-quality information for those with diagnosed dementia and their carers. Providing people with dementia and their carers with good-quality information on the illness and on the services available both at diagnosis and throughout the course of their care.

The National Dementia Strategy urges a need for the development and distribution of good-quality information sets on dementia and services available, of relevance at diagnosis and throughout the course of care, and local tailoring of the service information to make clear local service provision:

> The challenge is to generate an individually tailored comprehensive package of high-quality information. This should be developed nationally to include information on the nature of the condition, and then adapted locally to describe the treatment and the support available. Different materials might be needed as the disease progresses and to cover the evolution and management of different symptoms and situations. Equally, versions would be needed to work across the diverse populations affected by dementia (e.g. different language groups, minority ethnic groups, people with learning disabilities and people with early-onset dementia).

COMMUNICATION SKILLS FROM CARERS

Caring for and caring about people with dementia require specific communication skills. However, it seems that training for healthcare professionals and family caregivers usually to enable them to meet the communicative needs of people with dementia could be improved.

Eggenberger, Heimerl and Bennett (2013) searched MEDLINE, AMED, EMBASE, PsychINFO, CINAHL, The Cochrane Library, Gerolit, and Web of Science for scientific articles reporting interventions in both English and German. An 'intervention' was defined as communication skills training by means of face-to-face interaction with the aim of improving basic communicative skills. Both professional and family caregivers were included. The effectiveness of such training was analysed by the authors. Different types of training were defined. This review included 12 trials totaling 831 persons with dementia, 519 professional caregivers, and 162 family caregivers. Most studies were carried out in the United States, the UK and Germany. Eight studies took place in nursing homes; four studies were located in a home care setting. No studies could be found in an acute care setting.

This review found that communication skills training in dementia care significantly improved the quality of life and wellbeing of people with dementia and increased positive interactions in various care settings. Communication skills training showed significant impact on professional and family caregivers' communication skills, competencies, and knowledge.

Communication difficulties are distressing (Killick and Allen, 2001) and frustrating (Friedman and Tappen, 1991) for the person with dementia themselves, and represents one of the major problems for family carers (Touzinsky, 1998)). It is vital that communication continues (Moss *et al.*, 2002), both verbal and non-verbal, despite progression of the condition. As far as possible, communication strategies need to be individualised (Runci, Doyle and Redman, 1999) and to take into account differences between individuals and different degrees of cognitive ability. Similarly, allowance must be made for individual responses to attempts to improve communication (Hopper, Bayles and Tomoeda, 1998).

Communication is a reciprocal process in which messages are sent and received between two or more people (Riley, 2004), and can be defined as, *'person-to-person transmission of ideas through ... language or ... non-verbal media'* (Powell, 2000). Communication *'is a fundamental aspect of all human relationships'* (Richter, Roberto and Bottenberg, 1995), and is an essential element of good care (Allan, 2001). Effective communication can improve the quality of life for a person with dementia. However, experts highlight that people with dementia lack the opportunity to talk and express their feelings about the quality of their own life (Goldsmith, 1996) and services they receive (Bamford and Bruce, 2000).

Communication is a fundamental requirement for all human beings. It gives substance to individuals' lives, is essential for survival and growth, and enhances a sense of belonging. People learn how to communicate through life experiences and interaction with their social environment. Individuals acquire a unique lexicon that they use to interact with others. The act of communicating and expressing oneself is affected by the person's ability and may therefore be compromised by a disability. People communicate their needs, wishes and feelings as a means of maintaining quality of life and preserving a sense of identity. However, when this ability is compromised – for example, by dementia – it is important for the nurse to demonstrate sensitivity and encourage the person to communicate in whichever way suits him or her best. The way in which individuals communicate reflects who they are. Communication will also be influenced by the context in which the person interacts.

The process of communication can be complex in a care setting, especially when the nurse is interacting with a person who has dementia. Poor communication can compromise care by all health professionals, which can lead to undue anxiety and frustration on the part of the patient.

Northouse and Northouse (1998) stated that human communication has several identifiable properties. These properties represent the fundamental assumptions upon which theories of human communication are constructed.

BASIC COMPONENTS OF COMMUNICATION

At a basic level, communication is essentially an activity of daily living, but might come under the work of a speech and language therapist rather than an occupational therapist. During the activity of **communication**, a sender transmits a message through an appropriate channel to a receiver. The sender is responsible for the content and accuracy of the message. The sender will know that the message has been delivered accurately when the desired response is evident from the receiver, in other words the sender gets feedback. Where there is no feedback, the sender may presume that communication has failed. The sender must carefully consider the recipient when formulating the message. The person who formulates the message is known as the encoder. The person who receives the message and interprets it is known as the decoder (Arnold and Boggs, 2007).

For communication to be effective it is assumed that the sender is clear about the purpose of the message, what it is supposed to achieve and has carefully considered the recipient when encoding the message. It is also assumed that the listener is a willing participant in the interaction.

- *Communication is a process.* Individual sentences, words or gestures make sense only when they are viewed as part of the ongoing stream of events. Communication must be viewed as an ongoing dynamic process.
- *Communication is a 'transaction'.* During an interaction, both individuals are influenced by each other through what they say and do. Communication is thus a process by which meaning is assigned and conveyed in an attempt to create **'shared understanding'**. This process requires a vast repertoire of skills in intrapersonal and interpersonal processing, listening, observing, speaking, questioning, analysing and evaluating. It is through communication that collaboration and cooperation occur.
- *Communication is ever-changing and context-specific.* Different words are used in different situations. The way in which a person communicates is adapted to suit the other individual involved in the interaction and the environment in which the conversation takes place. Manning (1992) explained how a person's daily encounters are dictated by the social rules operating in a given environment, therefore influencing how he or she speaks.
- *Communication is multidimensional.* A spoken sentence may reflect more than a simple exchange of a message. It will reflect the relationship between the individuals who are interacting.

The basic requirements for effective communication are:
- **content** – refers to the topic or message to be sent

- **structure** – how the sender puts words together to make up the message
- **word structure** – based on English grammar to make sure the message is constructed accurately
- **appropriate language** – needs to be understood by both the sender and receiver.

THE IMPORTANCE OF SKILLED COMMUNICATION

According to McCabe and Timmins (2006), the term **'therapeutic'** relates to the art of healing, the effective treatment of medical disorders, the eradication of ill health and the improvement of general wellbeing.

Establishing a therapeutic relationship with patients hopefully allows them to feel comfortable enough to express their needs. It is commonly argued that, only through good communication and the development of the therapeutic relationship, can communicators can truly identify and meet the unique needs of the people they are caring for. However, there are many factors that influence this process, known as 'barriers' or 'filters' (Nelson, 2010).

COMMUNICATING WITH PEOPLE WITH DEMENTIA

Research suggests that simply defining dementia in terms of organic brain disease and linking the process with ageing may not be as straightforward as was once thought. Stokes and Holden (1990) adopted the view that dementia was not a disease in its own right but a collection of signs and symptoms requiring further investigation.

Walsh (2006) stated that dementia is a term used to describe a group of brain disorders that have a profound effect on an individual's life. A gradual decrease in cognitive ability means that the ability to think and communicate gradually decline and the person finds it difficult to process new information. The main common forms of dementia are progressive and irreversible, with symptoms gradually worsening. It affects each person in a unique way, and this must be borne in mind when developing a communication strategy for any person with dementia.

An early sign that a person's ability to communicate is compromised by the dementia of Alzheimer's type might be that he or she cannot find the right words, particularly names of objects. The person may substitute an incorrect word or may not find any word at all. This, however, can gradually progress to forgetting names of friends and family and confusion over family relationships. Sometimes an individual with dementia may not recognise their loved ones, which can be distressing. The declining communicative abilities of a person with dementia can create many barriers that can present unique challenges (Miller, 2002). Killick and Allan (2001) noted that every person with dementia is unique and that their behaviour cannot be attributed solely to this condition.

Communication deficits and other cognitive impairments associated with dementia mean that the patient may be unable to initiate a conversation. The responsibility to help the patient communicate lies with the nurse. Knowledge of how dementia affects communication will assist this process.

As discussed in detail in **Chapter 6**, the effect of dementia on the person's ability to communicate varies depending on the stage of the disease. A person-centred approach advocated by Kitwood (2001) and the Department of Health (2009) stresses the need to acknowledge the uniqueness and individuality of each person when assessing his or her ability to communicate.

Person-centred care is 'value-driven', meaning that it relates to the values of the individual caring for the person, and focuses on promoting empowerment, wellbeing and independence (Kitwood, 2001). It enables the nurse to identify the remaining communication ability rather than focusing on communication deficit, thus encouraging interaction centred on the person's ability. Effective communication improves the quality of life of people with dementia (Killick and Allan, 2001). It is essential that the nurse makes an effort to listen and understand the patient.

Engaging with patients who have dementia may be mutually satisfying or frustrating when difficulties are encountered. Killick and Allan (2001) gave a moving account of their frustration at being unable to engage with people with dementia, and how they altered their perceptions and attitudes to connect with this patient group in a more meaningful way. The gradual reduction in cognitive and expressive ability in people with dementia places demands on nurses. If not equipped with the necessary skills, engaging with patients can be uncomfortable. It may lead to misunderstandings and patients' needs not being fully met.

Finally, Perrin's (1997) study found that people with dementia were significantly deprived of human contact and much contact was superficial or brief. This can lead to a growing sense of deprivation, isolation and detachment. The problem of social isolation among those with dementia is significant and has been well documented (Department of Health, 2009).

COMMUNICATION STRATEGIES

Kitwood (2001) stressed the importance of listening to the person with dementia as well as family members and carers. Advice included: 'give us time to speak', 'don't rush us into something because we can't think or speak fast enough to let you know whether we agree' and 'avoid background noise if you can'.

'Talking mats' (www.talkingmats.com) can be used to improve the effectiveness of communication with people who have dementia. They comprise a low-technology communication aid developed at the University of Stirling to help people with communication difficulties express their views. They use a simple system of picture symbols and a textured mat that allows people to indicate their feelings about various choices within a topic by placing the relevant image below a visual scale. Murphy and colleagues (Murphy, Gray and Cox, 2007) found that people with dementia show improvements in the effectiveness of their communication when using talking mats. This is particularly significant in those with moderate and late-stage dementia.

THE DOCTOR–PATIENT CONSULTATION

The doctor–patient interview should be structured appropriately. Good communication skills will enable you to develop a collaborative partnership with the patient. The Calgary-Cambridge guide to consultations (Kurtz, Silverman and Draper, 1998) has made a massive impact in the conduct of the medical interview in the UK, and provides a reminder of the key stages in effective communication during your consultation with a patient. Here, a *'consultation'* could mean any planned, structured interaction with a patient, for example, an ante-natal booking visit, attending for the ultrasound scan, or discussing the outcomes of the scan. The **Calgary-Cambridge guide** suggests five stages for structuring this interview, which is extensively described elsewhere. Whatever your involvement with the patient, the principles of the model are valuable to integrate into your practice.

White, Levinson and Roter (1994) have looked specifically at closure and have attempted to separate out this element of the consultation from the explanation and planning phase. This study is the first description of how physicians and patients communicate during the closing of office visits. Notably, the patients raised new problems at the end of the visit in 21% of the cases. The findings suggest ways physicians might improve communication in the closing phase of the medical interview. Orienting patients in the flow of the visit, assessing patient beliefs, checking for understanding, and addressing emotions and psychosocial issues early on may decrease the number of new problems in the final moments of the visit.

A term that has been coined in the literature is that of **'hidden agendas'** to describe problems that only surface in the closing moments of the interview. These are often emotionally charged or psychosocial issues, and he surmised that such late presentations of problems may well relate to the failure of physician to facilitate disclosure earlier. Patients waited for the 'right' moment to present their 'real' problem and if it was not deliberately provided earlier on, the opportunity might not present itself until the very end of the interview.

VERBAL COMMUNICATION

Verbal communication is the use of words to express oneself, and is regarded as the key component in delivering a message (McCabe and Timmins, 2006).

Words are symbols that are used to convey a message. Communication allows individuals to share their perceptions of the world and express their feelings. The choice of words is influenced by the person's sociocultural background and the environment in which the interaction takes place. For accuracy of the message, the receiver needs to share a similar lexicon of words. This promotes mutual understanding and allows the communication process to flow. It is vital to make sure the receiver understands the message by evaluating any feedback.

From 'Communicating with people with dementia' from the 'NHS Choices' website.
- speak clearly and slowly, using short sentences
- make eye contact with the person when they're talking, asking questions, or having other conversations
- don't make them respond quickly, because they may feel pressured if you try to speed up their answers
- encourage the person to join in conversations with others where possible
- don't speak on behalf of the person during discussions about their welfare or health issues, as this can make them feel invisible and they may not speak up for themselves in other situations
- don't patronise the person you're looking after, or ridicule what they say
- don't dismiss what the person you're looking after says if they don't answer your question or it seems out of context – instead, show that you've heard them and encourage them to say more about their answer
- avoid asking the person to make complicated choices – keep it as simple as possible
- you may find that you'll need to use other ways to communicate, and you may have to rephrase questions because the person can't answer in the way they used to.

DIFFICULTIES IN VERBAL COMMUNICATION: A COGNITIVE PERSPECTIVE

A number of observations can be made specific to dementia in communication in particular types of dementia. However, one has to be careful not to make sweeping generalisations.

The ability to think of the right word may be noticeably worse in the early stages. Later, only everyday words may be used and other words lost completely. Word finding difficulties can be particularly characteristic of certain types of dementia. For example, as discussed by Ratnavalli (2010), primary progressive aphasia is a focal neurodegeneration of the brain affecting the language network. Patients can have isolated language impairment for years without impairment in other areas. Primary progressive aphasia is classified as primary progressive nonfluent aphasia, semantic dementia and logopenic aphasia, which have distinct patterns of atrophy on neuroimaging. Logopenic aphasics have word finding difficulties with frequent pauses in conversation, intact grammar, and word comprehension but impaired repetition for sentences.

Pronouncing letters and words is not affected until the very late stages. Even according to McGurn and colleagues (McGurn *et al.*, 2004) who reported relatively recently that pronunciation of irregular words is preserved in dementia (validating premorbid IQ estimation).

Putting sentences together is not much affected in the early and middle stages, but may get worse later. Small, Kemper and Lyons (2000) reviewed that sentence processing in dementia of the Alzheimer type is influenced by several grammatical and extragrammatical factors, including phrase structure and verb-argument relations, number of propositions or verbs, and processing resource capacity.

Furthermore, a person with dementia might say things which appear out-of-place in a particular conversation. This makes the person appear uninterested in what others are saying. He or she may fail to pick up humour or sarcasm or subtle messages. Comprehension of insincere communication is an important aspect of social cognition requiring visual perspective taking, emotion reading, and understanding others' thoughts, opinions and intentions.

According to Shanay-Ur and colleagues (Shanay-Ur *et al.*, 2012), behavioural variant frontotemporal dementia patients show uniquely focal and severe impairments at every level of theory of mind and emotion reading, leading to an inability to identify obvious examples of deception and sarcasm. This is consistent with studies suggesting this particular condition appears to target a specific neural network necessary for perceiving social salience and predicting negative social outcomes. (This was discussed in detail in **Chapter 9**.) What the person has to say is most affected. In the early stage, topics are fewer and the person does not try to explain original thoughts or insights. He or she may speak less and conversation is dull. Later he or she cannot keep to the topic and becomes vague and rambling. He or she may speak more but begins to make less sense.

Patients with dementia who confabulate retrieve personal habits, repeated events or over-learned information and mistake them for actually experienced, specific unique events. Although some hypotheses favour a disruption of frontal/executive functions operating at retrieval, the respective involvement of encoding and retrieval processes in confabulation is still controversial. Attali and colleagues (Attali *et al.*, 2009) have argued that poor encoding and over-learned information are involved in confabulation in dementia of the Alzheimer type.

NON-VERBAL COMMUNICATION

Current research suggests that the majority of communication is non-verbal.

According to Argyle (1988), only 7% of the message is communicated verbally by the words used during an interaction, while the remaining 93% is communicated non-verbally. Of the non-verbal communication, 38% involves the use of vocal tones and 55% is attributed to body language.

Non-verbal communication plays a central rôle in human social interaction. It is culture-specific and contextually bound. What is accepted in a given sociocultural context might be inappropriate in another. When communicating with a patient from a different culture, it is necessary to be aware of and acknowledge the unique way in which non-verbal communication can have different connotations.

Expressions of pain or discomfort such as crying are specific to various cultures; some cultures may value a more stoic attitude while others may encourage a more emotive state (Helman, 2007). Non-verbal communication conveys powerful messages (Argyle, 1994), and should ideally be given special attention in all professional interactions. It should complement and reinforce verbal communication. Non-verbal communication includes facial expressions, eye contact, posture, appearance, gestures, and personal space and bodily contact. Most of these factors help to regulate how the communication process evolves. For example, eye contact and close proximity may indicate interest, concern and warmth.

Egan (2002) suggested using the acronym **SOLER** when engaging in non-verbal communication:

- **S** – sit facing the patient Squarely
- **O** – maintain an Open posture
- **L** – Lean slightly forward
- **E** – establish and maintain Eye contact
- **R** – adopt a Relaxed posture.

This technique can be useful when communicating with people who have dementia. However, it may not be suitable for those with late-stage dementia who may be experiencing psychotic symptoms.

Paralinguistic features of communication refer to the individual way of speaking or the individual characteristics of a person's voice. These include (McCabe and Timmins, 2006):

- *volume* – a change of volume can express how the person is feeling; volume can be changed to suit different situations
- *intonation and pitch* – range of frequencies (low to high) used to suit meaning
- *rate of speech* – slow or fast delivery can be used to express different emotions and attitudes

- *tone of voice* – combination of volume, intonation and rate of speech to convey different messages
- *conversational cues* – such as 'mmm', 'hmm', 'I see', 'right', 'really' – these indicate the degree of interest of the listener, whether or not they are agreeing, are generally known as social reinforcers
- *choice of words* – and how these are emphasised – this may indicate the degree of interest.

The paralinguistic features expressed by the sender and the receiver influence the flow of the conversation (Northouse and Northouse, 1998).

'NHS Choices' currently emphasises that communication is not just talking. It also involves gestures, movement, facial expressions and other non-verbal means. Body language and physical contact become more significant when communication is difficult.

From 'Communicating with people with dementia' from the 'NHS Choices' website.
There are several ways to make communication easier:
- being patient and remaining calm can help the person communicate more easily
- keep your tone of voice positive and friendly where possible, because tone is also a means of communication
- don't stand too close to the person while talking as it can intimidate them – either be on the same level or lower than they are, which is less intimidating
- patting or holding the person's hand while talking to them can help to reassure them and make you feel closer – watch their body language and listen to what they say to see whether they're comfortable with you doing this.

Reading the non-verbal cues of patients is essential to understand patient's feelings, but you need to need to check them out: for example, *'You seem upset – would you like to talk about it?'* You could try to transmit your own non-verbal cues, remembering the general principle that non-verbal cues win out over verbal cues, and you should try to adopt appropriate eye contact, posture, position, movement, facial expression, timing and voice. Use of notes, records, computer may lose eye contact: can cause problems; therefore, postpone using records until the patient has completed his or her opening statement, wait for opportune moment before looking at the notes and separate listening from note reading by verbal signposting.

MEANS OF NON-VERBAL COMMUNICATION
- *Posture*: sitting, standing, relaxed
- *Proximity*: use of space, physical distance between communicators

- *Touch*: handshake, pat, physical contact during physical examination
- *Body movements*: hand and arm gestures, fidgeting, nodding, foot and leg movements
- *Facial expression*: raised eyebrows, frown, smiles, crying
- *Eye behaviour*: eye contact, gaze, stares
- *Vocal cues*: pitch rate, volume, rhythm, silence, pause, tone, speech errors, affect, responsiveness
- *Use of time*: early, late, on time, overtime, rushed, slow to respond
- *Physical presence*: race, gender, body shape, clothing, grooming
- *Environmental cues*: location, furniture placement, lighting, temperature, colour

ACTIVE LISTENING

'NHS Choices' makes some very useful recommendations, shown in the Table 12.1 below.

TABLE 12.1 Adapted from the 'NHS Choices' website on communication

- Use eye contact to look at the person, and encourage them to look at you when either of you are talking
- Try not to interrupt them, even if you think you know what they're saying
- If possible, stop what you're doing so you can give the person your full attention while they speak
- Minimise distractions that may get in the way of communication, such as the television or the radio playing too loudly, but always check if it's OK to do so
- If you're not sure what's being said, repeat what you heard back to the person and ask if it's accurate, or ask them to repeat what they said
- Speak clearly
- You may need to speak more slowly
- 'Listen' in a different way – shaking your head, turning away or murmuring are alternative ways of saying no or expressing disapproval
- Sometimes the person may feel unhappy that they can't communicate in the way they would like to – being able to express these feelings may be very important to them, and they may find it reassuring if you just listen rather than try to cheer them up
- Try not to finish the person's sentences – instead, look for clues in their body language, expression and tone to suggest words, and check with them to see whether you've understood them correctly
- If you are looking after someone with dementia, you probably know people with dementia better than others already. These are only a few tips that you can build upon based on your own knowledge and experience.

This website (www.nhs.uk/Conditions/dementia-guide/Pages/dementia-and-communication.aspx) includes invaluable information about communication; this factsheet encourages all immediates of individuals with dementia to initiate conversations, especially if it seems that such individuals are initiating fewer conversations themselves.

THE IMPORTANCE OF THE CARER

It has been remarked previously that carers too have substantial communication needs.

For example, Stilgoe and Farook (on behalf of Demos) (2008) provide the following:

As with patients, carers needs are often assumed or overlooked. Although their role is crucial to the health and wellbeing of patients, the same Rethink research showed that a third of carers felt they weren't given enough information to play their part. This has serious implications for patients' care but also for the wellbeing of the carer. Even where consent hasn't been given by patients, there is still the opportunity to offer carers generalised information about treatments, conditions and the intricacies of the health system. One Rethink member talked about her experience:

> I need to know what you are trying to achieve for my son and how you are planning to do it. I need to understand the treatment that he is receiving so that I can play my part in his recovery programme. What I do not need to know are the personal details of what takes place between him and the professionals concerned.

The role of the carer, like that of the patient, is highly personal. Carers need time and space to discuss their thoughts and worries. But lack of time is the reason most psychiatrists give for not sharing information. Finding the time to develop a collaborative, conversational approach helps build a shared understanding and agree a way forward. As the president of the Royal College of Psychiatrists says, 'Good practice is built on partnerships – not only between doctor and patient, but between patient and carer and between carer and doctor.'

FACILITATING COMMUNICATION

The starting point for facilitating communication must be that it is centred on the person with dementia in his or her uniqueness.

Any barriers to communication, such as physical disability, the effects of medication and the environment and lack of staff time, need to be tackled robustly. The two types of method used to improve communication – practical day-to-day practices and more formal projects must include a desire on the part of professionals (and carers) to listen more and talk less.

A number of strategies are both simple and cost-effective such as planned walking, the use of a mirror and toy stimulation. Training for carers is an accepted part of care and this must also include informal carers.

A team approach can be used to develop and implement communication strategies: multidisciplinary teams, including speech-language therapists and dental staff where appropriate. Those assessing and providing personal care to people with dementia need to recognise that, with time and care, individuals can be helped to express themselves more clearly and also contribute to discussions about service evaluation and development.

WEBSITES

● Talking Mats: www.talkingmats.com

REFERENCES

Allan, K. (2001) *Exploring Ways for Staff to Consult People with Dementia about Services.* Bristol: Policy Press and Joseph Rowntree Foundation, available at: www.jrf.org.uk/publications/exploring-ways-staff-consult-people-with-dementia-about-services

Argyle, M. (1988) *Bodily Communication.* Second edition. London: Routledge.

Argyle, M. (1994) *The Psychology of Interpersonal Behaviour.* Fifth edition. London: Penguin Books.

Arnold, E., and Boggs, K.U. (2007) *Interpersonal Relationships: Professional Communication Skills for Nurses.* Fifth edition. St Louis, MO: Saunders Elsevier.

Attali, E., De Anna, F., Dubois, B., *et al.* (2009) Confabulation in Alzheimer's disease: poor encoding and retrieval of over-learned information, *Brain,* **132**(Pt. 1), pp. 204–12.

Bamford, C., and Bruce, E. (2000) Defining the outcomes of community care: the perspectives of older people with dementia and their families, *Ageing Soc,* **2**, pp. 543–70.

Department of Health (2009) *Living Well with Dementia: A National Dementia Strategy; Putting people first.* London: The Stationery Office, available at: www.gov.uk/government/uploads/system/uploads/attachment_data/file/168221/dh_094052.pdf

Department of Health (2013) *Dementia Challenge: About Dementia,* available at: http://dementiachallenge.dh.gov.uk/2012/05/22/about-dementia/

Egan, G. (2002) *The Skilled Helper: A Problem-Management and Opportunity-Development Approach to Helping.* Seventh edition. Pacific Grove, CA: Brooks/Cole.

Eggenberger, E., Heimerl, K., and Bennett, M.I. (2013) Communication skills training in dementia care: a systematic review of effectiveness, training content, and didactic methods in different care settings, *Int Psychogeriatr,* **25**(3), pp. 345–58.

Friedman, R., and Tappen, R.M. (1991) The effect of planned walking on communication in Alzheimer's disease, *J Am Geriatr Soc,* **39**(7), pp. 650–4.

Goldsmith, M. (1996) *Hearing the Voice of People with Dementia: Opportunities and Obstacles.* London: Jessica Kingsley.

Helman, C.G. (2007) *Culture, Health and Illness.* Fifth edition. London: Hodder Arnold.

Hopper, T., Bayles, K.A., and Tomoeda, C.K. (1998) Using toys to stimulate communicative function in individuals with Alzheimer's disease, *J Med Speech Lang Pathol,* **6**(2), pp. 73–80.

Killick, J., and Allan, K. (2001) *Communication and the Care of People with Dementia.* Buckingham: Open University Press.

Kitwood, T. (2001) *Dementia Reconsidered: The Person Comes First.* Buckingham: Open University Press.

Kurtz, S.M., Silverman, J.D., and Draper, J. (1998) *Teaching and Learning Communication Skills in Medicine*. Oxford: Radcliffe Medical Press.

Manning, P. (1992) *Erving Goffman and Modern Sociology*. Cambridge: Polity Press.

McCabe, C., and Timmins, F. (2006) *Communication Skills for Nursing Practice*. Basingstoke: Palgrave Macmillan.

McGurn, B., Starr, J.M., Topfer, J.A., *et al.* (2004) Pronunciation of irregular words is preserved in dementia, validating premorbid IQ estimation, *Neurology*, **62**(7), pp. 1184–6.

Miller, L. (2002) Effective communication with older people, *Nurs Stand*, **17**(9), 45–50.

Moss, S.E., Polignano, E., White, C.L., *et al.* (2002) Reminiscence group activities and discourse interaction in Alzheimer's disease, *J Gerontol Nurs*, **28**(8), pp. 36–44.

Murphy, J., Gray, C.M., and Cox, S. (2007) *Using 'Talking Mats' to Help People with Dementia to Communicate*. York: Joseph Rowntree Foundation, available at: www.jrf.org.uk/publications/using-talking-mats-help-people-with-dementia-communicate

National Institute for Health and Care Excellence (NICE) (2013) *Supporting people to live well with dementia (Quality Standard 30)*, statement 1, available at: http://publications.nice.org.uk/quality-standard-for-supporting-people-to-live-well-with-dementia-qs30/quality-statement-1-discussing-concerns-about-possible-dementia

Nelson, L. (2010) *Filters and Barriers to Communication*. eHow, available at: www.ehow.com/about_6301288_filters-barriers-communication.html

NHS (2012) NHS Choices: *Communicating with People with Dementia*, available at: www.nhs.uk/conditions/dementia-guide/pages/dementia-and-communication.aspx?tabname=Living%20with%20dementia [Page last reviewed: 08/08/2012]

Northouse, L.L., and Northouse, P.G. (1998) *Health Communication: Strategies for Health Professionals*, Third edition, London: Pearson (Prentice Hall).

Perrin, T. (1997) Occupational need in severe dementia: a descriptive study, *J Adv Nurs*, **25**(5), 934–41.

Powell, J.A. (2000) Communication interventions in dementia, *Rev Clin Gerontol*, **10**(2), pp. 161–8.

Proctor, G. (2001) Listening to older women with dementia: relationships, voices and power, *Disabil Soc*, **16**(3), pp. 361–76.

Ratnavalli, E. (2010) Progress in the last decade in our understanding of primary progressive aphasia, *Ann Indian Acad Neurol*, **13**(Suppl. 2), pp. S109–15.

Richter, J.M., Roberto, K.A., and Bottenberg, D.J. (1995) Communicating with persons with Alzheimer's disease: experiences of family and formal caregivers, *Arch Psychiatr Nurs*, **9**(5), pp. 279–85.

Riley, B. (2004) *Communication in Nursing*. Fifth edition. St Louis, MO: Mosby.

Runci, S., Doyle, C., and Redman, J. (1999) An empirical test of language-relevant interventions for dementia, *Int Psychogeriatr*, **11**(3), pp. 301–11.

Social Care Institute for Excellence (SCIE) (2004) *SCIE Research Briefing: Aiding Communication with People with Dementia*. London: SCIE, available at: www.scie.org.uk/publications/briefings/files/briefing03.pdf

Shany-Ur, T., Poorzand, P., Grossman, S.N., *et al.* (2012) Comprehension of insincere communication in neurodegenerative disease: lies, sarcasm, and theory of mind, *Cortex*, **48**(10), pp. 1329–41.

Small, J.A., Kemper, S., and Lyons, K. (2000) Sentence repetition and processing resources in Alzheimer's disease, *Brain Lang*, **75**(2), pp. 232–58.

Stilgoe, J., and Farook, F. (2008) *The Talking Cure: Why Conversation is the Future of Healthcare.* London: Demos, available at: www.demos.co.uk/files/Talking%20cure%20 final-web.pdf

Stokes, G., and Holden, U. (1990) Dementia: causes and clinical syndromes. In: Stokes, G., and Gouldie, F. (eds) *Working with Dementia*, Oxford: Winslow Press, pp. 16–28.

Sugden-Best, F. (2002) *Assessing and Maintaining Communication.* London: Speechmark Publishing.

Touzinsky L. (1998) Validation Therapy: restoring communication between persons with Alzheimer's disease and their families, *Am J Alzheimers Dis*, **13**(2), pp. 96–101.

Walsh, D. (2006) *Dementia Care Training Manual for Staff Working in Nursing and Residential Settings.* London: Jessica Kingsley Publishers.

White, J., Levinson, W., and Roter, D. (1994) 'Oh, by the way …': the closing moments of the medical visit, *J Gen Intern Med*, **9**(1), pp. 24–8.

CHAPTER 13

Home and ward design to promote living well with dementia

Statement 8. People with dementia have opportunities, with the involvement of their carers, to participate in and influence the design, planning, evaluation and delivery of services.

> Good design allows people to live fulfilling and productive lives. Bad design can cramp lifestyles and educational attainment, cause tensions within the household and damage communities.
>
> Angus Kennedy, quoted in *The Future Homes Commission: Building Homes and Communities Britain Needs*

The previous chapters have focused on the critical understood of '**personhood**' in perception of the needs of an individual with dementia, particularly in relation to wellbeing. I have also considered how certain types of dementia may bring specific issues, including how the physical health of an individual for dementia must be cared for. I then went on to discuss how individuals with dementia might enjoy leisure activities and other activities as part of a healthy lifestyle. The success of such approaches appears to depend on individuals having 'choice and control' over decisions that affect them, but the previous chapter considered also, in particular, how independent advocacy services can be helpful for living well with dementia. This is, of course, only part of the story. The rest of the story concerns the **environment** of that individual, and those closest to him or her.

A 'personhood' will have a genetic component, but that, of course, is only half of the story. Huppert (2014) reviews that there are two general statements that can be made concerning the link between genes and subjective wellbeing. First, for any complex outcomes such as mental health and wellbeing, there will be the involvement of multiple genes, each with a small effect. Second, the effects of these genes, even if they are all added together, do not determine wellbeing outcomes – they simply predispose individuals to certain outcomes depending on their environments and experiences, particularly the early environment and the quality of the nurturing that the infant has experienced.

This book now takes a shift of gear in thinking about how the immediate environment can enhance the quality of life for an individual with dementia, including home and ward design, assistive technologies and innovations of ambient assisted living. This chapter considers first home and ward design.

GENERAL ISSUES OF DESIGN

Up to 70% of acute hospital beds are currently occupied by older people (Department of Health, 2001), and up to a half of these may be people with cognitive impairment, including those with dementia and delirium (Royal College of Psychiatrists, 2005). The majority of these patients are not known to specialist mental health services, and are indeed undiagnosed. General hospitals are particularly challenging physical environments for people with memory and communication problems, with cluttered ward layouts, poor signage and other hazards. People with dementia in general hospitals have worse outcomes in terms of length of stay, mortality and institutionalisation. This impact is not widely appreciated by clinicians, managers and commissioners. The National Audit Office has estimated the excess cost to be more than £6 million per year in an average general hospital (National Audit Office, 2007).

There is no 'cure' for dementia, at present, and as previously described in **Chapter 5** it would be extremely reckless for anybody, whether a clinician or not, to overstate the impact of the pharmacological interventions given the current state of the evidence basis at the time of writing this book. Therefore any potential for the improvement of the environment must be considered, to maximise wellbeing and reducing disability. The living environment does not just include where the person lives, but also includes the wider environment of gardens, shops, transport, leisure and community services, such as cafés, clubs, pubs, schools and theatres.

'**Therapeutic design**' has the primary aim of improving independent functioning, and improving wellbeing of individuals with dementia and their immediates. As explained by Mary Marshall at the beginning of her book *Designing Balconies, Roof Terraces, and Roof Gardens for People with Dementia* (Marshall, 2010), there are a number of impairments that most people with dementia experience:

- impaired working and episodic memory

- disorientation and impaired attention
- poor concentration
- difficulty in naming and use of language
- impaired learning and recall of information
- impaired reasoning
- high levels of stress
- difficulty adjusting to the sensory and mobility demands of ageing
- difficulty with motor skills and concentration
- difficulty with planning and performing of sequences
- impaired decision-making.

In English health policy, it is essential that hospital managers do not exacerbate the functional impairments of individuals with dementia through improving 'flow' of patients through their hospitals. The policy of '**boarding**' of patients out of their own base specialty ward to other wards to accommodate influxes of new patients, has correctly come scrutiny (McMurdo and Witham, 2013).

The implications for this are enormous. Andrea Gillies, author of the Orwell Prize–winning novel *Keeper* (Gillies, 2010), writing in the *Guardian* explains about how an individual with dementia may interact with his or her environment in an unhelpful way.

This extract is from a very moving article called 'Dementia patients deserve better', also written by Andrea Gillies, but this time published in the *Guardian* newspaper (Gillies, 2011):

> Not only do people with dementia suffer memory loss, they are no longer able to make memory. Thus somebody with dementia in any new environment is going to have spectacular difficulty. In my memoir about looking after my mother-in-law, who has Alzheimer's, I describe how she woke every morning with no idea where she was, with apparent absolute amnesia; she wasn't able to learn her new surroundings and map them. She'd been hospitalised because she forgot to drink and became dehydrated, and all her efforts, once admitted, were devoted to escaping and getting home, despite having little idea where home was.
>
> Disorientation causes fear, and fear can make a person turn inward. It can also make people lash out, which isn't going to endear them to staff. In institutions operating with a siege mentality, speak up or risk being overlooked.

In October 2012, the Department of Health announced dedicated funding to create **care environments for people with dementia**, which aid treatment by helping avoid confusion and keeping patients calm. Up to £50 million has apparently now made available to NHS Trusts and local authorities, working in partnership with social care providers, to help tailor hospitals and care homes to the needs of those with dementia. Improved designs of this kind have previously been shown to help dementia patients manage their condition better, by helping to reduce agitation and confusion. It was proposed that the funding could be used for specially designed rooms and spaces that might include:

- hi-tech sensory rooms using lighting, smells and sound to stimulate those with dementia
- large print photos of local scenes from years gone by to help people with dementia feel connected to their past
- specially adapted outside space to prevent patients from wandering, by helping them keep busy and active with activities such as gardening
- technology such as day/night clocks and controllable mood lighting to emulate day and night, which help people with dementia stay independent and well-cared for
- simple changes such as the use of calming colours, non-reflective surfaces, large-print signs and the creation of zones to help residents know where they are and find their way back to their room.

Every project would involve dementia patients, their families and carers in the design, to ensure they fully meet the needs of those with the condition.

A major thrust in policy has been to encourage independent living through optimal design of environments for people affected by dementia, and thus to encourage wellbeing. For example, *Homes for Our Old Age: Independent Living by Design*, published by the Commission for Architecture and the Built Environment (Ongeri, 2009), identifies the following aspects:

All [these] buildings are successful, modern social care environments and meet their objectives of enabling independence and a good quality of life. Lessons can be identified for those involved in the commissioning and design of home care:

> Design for home care or support must recognise that each building is someone's home, not just a place for social care

> Those delivering the schemes need to be aware of the experiences of the ageing and disabled population – poverty and affluence, discrimination and equality, isolation and inclusion, and the needs and requirements of a diverse society

> Internal house design and layout needs to be flexible to accommodate changing care or support needs

> Independence and quality of life require high-quality design, management and services

Design for social care means future-proofing the buildings we already have so that a resident knows they can remain in their home as their needs change

Schemes need to be seen as community assets which allow residents to mix with local people but also enable them to feel their home is secure and private

Developers and providers should talk to, and involve, residents, both before and after development and occupancy.

THE CHALLENGE

Desai, Schwartz and Grossenberg (2012) identify that **behavioural disturbances** are frequently the most challenging manifestations of dementia and are exhibited in almost all people with dementia.

Common behavioural disturbances can be grouped into four categories: (1) mood disorders (e.g. depression, apathy, euphoria); (2) sleep disorders (insomnia, hypersomnia, night-day reversal); (3) psychotic symptoms (delusions and hallucinations); and (4) agitation (e.g. pacing, wandering, sexual disinhibition, aggression). They are often persistent, greatly diminish quality of life of patients and their family caregivers, cause premature institutionalisation, and pose a high economic burden on the patient, family and society. Behavioural disturbances can be prevented and treated with a multifaceted approach that supports dignity and promotes comfort and quality of life of persons with dementia and their family members.

Principles of management include prompt treatment of reversible factors and management of symptoms using primarily individualised non-pharmacological interventions. Pharmacological interventions need to be restricted to behavioural emergencies and for short-term treatment of behavioural disturbances that pose imminent danger to self or others.

PUBLIC SPACES

Life appears to be easier for people with dementia when their surroundings make sense and facilities are clearly marked. The use of contrast plays a vital rôle in signposting areas for people with dementia. Flooring should be in plain colours with the edge of each step in a contrasting primary colour. Light switches are easily recognised if the surrounding wall is painted a different colour. Toilet doors stand out if they are painted to contrast against their background.

DEMENTIA-FRIENDLY GARDENS

At the University of Stirling, the dementia-friendly garden at the Iris Murdoch Building is said to *combine beauty with practicality*. Their garden has been designed to demonstrate some of the important features that should be incorporated into a garden space for people with dementia. Each door to the garden is a different colour and features a matching coloured cue for people with dementia to find their way back to the door they left the building by.

The **garden** provides a safe and secure environment with barrier-free access and no steep gradients. Seating is provided away from the building to prompt movement and fragrant ground-covering plants encourage visitors to bend and take more exercise. This is a garden designed to provide a feast for the senses. Plants such as rustling bamboo have been selected to provide sensory stimulation. Similarly, the intense red foliage of a Japanese maple guides the eye to a central focal point. This versatile space is an excellent focus for meaningful activities for people with dementia.

DECORATING ROOMS: GENERAL PRINCIPLES

One of the best ways to decorate rooms well for a person with dementia is to furnish the space with personal belongings, an approach that is strongly encouraged by many assisted living homes.

It is generally recommended that 'rules' should not stifle creativity and design, but here are some considerations that have been suggested:
- decorate the walls
- make the environment 'cozy'
- add some special finishing touches
- have toys, books, and games available
- put up a bookshelf.

SPECIFIC PARTS OF THE HOUSE

Balconies

There are a number of good reasons for why balconies can be desirable in design of the home for an individual with dementia.

These include fresh air (and escaping from unpleasant smells trapped within a house), the right to a private life enshrined in article 8 of the European Convention of Human Rights, an atmosphere where individuals can hear more easily (40%–50% of people over the age of 75 have some sort of hearing loss), encouraging a connect with the outside environment and nature, and improved serenity in mental health (Marshall, 2010).

Notwithstanding this, there is very specific help on the safety aspects, such as the Health and Safety Executive's **'Health and Safety in Care Homes'** (HSE, 2011). Disinhibition–impulsivity has been identified as an important feature of some presentations of frontotemporal dementia (Mendez *et al.*, 1998; Mendez *et al.*, 2008). Individual safety is therefore a policy consideration for some patients presenting with dementia. Specific design features to encourage wellbeing include consideration of exposure to sun, wind, rain or snow; views; flooring; access; lighting; and balustrades. You may find the book from the Stirling group on balconies helpful (Marshall, 2010).

Furthermore, beneficial effects of exposure to sunlight thereby activating vitamin D_3 and warding against osteoporosis cannot be underestimated. Vitamin D_3 has a clear rôle in preserving bone strength, and all tissues have vitamin D receptors (McNair *et al.*, 2013). A further crucial neuroscientific effect is light has an essential rôle in setting the 'body clock' or 'circadian rhythmicity'. Detailed research is ongoing as to the quality of sleep in individuals with dementia, and this may involve mechanisms not just related to sunlight. Notwithstanding, if circadian rhythmicity can be positively influenced then persons might be able to live more independent lives for longer.

Bathroom design for people with dementia

The bathroom can be a dangerous place for people with dementia.

It is generally recommended that general lighting is provided from a minimum of two ceiling-mounted lights. Hot water, taps left running and slippery surfaces are all hazards. Contrasting colours will improve bathroom facilities, and lighter colours should be used for wall tiles and vinyl floors. Toilet seats, handrails and towels should all be easily identifiable. Even something as simple as soap should be a different colour from the sink it sits on. Specifically, if showers do not have clear acrylic sides, light-coloured screens are advised which transmit more light. To maintain an optimised acoustic environment, usual recommendations are that alternative finishes are used wherever possible – for example, slip-resistant lino and attenuation of extractor fans.

Kitchen design for people with dementia

For general lighting, the use of long-light sources, such as fluorescent tubes, is generally recommended; spotlights are thought to be best avoided. Making things clear very often helps a person with dementia. Glass jars for tea and coffee, clear-fronted cookers and even fridges with glass doors can make a difference. You can also help people with dementia make sense of identical looking cupboards by installing glass doors on units; or alternatively, it might be worth improving the overall appearance of cupboards by improving low-profile fluorescent tubes mounted on top of wall-mounted cupboards.

Bedroom design for people with dementia

The bedroom is often the only defensible 'personal space', and can be a place of refuge for an individual with dementia.

A bedroom can be a place to watch TV or radio, or listen to music, and these activities can make a vital contribution to somebody's quality of life. For example through TV and radio, a person with dementia can keep up to date with interests and current affairs. A light switch should be readily accessible adjacent to the bed, bedrooms should be shielded from light at night by the use of light-absorbing curtains. Design considerations, from an acoustic perspective, include appropriate ceiling heights, use of soft furnishings, appropriate floor coverings and, where necessary, appropriate control buzzer mechanisms.

Helping a person with dementia get a good night's sleep is vital. Finding their bed may be confusing, so use contrasting bed linen and sheets to clearly define their sleeping area. Raised edges not only help prevent people falling out of bed but also provide psychological support for those who had shared a bed with a partner for many years. People with dementia can be confused when they see their reflection in a mirror, as they may not recognise the person who is looking back at them. The use of mirrors that can be covered or easily removed can help prevent such distress.

Living room design for people with dementia

Living rooms, avoiding dark carpets, are frequently used as communal spaces where many people are gathered.

Often the furniture is oriented towards the television, which remains on constantly and at high volume. From a visual perspective, it makes sense to use plug-in table lights to increase lights at task areas such as reading seats or games tables. An individual with dementia may have no say on what is on, the volume, etc.

There are a number of useful design features to soften noise, which will help people with hearing loss and dementia to hear appropriate sounds, and improve communication in living rooms. Lower ceilings made of absorbent materials will help to attenuate unnecessary noise. Also, designers are encouraged to choose a floating floor that will minimise the impact of noise from footsteps, trolleys, and so forth.

Technology has revolutionised living room design for people with dementia. Seats fitted with pressure pads can turn on lights as you get up or sit down. Fireplaces with flame effect fires can be made from wipe-clean materials and programmed to operate at specific temperatures.

Dining room design for individuals with dementia

There are many aspects of optimising dining room design for individuals with dementia; even the way in which you set a table can improve the life of someone with dementia.

Professional designers often use contrasting colours for cutlery, crockery and tablecloths. Heavier plates with lips are less likely to slip or spill. Ceramic or porcelain mugs and cups make drinking more pleasurable than from plastic.

People with dementia need quality eating and drinking time to live a healthy lifestyle.

There are simple ways in which the acoustic environment can be modified to make the experience of dining more pleasurable. This includes avoiding the use of metal shutters between the main catering kitchen and the dining area; avoiding clustered tables to help individuals with dementia see the people they are conversing with; and consideration to furnishings, table settings and background noise (e.g. TV or music).

IMPORTANT SENSORY CONSIDERATIONS

Lighting and vision

It is unlikely for dementia to affect visual areas of the brain (or cerebral cortex) at all, or even towards the end, and therefore higher-level perception deficits are unlikely to be realised by the individual with dementia (such as colour constancy problems, movement detection). However, peripheral vision problems can occur easily with ageing (such as with cataracts, glaucoma, age-related macular degeneration).

The University of Stirling's publication entitled *Light and Lighting Design for People with Dementia* (McNair *et al.*, 2013), offers important explanations for why the visual environment is important for wellbeing:

- help to see what is around them, what they need and where they want to go
- prompts from familiar sights – furniture, objects, plants and pets
- to use landmarks to find their way
- to see spaces, rooms, equipment and signs to find their way – for example, to go to the toilet or to the dining room
- to enjoy the sights of changing seasons – snow, sunshine, rain, frost – all of which can stimulate memories and aid enjoyment and pleasure for its own sake
- to see other people's faces, gestures and body language, as well as their locations
- to enjoy recreational activities
- to join in ordinary routines – laying the table, washing up, sorting clothes, getting dressed and washed, shaving, putting on make up, brushing hair.

There are many different types of lamps, with different characteristics, including price, lifespan, quality of life, and energy efficiency. Brawley (2009) argued that good lighting is perhaps the *most important* and least understood element in designing healthcare environments. Too often, when one moves beyond the lobby to the patient or resident care areas, the vibrant daylight and lighting systems that created the inviting, pleasant, and visually comfortable environment in the lobby reverts back to the same old familiar, institutional glare-producing ceiling fixtures – a poor strategy for rehabilitation or adaptive healthcare environments that should communicate the message of a caring, healing environment.

Much recent research has focused on the impact of bright light on nighttime sleep and daytime engagement and agitation. In these studies, bright light is delivered at different times (morning, midday and/or evening), may have different colour temperature (cooler or warmer), may be natural light (sunlight) or electric, exposure ranges from 20 minutes to 2 hours, and outcomes generally include either quality of sleep or presentation of challenging behaviours (please see Kim, Song and Yoo, 2003, for a brief review of research conducted prior to 2003).

Despite earlier research that showed positive results on nighttime sleep with evening bright light (Satlin *et al.*, 1992, Van Someren *et al.*, 1999), Ouslander and colleagues (Ouslander *et al.*, 2006) found no impact on nighttime sleep of an intervention that included evening bright light exposure (2 hours at approximately 1500 lux) reduced nighttime noise and disruption reduction routines. Thorpe and colleagues (Thorpe *et al.*, 2000) used brighter light (at approximately 10 000 lux) in the morning, and found a modest impact on reduction of agitation.

Lighting is frequently taken for granted, creating problems for residents, patients and staff. The decline in both visual acuity and visual performance is a fact of life for older adults. Normal changes impact visual ability and age-related eye diseases can cause further impairment. The combined changes for a 65-year-old cause a slower adaptation to changes in light levels, increased sensitivity to glare and decreased sensitivity to contrast. These changes are a lot for any person to adjust to. Though vision impairments may vary they also affect many younger persons as well. Many disorders, including depression, epilepsy, cognitive disorders and the medications used to treat them produce increased sensitivity to light and poor lighting.

Lighting is a powerful design tool that can be used to support individuals of any age to engage in the normal activities of their daily lives. Higher-quality and increased quantities of appropriate lighting help to maximise abilities and minimise challenges for many individuals with compromised vision. The challenge becomes adapting the environment to support the needs of the users and to help compensate for vision changes, no matter the cause.

Brawley (2009)indeed concludes:

Greater efforts must be made to provide adequate/safe interior lighting in adaptive healthcare environments, rehabilitation, and living environments for older adults. Good lighting design today comprises energy efficient, indirect electric lighting and light controls, combined with greater use of large skylights and larger windows for daylighting. Research has confirmed that light not only enhances vision but contributes to overall good health. Increased access to safe, healthy outdoor environments can encourage residents and patients outdoors into the sunlight for healthy bright light exposure to reset circadian cycles, for bone health, exercise and to provide a general sense of increased wellbeing. These minimally invasive interventions may prove to be one of the most affordable prescriptions for fewer fractures, better sleep quality, reduced depression and an increased sense of well being.

Torrington and Tregenza (2007) reviewed the background to the discussion of lighting in dementia wellbeing at the time. Their discussion had arisen from two multidisciplinary research projects.

The first, which ran from 2000 to 2004 and was called Design in Caring Environments (DICE), examined standards and guidelines for the design of care homes for older people. The work included a literature review; a comprehensive survey of 38 residential care homes in Sheffield and Rotherham in the UK; quality of life measures of around 400 residents in these homes; and assessment of staff and management attitudes and practices. The buildings and the way they were used were recorded on the Sheffield Care Environment Assessment Matrix, and multivariate analyses were applied to the data.

The second project, which ran from 2003 to 2006 and was called INDEPENDENT, examined the rôle of technology in enhancing the wellbeing of people with dementia. The programme involved focus groups and interviews with dementia sufferers and their carers, discussing their needs and wishes, which led to design and testing of prototype applications.

An attractive or interesting view from windows can have a therapeutic effect or can reduce discomfort. In a comprehensive literature review, Farley and Veitch (2001) report that windows with views onto nature may enhance working and wellbeing in a number of ways, including life satisfaction. They conclude also that a view outside is important, not only for its restorative quality, but as a means of enhancing control over the environment. The wellbeing of a person with dementia can be substantially improved by increasing the number of enjoyable activities undertaken. Widely used methods of quantifying the quality of life of people with dementia, such as Dementia Care Mapping, and the Pleasant Events Schedule–Alzheimer's Disease, are based on person-centred care, and have an underlying assumption that engaging in a range of activity is beneficial. In general, there exists a strong association between activity and quality of life while ageing (Menec, 2003).

Increasing the range of possible activities open to people with dementia is likely to enhance their wellbeing, especially when they are provided with the opportunity to continue activities that they have enjoyed for many years. The opportunity for these can be influenced by a building's characteristics on two levels. First, the overall form of the interior planning can determine the way in which people may form groups, have privacy, enjoy daylight. For instance, long narrow corridors can inhibit conversational groups, and deep building forms tend to reduce the proportion of the interior that has an external view. Second, the detailed design of building elements can determine accessibility, physical support and safety. An example is the way in which fire doors hinder mobility and social interaction.

Widening the scope of activities implies the provision of any physical support needed; it is clear that not only should users be safe, but that they are helped by feeling that they are safe. Safety should not be a reason for restricting desired activities, but one of the objectives of creative design. That dementia is not a homogenous condition is important in a consideration of different types of dementia and wellbeing. The presentation of dementia of Lewy bodies is typically one of cortical and subcortical cognitive impairments, with worse visuospatial and executive dysfunction than dementia of the Alzheimer type (Weisman and McKeith, 2007). There may be relative sparing of memory especially in the early stages. Core clinical features of Lewy body dementia include fluctuating attention, recurrent visual hallucinations, and Parkinsonism. This might have important safety implications. Also, it might be worth being mindful of the potential danger posed by high balconies for individuals who are impulsive, such as in the behavioural variant of frontotemporal dementia (Health and Safety Executive, 2007).

Colours

It has become more commonplace to hear of new care homes and hospitals being built with a **'dementia-friendly colour scheme'**. Colour affects people both perceptually and emotionally. It anecdotally appears to trigger memories, encourage social activity and eating, and may even help people find their way around. The neuroscientific basis for these phenomena is likely to be better known with time, for individuals with and without dementia.

Colour contributes enormously to one's enjoyment of the environment. Many dementia-friendly colour schemes are possible. The key design issues are colour, fixtures and fittings, furniture and furnishings, and surfaces. Good design around all these can help people with dementia, and make also improve the wellbeing for all those present in the 'caring environment'.

In keeping with the 'person-centred approach', ideally colours should reflect people's religious and spiritual needs, as well as their cultural and socio-economic backgrounds. Where there can be personalisation, colour should reflect personal wishes.

The ageing process can lead to deteriorated visual perception, mainly due to peripheral problems such as changes in the eye lens, rather than central cortical problems due to the neuropathology of the dementia process. However, it is possible that one day peripheral changes in the retina might be found to be a useful peripheral marker for cortical dementias, and this could prove to be a powerful diagnostic tool in the future. Nerve cell death is the key event in all neurodegenerative disorders, with apoptosis and necrosis being central to both acute and chronic degenerative processes. Results from Cordeiro and colleagues (Cordeiro *et al.*, 2010) help directly to observe retinal nerve cell death in patients as an adjunct to refining diagnosis, tracking disease status and assessing therapeutic intervention (much more distally).

Vision perception problems can include impaired depth perception, spatial disorientation, altered colour perception and reduced ability to perceive contrasts. Like many older people, people with dementia may have cataracts, macular degeneration, diabetes retinopathy, colour-blindness (particularly in men) and glaucoma. Blurred vision and loss of central and peripheral vision are the most serious effects of such impairments.

The State Government of Victoria, Australia, Department of Health (2011) provides the following useful 'tips for colour selection'.

- Colour awakens emotional responses related to past experiences and cultural background.
- Colour can be used to increase and reduce visibility.
- Colour contrast and good lighting help people's navigation, orientation, mobility, independence and involvement.
- Too many colours together can be distracting.
- Older people are best able to discriminate strong colours at the warm end of the spectrum.
- Colours with a high degree of brightness, such as yellow, are highly visible.
- Colours such as peach, coral and soft apricot tones flatter skin tones and add warmth to any setting.
- Pastel blues and lavenders are hard for older people to see and often look grey.
- People with colour vision issues are less sensitive to colours on either end of the colour spectrum. Reds and blues will look darker.
- As colour preferences are personal, giving people the chance to personalise private spaces is important.

Calkins (2010) suggests the following four principles for the use of colour for individuals living well with dementia. They are as follows.

- **Principle #1:** Emphasise what's important. Within any setting, there are some elements that carry important information, such as orientation cues, or views to interesting activity areas. Pay close attention to those elements that have the potential to provide useful information to the cognitively impaired individual, and give these more emphasis with brighter colours (using hue, value and chroma), higher contrast with the background, and more light.
- **Principle #2:** De-emphasise what's *not* important. People with dementia can struggle to make sense of their environments, and should not have their attention unnecessarily drawn to elements that do not convey meaningful information

- **Principle #3:** People with dementia have impaired contrast perception, which makes it harder to see the edges of objects, particularly when the foreground (object) and background are similar colour and value. This is particularly important when designing to support functional independence.
- **Principle #4:** People with dementia may have some unique needs, but they are still people, and no research has yet suggested they respond differently emotionally/visually to colors than the general population.

The acoustic environment

The publication published by the University of Stirling entitled *Hearing, Sound and the Acoustic Environment for People with Dementia* (McManus and McClenaghan, 2010), offers important explanations for why the acoustic environment is important for wellbeing:

- aids communication
- ensures inclusion
- reduces the impact of impairments and enable the person with dementia to participate and optimise his or her ability to function
- reduces the risk of further confusion for the person with dementia that is precipitated by an environment which is too noisy and overstimulating
- reduces the risk of including behaviours such as anger, frustration and aggression that can be in response to the environment which is too noisy and overstimulating
- reduces the risk of falling.

Falls management is a recurrent theme in the management of individuals with dementia. Problems with falls can be precipitated by visual problems. For example, in 1999 some 189 000 falls requiring hospital treatment occurred in individuals with visual impairment, of which 89 500 were attributed to the visual impairment itself (Scuffham *et al.*, 2002).

The acoustic environment for older people can be improved by:

- regular hearing assessments to identify the individual needs and risks for each person
- specific training and increased awareness for care staff
- reducing unnecessary noise
- supporting the person to hear as well as possible so he or she can function as well as possible
- being aware of the strengths and limitations of hearing aids.

The following practical interventions will improve the acoustic environment:

- turning off unnecessary sources of noise such as televisions, radios and stereos
- establishing a basic understanding of how hearing and hearing aids work

- fitting the appropriate finishes to hard and soft surfaces, such as floors, window dressings, ceilings
- considering the layouts of buildings, how rooms relate to each other, and how sound and noise will carry them
- promoting sound and minimising noise
- managing peak noise times such as meal times and managing visiting times effectively
- constructing the building to manage actively noise which comes from lifts, laundry rooms, kitchens, and so on.

CARE HOMES

Typically, 70% of care home residents exhibit significant confusion and other cognitive impairments. The basic belief is that a well-designed environment can provide better support through familiarity, clarity of purpose and minimising distraction.

The RCA/Helen Hamlyn project addressed two important areas in the care home – dining spaces and bedrooms – both of which host activities fundamental to daily living (Timlin and Rysenbry, 2010). The aim was to create environments and products that maximise the existing abilities of the residents, promoting independence and improving their experience of living within the building.

An **'immersive research method'** was adopted, which recognised the difficulties of studying people affected by dementia and allowed the researchers to become part of the everyday routine. Numerous care homes were visited, where residents and staff were interviewed and observed. Focus groups were held with people in the early stages of dementia. Best practice and emerging theories in dementia care were researched in order to establish which elements of the designed environment could be used to reinforce good practice. A key insight was that the design of care environments directly impacts on a resident's ability to care for themselves and on their dependency on staff. By designing to help them complete basic tasks such as dressing or eating, their quality of life could be improved and staff workload reduced, thereby allowing time for more meaningful engagement between carers and residents.

Bedrooms

Dressing is an intensely private experience. Often with the progression of dementias, a person's cognitive and physical abilities may decline to the point at which a person is obliged to accept assistance from others, dress in the presence of another person, or even have a carer dress them. This process can be stressful and frustrating. Numerous care strategies have been developed to help people adjust to the new realities of assistance with dressing. However, relatively little attention has been given to the design of the environment or products that a carer uses to perform this assistance, resulting in a make do approach by both carers and residents.

Gardens

Ensuring that residents can access the garden without risk to themselves is essential for their independence and wellbeing. Gardens that are unsafe will require staff supervision, restricting access, adding an unnecessary duty for staff and reducing resident choice.

WARD SETTINGS: THE 'ENHANCING THE HEALING ENVIRONMENT' INITIATIVE FROM THE KING'S FUND

At least one in four people accessing acute hospital services are likely to have dementia and the number of people with dementia is expected to double over the next 30 years. The health departments of the four UK countries have produced dementia strategies with the aim of ensuring that people with dementia receive high-quality care in all healthcare settings. Hospital stays in particular are well recognised to have detrimental effects on people with dementia.

The evidence from the Enhancing the Healing Environment programme is that relatively straightforward and inexpensive changes to the design and fabric of the care environment can have a considerable impact on the wellbeing of people with dementia, as well as improving staff morale and reducing overall costs. However, the *Report of the National Audit of Dementia Care in General Hospitals* (Royal College of Psychiatrists, 2011) suggested that most hospitals had yet to implement such changes. These design principles are offered as a practical resource to help healthcare organisations develop dementia-friendly healthcare environments.

Simple practical questions in assessment of ward settings overall include the environment 'promoting' the following:
- meaningful interaction between patients, their families and staff
- wellbeing
- eating and drinking
- mobility
- continence and personal hygiene
- orientation
- calm and security.

RECOMMENDED READING

Dementia Services Development Centre (2010a) *Designing Balconies, Roof Terraces and Roof Gardens for People with Dementia*. Dementia Design Series. Stirling: University of Stirling.
Dementia Services Development Centre (2010b) *Hearing, Sound and the Acoustic Environment for People with Dementia*. Dementia Design Series. Stirling: University of Stirling.

Dementia Services Development Centre (2010c) *Light and Lighting Design for People with Dementia*. Dementia Design Series. Stirling: University of Stirling.

RECOMMENDED WEBSITES

- University of Stirling: Dementia Services Development Centre 'Buildings and gardens': www.dementia.stir.ac.uk/housing-dsdc/design-housing
- *Environments of Care for People with Dementia* (The King's Fund): www.kingsfund.org.uk/projects/enhancing-healing-environment/ehe-in-dementia-care
- The 'Dementia Enabling Environment Project' (Alzheimer's Australia): www.enablingenvironments.com.au
- Department of Health (2012) *£50 Million Investment to Give People with Dementia Specially Designed Care Homes and Wards*. Press release, 25 October. London: Department of Health, available at: www.gov.uk/government/news/50-million-investment-to-give-people-with-dementia-specially-designed-care-homes-and-wards

REFERENCES

Brawley, E.C. (2009) Enriching lighting design, *NeuroRehabilitation*, **25**(3), pp. 189–99.

Commission for Architecture and the Built Environment (CABE) (2009) *Homes for Our Old Age: Independent Living by Design*. London: CABE, available at: www.designcouncil.org.uk/Documents/Documents/Publications/CABE/homes-for-our-old-age.pdf

Calkins, M.P. (2010) *Using Color as a Therapeutic Tool*, on the Ideas Institute website, available at: www.ideasinstitute.org/article_021103_b.asp

Cordeiro, M.F., Guo, L., Coxon, K.M., *et al.* (2010) Imaging multiple phases of neurodegeneration: a novel approach to assessing cell death in vivo, *Cell Death Dis*, 1, p. e3.

Department of Health (2001) *National Service Framework for Older People*. London: The Stationery Office.

Department of Health (2011) *Living Well with Dementia: A National Dementia Strategy Good Practice Compendium*, London: TSO, available at: www.gov.uk/government/publications/living-well-with-dementia-a-national-dementia-strategy-good-practice-compendium

Desai, A.K., Schwartz, L., and Grossberg, G.T. (2012) Behavioral disturbance in dementia, *Curr Psychiatry Rep*, **14**(4), pp. 298–309.

Farley, K., and Veitch, J. (2001) *A Room With a View: A Review of the Effects of Windows on Work and Wellbeing*. Ottawa, Canada: Institute for Research in Construction, available at: http://archive.nrc-cnrc.gc.ca/obj/irc/doc/pubs/rr/rr136/rr136.pdf

Future Homes Commission (2012) *Building Homes and Communities Britain Needs*, available at: www.architecture.com/Files/RIBATrust/FutureHomesCommissionLowRes.pdf

Gillies, A. (2010) *Keeper: A Book About Memory, Identity, Isolation, Wordsworth and Cake*. London: Short Books.

Gillies, A. (2011) 'Dementia patients deserve better' (18th December 2011), from the *Guardian*, available at: www.theguardian.com/commentisfree/2011/dec/16/dementia-alzheimers-postal-lottery-nhs-patients

Health and Safety Executive (2007) *Falls from Windows and Balconies in Health and Social Care*, available at: www.hse.gov.uk/pubns/hsis5.pdf

Health and Safety Executive (2011) *Health and Safety in Care Homes*, available at: www.hse. gov.uk/pubns/books/hsg220.htm

Huppert, F. (2014) The state of well-being science: concepts, measures, interventions and policies. In: Huppert, F.A., and Cooper, C.L. (eds) *Interventions and Policies to Enhance Well-being*, vol. 6. Oxford: Wiley-Blackwell. pp. 1–49.

Kim, S., Song, H.H., and Yoo, S.J. (2003) The effect of bright light on sleep and behavior in dementia: an analytic review, *Geriatr Nurs*, **24**(4), 239–43.

Marshall, M. (2010) *Designing Balconies, Roof Terraces and Roof Gardens for People with Dementia*. Stirling: Dementia Services Development Centre, University of Stirling.

McManus, M., and McClenaghan, M. (2010) *Hearing, Sound and the Acoustic Environment for People with Dementia*. Stirling: Dementia Services Development Centre, University of Stirling.

McMurdo, M.E.T., and Witham, M.D. (2013) Unnecessary ward moves, *Age Ageing*, Epub July 28, available at: http://ageing.oxfordjournals.org/content/early/2013/07/25/ageing. aft079.short?rss=1

McNair, D., Cunningham, C., Pollock, R., *et al.* (2013) *Light and Lighting Design for People with Dementia*. Third edition. Stirling: Dementia Services Development Centre, University of Stirling.

Mendez, M.F., Lauterbach, E.C., and Sampson S.M.; ANPA Committee on Research. (2008) An evidence-based review of the psychopathology of frontotemporal dementia: a report of the ANPA Committee on Research, *J Neuropsychiatry Clin Neurosci*, **20**(2): 130–49.

Menec, V.H. (2003) The relation between everyday activities and successful ageing: a 6-year longitudinal study, *J Gerontol B Psychol Sci Soc Sci*, **58**(2), pp. S74–82.

National Audit Office (2007) *Improving Services and Support for People with Dementia*. London: The Stationery Office.

National Institute for Health and Care Excellence (NICE) (2013) *Supporting people to live well with dementia (Quality Standard 30)*, statement 8, available at http://publications. nice.org.uk/quality-standard-for-supporting-people-to-live-well-with-dementia-qs30/ quality-statement-8-planning-and-evaluating-services

Ongeri, S. (2009) *Homes for our Old Age: Independent Living by Design*. London: Commission for Architecture and the Built Environment, available at: www.designcouncil.org.uk/ Documents/Documents/Publications/CABE/homes-for-our-old-age.pdf

Ouslander, J.G., Connell, B.R., Bliwise, D.L., *et al.* (2006) A non-pharmacological intervention to improve sleep in nursing home patients: results of a controlled clinical trial, *J Am Geriatr Soc*, **54**(1), 38–47.

Royal College of Psychiatrists (2005) *Who Cares Wins: Improving the Outcome for Older People Admitted to the General Hospital*. London: Royal College of Psychiatrists.

Royal College of Psychiatrists (2011) *Report of the National Audit of Dementia Care in General Hospitals*. London: Healthcare Quality Improvement Partnership.

Satlin, A., Saitlin, A., Volicer, L., *et al.* (1992) Bright light treatment of behavioral and sleep disturbances in patients with Alzheimer's disease, *Am J Psychiatry*, **149**, 1028–32.

Scuffham, P.A., Legood, R., Wilson, E.C.F., *et al.* (2002) The incidence and cost of injurious falls associated with visual impairment in the UK, *Vis Impair Res*, **4**(1), pp. 1–4.

State Government of Victoria, Australia, Department of Health (2011) *Dementia-Friendly Environments: A Guide for Residential Care (Interior Design)*, available at: www.health.vic. gov.au/dementia/changes/interior-design.htm

Thorpe, L, Middleton, J, Russell, G, *et al.* (2000) Bright light therapy for demented nursing home patients with behavioral disturbance, *Am J Alzheimers Dis*, **15**, 18–26.

Timlin, G., and Rysenbry, N. (2010) *Design for Dementia: Improving Dining and Bedroom Environments in Care Homes*, available at: www.hhc.rca.ac.uk/2988-3029/all/1/Design-and-Dementia.aspx

Torrington, J.M., and Tregenza, P.R. (2007) Lighting for people with dementia. *Lighting Res Technol*, **39**, pp. 81–97.

Van Someren, E.S., Colenda, C.C., Cohen, W., *et al.* (1999) Bright light therapy: improved sensitivity to its effects on rest-activity rhythms in Alzheimer patients by application of nonparametric methods, *Chronobiol Int*, **16**(4), pp. 505–18.

Weisman, D., and McKeith, I. (2007) Dementia with Lewy bodies, *Semin Neurol*, **27**(1), pp. 42–7.

CHAPTER 14

Assistive technology and living well with dementia

Statement 7. People with dementia live in housing that meets their specific needs.

It is widely propagated in the media that the two major drivers for 'increased costs of caring' for the NHS comprise the ageing population, as well as the increasing rôle that technological advances will play. Both factors are of course subject to ferocious debate regarding the economic sustainability for the NHS, but certainly one potent myth is that assistive technologies are always expensive. This is not true, and the field of assistive technologies is ever expanding.

David Gems (2011) argues that **gerotechnology** is at the heart of living well in the context of ageing:

> [Another] goal of research on ageing is to improve the health of older people. Here, bio-gerontology is akin to other biomedical research topics, sharing with them the goal of understanding the biological mechanisms that underlie pathology. The particular value of such understanding is that it enables the development of therapeutic treatments, leading to improved health and wellbeing.

A formidable challenge still remains in the relative lack of evidence for pursuing good design principles as well as assistive technologies in improving living well with dementia. For example, the National Dementia Strategy (Department of Health, 2009) provides the following.

The evidence base on design principles is sparse, but there is consensus on key principles and a number of good practice checklists are available. There is a more substantial evidence base to show the opportunities offered by assistive technology and telecare to enable people with dementia to remain independent for longer, and in particular to help the management of risk. But the data on newer approaches are still sparse and inconclusive. An evaluation of one scheme demonstrated cost effectiveness and reports of improved quality of life. Large-scale [Department of Health] field trials of such technology are currently under way.

Dementia conditions have the potential to make day-to-day life more difficult. It is clearly very difficult to 'know' what an individual feels in terms of his or her wellbeing, even if he or she is unaffected by dementia, though a conceptual framework of general **consciousness** is now under way (see, for example, Crick and Koch, 2003). Indeed, as Greenfield (2002) explains, the relationship between the words 'consciousness' and 'mind' merit attention.

Emotions play a critical rôle in the evolution of consciousness and the operations of all mental processes (Izard, 2009). Little things like mislaying keys, forgetting to turn off the taps or leaving the gas unlit can prove frustrating or even create hazards.

Orpwood (2007) has argued that mechanisms underlying consciousness and qualia are likely to arise from the information processing that takes place within the detailed micro-structure of the cerebral cortex. Orpwood's framework looks at two key issues: first, how any information processing system can recognise its own activity, and second, how this behaviour could lead to the subjective experience of qualia. In particular, it explores the pattern processing capabilities of attractor networks, and the way that they can attribute meaning to their input patterns and goes on to show how these capabilities can lead to self-recognition. That paper suggests that although feedforward processing of information can be effective without attractor behaviour, when such behaviour is initiated, it would lead to self-recognition in those networks involved. It also argues that attentional mechanisms are likely to play a key rôle in enabling attractor behaviour to take place.

There has become a growing feeling that 'assistive technologies' (ATs) may provide more support for the carer than for the individual with dementia (McKinney et al., 2004), or to ease service provision. However, there have been some noteable exceptions to this focus on security and safety, such as the work of Topo and colleagues (Topo et al., 2004) on the enjoyment of music, and Alm and colleagues (Alm et al., 2005) on general reminiscence.

However, the influence of engineering on the quality of life research has come to a fore in most recent years (e.g. Orpwood et al., 2007). The INDEPENDENT study has been specifically aimed at designing technology to support quality of life. This collaborative project involved academic engineers, social scientists and architects, together with representatives of user groups and a manufacturer. The design work was based on a comprehensive user survey in which people with dementia themselves highlighted the factors that affected their quality of life. These data were analysed through a series of multidisciplinary workshops through the whole consortium.

There have been, nonetheless, a number of concerns raised about the assistive technology. Prof Roger Orpwood submitted the following comment to the consultation held by the Nuffield Council on Bioethics (2009) summarised in *Dementia: Ethical Issues* between May and July 2008.

> Care professionals often express concern about the use of assistive technology because they see it as something to replace human care. There is no doubt that there is a real danger that some purchasers may see it in this way, either to save money on the part of local authorities, or to reduce the need for direct support on the part of relatives. Those of us involved in developing such equipment see it more as augmenting human care rather than replacing it. However there are some things technology can do that is better than human support. It doesn't get tired or frustrated, it can operate 24 hours a day, and it clearly doesn't get upset by the behaviour of the person with dementia. There is evidence from our own work that technology can provide a much clearer picture of how the user is getting on than can care staff. Our last client in London had a major sleep problem that no-one had picked up, but as soon as our sensor network was turned on the problem shouted at us. So technology has an important role to play, and can do some things better than human carers, but it cannot be a replacement for human care, and all the expression of feeling, empathy and understanding that humans can provide. There are major ethical concerns if it is viewed as a replacement.

WHAT IS ASSISTIVE TECHNOLOGY?

The term 'assistive technology' can be defined as:

> any device or system that allows an individual to perform a task that they would otherwise be unable to do, or increases the ease and safety with which the task can be performed. (Royal Commission on Long Term Care, 1999)

AT encompasses community equipment, housing adaptations, community alarms and the burgeoning variety of devices associated with 'smart' and 'telecare' (see Tinker, 2003, for a discussion of the changing terminology in the context of housing policies). According to Professor Sixsmith and colleagues (Sixsmith *et al.*, 2012), '*the future landscape of assistive technologies is largely dependent on the R&D process and is shaped by the ideas, approaches, concepts, and methods that are utilized [sic] in the process.'*

These technologies generally help with the following functions:

- speaking
- eyesight
- hearing
- moving about
- cognition (thought processes and understanding)
- activities of daily living, such as dressing and preparing meals
- socialising.

AT ranges from very simple tools, such as calendar clocks and touch lamps, to high-tech solutions such as satellite navigation systems to help find someone who has gone missing.

BENEFITS OF ASSISTIVE TECHNOLOGY

AT can:

- promote independence and autonomy, both for the person with dementia and those around him or her
- help mitigate potential risks in and around the home
- possibly reduce early entry into care homes and hospitals
- facilitate memory recognition and recall
- reduce the stress on carers, improving their quality of life, and subsequently that of the person with dementia.

LIMITATIONS OF ASSISTIVE TECHNOLOGY

AT may not be the right answer for everybody. People have different needs, abilities and preferences and *one size does not fit all*. Some people may benefit from additional carer support or services rather than using technology at all.

If AT does not meet the individual needs and preferences of the person, it may be ineffective or may even cause additional confusion or distress.

For example, AT and telecare may not be the answer if:

- the person switches off or unplugs the equipment
- the person is confused or distressed by any alarm sounds or recorded messages
- there are insufficient carers or care workers to respond to an alert.

AT on its own cannot provide human contact and personal care. Many older people experience loneliness and social isolation. Technology should only be provided as an addition to contact and care, not as a replacement.

WHAT ASSISTIVE TECHNOLOGY IS AVAILABLE?

There are many different technologies that can be adapted to the needs of someone with dementia.

AT products can be divided into different segments, one common classification based on the health conditions they address is the following.

- *Beds, seating systems, and ergonomic aids*: devices designed to enable the physically and cognitively impaired to sit or sleep safely and comfortably, or position themselves to perform several tasks.
- *Communication aids*: devices to help to communicate to persons with impaired speech, hearing or writing abilities.
- *Daily living aids*: devices that provide self-help to support daily living activities (dressing, bathing, eating, personal hygiene, etc.).
- *Vision and reading aids*: designed to assist the visually impaired and the blind (electronic reading machines, Braille translators, magnifiers, accessible books devices).
- *Environment aids*: such as electronic systems that enable a person with limited mobility to control several appliances (telephone, lights, etc.).

The European Union market for AT is huge and markets are geographically and sectorally rather fragmented. Manufacturers and distributors are mostly medium to small enterprises, with the exception of some mass production items (such as basic hearing devices or basic wheelchairs). The market within the European Union can be considered as an open market, but what can be difficult is getting a product 'allowable' within the provision of public health services.

Adaptations

There are many different types of equipment that may enable people with dementia to remain independent for longer or make it easier for others to give support. Adaptations and improvements to the home may also help a person to stay at home for longer. Of course, each person is different. What may be useful for one person at a particular stage may not be appropriate for another.

The following professionals can guide on acquisition of AT devices.

- **An occupational therapist** can advise on equipment and useful strategies to help someone with dementia with everyday activities, such as washing and dress.
- **A qualified physiotherapist** can advise on mobility aids, such as walking frames and wheelchairs, and on safe ways of helping someone with dementia to move.
- **A district nurse** can advise on the kind of equipment needed for nursing someone at home. Contact the district nurse through your GP surgery or health centre.

- A **continence adviser** can advise on problems relating to incontinence and give information on a range of aids.

IMPROVING WELLBEING

Innovative products that can help with the difficulties that people with dementia experience include:

- **memory aids**, such as clocks with large faces or notice boards for messages
- **equipment for washing and for using the toilet**, such as bath seats or raised toilet seats
- **equipment for maintaining continence and personal dignity**, including commodes, continence aids and dressing aids
- **equipment for eating and drinking**, such as specially adapted cutlery or non-spill cups
- **equipment to help people to continue to participate in household activities** such as cooking and cleaning, including kettle tippers and adapted kitchen tools
- **transfer aids** such as bed sticks, transfer turntables and hoists, which help people to move from a bed to a chair, for example
- **mobility aids**, including walking frames and wheelchairs
- **adaptations** to seating and beds, such as chair or bed raisers
- **equipment to help the individual take medication**, such as boxes with a pill compartment for each day of the week
- **nursing equipment**, including bedpans or pressure relief mattresses
- **safety devices**, such as gas detectors and water-level alerts.

It is perhaps useful also to keep in mind that equipment is not always the answer. It may be enough to make small changes in the way that daily activities are organised.

A FRAMEWORK FOR QUALITY OF LIFE AND ASSISTIVE TECHNOLOGIES: THE INDEPENDENT PROJECT

Chapters 3 and 4 have already considered the basic theoretical constructs for quality of life and wellbeing in dementia.

Figure 3.2 in **Chapter 3** demonstrates a proposed ecological model that has been developed to facilitate structured applied research in this area.

As explained in Sixsmith, Orpwood and Torrington (2007), **INDEPENDENT** was the UK government-funded project to explore the potential of technology to enhance the quality of life of people with dementia, to help them to live independently, and to empower them without compromising their rights or privacy. The project's specific aim was to consider the needs of people with dementia and to harness the potential of new technologies for a group that had been previously marginalised in society.

The project considered a *'wish list'* of issues to improve quality of life (Orpwood *et al.*, 2008), described in **Table 14.1**.

TABLE 14.1 INDEPENDENT workshops and a wellbeing 'wish list'

Theme	Description
1. Oral/personal histories	Promoting reminiscence both when alone or with others.
2. Social participation	Assisting people with forming new or continuing relationships with friends and family. Encouraging assisting with family visits.
3. Conversational prompting	Supporting the act of conversation with others.
4. Encouraging use of music	Promoting the enjoyment and use of music, either as a specific activity or through passive enjoyment.
5. Encouraging community relationships	Promoting relationships, with helping participation in the local community.
6. Supporting sequences	Supporting activities that involve a series of steps.
7. Exercise/physical activity	Encouraging and supporting physical activity.
8. Encouraging access to nature.	Encouraging and assisting access to outer spaces and nature.
9. Sharing experiences of care and caring	Providing support with physical care tasks to free quality time between carer and person-with-disability.
10. Creative activities	Supporting people to take part in hobbies, pastimes and creative activities.
11. Pottering in the house	Participation in minor tasks and household chores.

Source: Sixsmith, *et al.* (2007). The INDEPENDENT project aimed to address an agenda of developing technologies to enhance positively quality of life. As part of the project, workshops were established to create a 'wish list' of potential areas for the development and implementation of technological solutions. During the workshops, a long-list of 69 specific ideas for individual design technologies was developed, forming the basis for further work.

As Orpwood and colleagues describe (Orpwood *et al.*, 2007; Sixsmith, Orpwood and Torrington, 2007), 69 designs were considered, **four** of which were selected for the initial design work within the project:

1. *A simple music player.* This should be a relatively simple device to enable someone with dementia to select and play any music they like through a player that looks like a typical musical playing device, but which uses very simple controls such as a single button to operate it.
2. *Window on the world.* The window on the world combines two ideas by using web-based technologies to provide remote images within the user's home in order to enhance engagement with the family and wider community.
3. *Conversation prompter.* When the user loses his or her train of thought the

device would prompt, through replaying the last few seconds of the user's speech or providing keywords or topics.

4. *Sequence assisting device.* The device would break simple tasks into separate clearly defined, and easily understandable stages, and prompt the user to enact each stage in turn.

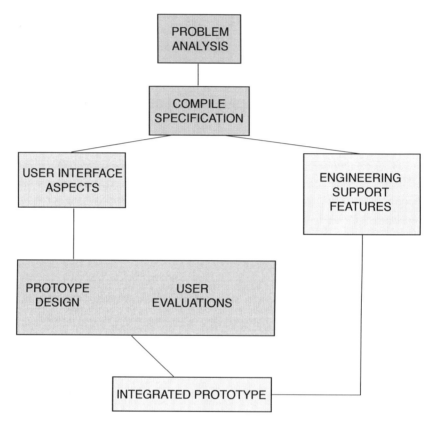

FIGURE 14.1 An assistive technology design methodology to deal with the complex user-interface (the methodology is based on the recognition that most of the difficulties and unforeseen circumstances occur with the user interface aspects of the design rather than the supporting technology; as a consequence, the methodology aims at evolving solutions for these aspects by working on them in isolation in an iterative fashion with typical end users (*see* Orpwood *et al.*, 2005))

Professor Roger Orpwood (2009) has been instrumental in mapping out a new design methodology for assistive technologies in dementia. Orpwood (2009) highlights that the designer needs to make close observations about how the user has reacted, and in some cases make measurements of their responses. Having tested an initial prototype, Orpwood proposes that the design can then be amended to take into account any problems or concerns that arose, with the testing repeated. This is shown schematically in Figure 14.1.

Orpwood and colleagues (Orpwood *et al.*, 2005) suggest that the design process can be improved, thereby improving wellbeing, by acknowledging a need for carer emulation, a need for familiarity, a need for prompts and reminders, and a need to monitor on-going behaviour. The view of Orpwood and others (Orpwood *et al.*, 2008), that ATs should be **'user led'**, is reflected in the National Dementia Strategy (Department of Health, 2009):

> The needs of people with dementia and their carers should be included in the development of housing options, assistive technology and telecare. As evidence emerges, commissioners should consider the provision of options to prolong independent living and delay reliance on more intensive services.

THE ENABLE PROJECT

The aim of the **ENABLE** project, funded by the European Commission, was to evaluate a series of items of support equipment with dementia. Indeed, a complete smart home system has been installed in a sheltered housing scheme in Deptford run by Housing 21 (Orpwood *et al.*, 2005). The overall aim was to investigate whether it is possible to facilitate independent living of people with dementia and to promote their wellbeing through access to enabling technological systems and products.

Key objectives were to:

- develop prototype technologies designed to provide stimulation, facilitate communication and promote safety
- develop a methodology for assessment and analysis
- develop a methodology for cost/benefit assessment
- examine the use and usefulness of assistive technologies by both people with dementia and their family carers.

Löfqvist and colleagues (Löfqvist *et al.*, 2005) provide a very useful review of assistive technologies in five European countries. The aim of this study was to investigate the use and need of assistive devices (ADs) in a cross-national European sample of very old persons, focusing on national similarities and differences as well as similarities and differences according to age and level of health status. Data from the ENABLE-AGE research project were utilised involving very old persons in Sweden, Germany, Latvia, Hungary and the UK. Personal interviews with single-living old persons were conducted. Of the total sample, 65% reported that they had and used one or more ADs, and 24% reported unfilled need.

The most commonly used examples of AT were devices for communication, followed by devices for mobility. Participants in Hungary and Latvia used a lower total number of ADs. Comparisons among subgroups according to age between the Western and the Eastern European national samples showed significant differences. The result can, to some extent, be explained by different welfare systems and presumably differences in knowledge and awareness of ADs, and further research is called for. However, the result can serve as input for future planning and development of information, services, and community-based occupational therapy, to improve healthcare and social services for older people.

THE ROSETTA PROJECT

ROSETTA ('RObot control for Skilled ExecuTion of Tasks' in natural interaction with humans; based on Autonomy, cumulative knowledge and learning) develops 'human-centric' technology for industrial robots that will not only appear more human-like, but also cooperate with workers in ways that are safe and perceived as natural.

Such robots will be programmed in an intuitive and efficient manner, making it easier to adapt them to new tasks when a production line is changed to manufacture a new product. The project aims at supporting industry through developing technologies that make it easier to utilise and integrate industrial robots into otherwise manual assembly lines.

It is thought that today's marketplace is characterised by products that come in many variants or configurations, but have short lifetimes. This appears to call for flexible manufacturing systems that allow for frequent product changes. Industrial robot automation is the automation method of choice to meet with those demands, but this application requires the ability to adapt even more quickly to new tasks.

DISCRETIONARY POWERS TO ASSIST WITH HOUSING REPAIRS, ADAPTATIONS AND IMPROVEMENTS

The National Dementia Strategy (Department of Health, 2009) emphasises the importance of good housing for living well in dementia, emphasising for example, monitoring the development of models of housing, including extra care housing, to meet the needs of people with dementia and their carers; nurturing staff working within housing and housing-related services so that they may develop skills needed to provide the best quality care and support for people with dementia in the rôles and settings where they work; and maintaining a watching brief over the emerging evidence base on assistive technology and telecare to support the needs of people with dementia and their carers to enable implementation once effectiveness is proven.

TELECARE

Within many healthcare systems, there has been a growing focus on the value of telehealth and telecare interventions for improving quality and cost-effectiveness of care for people with long-term complex health and social care needs (Gaikwad and Warren, 2009).

Telecare has many definitions and the Social Care Institute for Excellence recognises there is quite a complicated terminology debate in this field.

This briefing and the main report use the following description of telecare:

> Equipment [that] is provided to support the individual in their home and tailored to meet their needs. It can be as simple as the basic community alarm service, able to respond in an emergency and provide regular contact by telephone.
>
> (Department of Health, 2005)

Telecare and telehealth services use technology to help you live more independently at home. They include personal alarms and health-monitoring devices.

Telecare and telehealth services are especially helpful for people with long-term conditions, as it gives the person and his or her closest peace of mind about safety and relatively stable personal health.

The term 'telecare' refers to devices that continuously, automatically and remotely monitor real-time emergencies and lifestyle changes over time to manage the risks associated with living alone. Sensors around the home can be linked via a telephone line to a nominated person or call centre. The system monitors a person's activities and, if a problem occurs, triggers an alarm to a relative, keyholder or call centre.

Sensors can be used to detect a range of situations that could indicate a potential hazard, including the following.

- *Floods*: sensors can be fitted on skirting boards or floors in the kitchen or bathroom. If the taps have been left running and cause a flood, the system will shut off the water and raise the alarm. Specially designed plugs can also be used to prevent floods from taps that have been left running.
- *Extreme temperatures*: sensors will send a warning signal if the temperature is very low, very high, or if there is a rapid rise in temperature. This can be useful in the kitchen, for example to detect a pan that has boiled dry, and can also detect if the temperature in a room is low enough to pose a risk of hypothermia.
- *Gas*: sensors detect if someone forgets to turn the gas off, and a device will automatically shut off the gas and raise the alarm.
- *Falls*: sensors worn on the hip can detect the impact of a person falling.
- *Absence from a bed or chair*: if a person gets up and doesn't return within a

pre-set time, or if they don't get up in the morning, a bed or chair occupancy system can raise an alarm.

- *Getting up in the night*: bed occupancy sensors or pressure-mat sensors placed by the bed can be used to activate an alarm when the person gets up in the night, to alert someone to help them get to the toilet. Similarly, lights with movement sensors can be fitted to switch on if a person gets out of bed or enters a room.
- *Leaving the home*: the system may be set up to trigger a response if the front door is opened, perhaps during specified times – for example, at night, or if a person does not return within a specified time. Door systems such as these use passive infra-red or door contacts, and can help to reduce risk and retain the person's independence.

AT Dementia is an organisation that provides information about telecare support and also produces a self-assessment guide that can help people identify which ATs may be of use to them.

Devices to enable safer walking

Tracking devices use satellite technology to help trace someone who has gone missing. A person's location can be viewed on a computer or mobile phone. Most devices have the facility for the person carrying the device to press a panic button if they get lost. A mobile phone with location finder technology could also be considered instead of a stand-alone tracking device. When purchasing a device to enable safer walking it is important to consider how reliable it is – for example, whether it works when the person is indoors, and how often the device will need charging.

Research suggests that tracking devices give both people with dementia and carers an enhanced sense of independence and help carers feel more reassured.

As with other technologies, there are ethical issues to consider if a person is unable to give their informed consent to carrying (or wearing) this sort of device. Other things to consider are what items the person should carry in case he or she gets lost – for example, personal information and contact details of someone who can help him or her. There are clearly, therefore also, valid legal concerns about whether such measures can be legal as regards universal human rights, in being both necessary and proportionate.

Devices to oversee daily activity

It is possible to install sensors to monitor a person's activity in their own home over a period of time. This can sometimes help relatives or community services get a better idea of a person's activity during the day and night. A system such as this can allay fears that the person with dementia is not coping well, and may help those around them to step back and not take over unless it is absolutely necessary.

Other aids

Other problems associated with dementia include mobility problems, incontinence and difficulties with sight or hearing.

INNOVATIONS FROM THE DESIGN COUNCIL

The Design Council has recently featured five interesting innovations to contribute to an aspiration for individuals with dementia to live well.

The teams behind these solutions include designers, entrepreneurs and service providers, as well as experts in nutrition, dog training and olfaction. The concepts are all focused on and around the point of diagnosis, aiming to be preventative measures that improve quality of life in the early stages of dementia for the increasing numbers of people being diagnosed.

The five solutions given here are examples of the vast potential of innovative ideas in an under-served market and show how design can play a key rôle in confronting a major social challenge.

1. *'Buddie'*: attractive wristband personal alarm that can send alerts from anywhere to Buddie's support services.
2. *Grouple*: a secure, private online social network helping people share the responsibilities of caring for someone with dementia.
3. *Trading Times*: an online service that matches carers with local businesses for flexible paid work
4. *Dementia Dog*: assistance dogs helping people with dementia lead more fulfilled, independent and stress-free lives.
5. *Ode*: a fragrance-release system designed to stimulate appetite among people with dementia.

TELEHEALTH

Special **telehealth** equipment can also monitor your health in your own home. It can be equipment to measure your blood pressure, blood glucose levels or your weight. This can reduce the number of visits you make to your GP and also the number of unplanned visits to the hospital you make. You're taught how to do the tests on yourself, and the measurements are automatically transmitted to your doctor or nurse, who can then see the information without you having to leave home. They can let you know if they have any concerns.

It is well known in innovation that individuals react differently to different products. For example, some people might find it helpful to have a recorded message that plays when they open the front door, reminding them to take their keys, while other people might find this confusing and obtrusive. However, some people may also be wary of trying new things or find it difficult to learn new skills. Choosing the right device is therefore not always an easy task.

If an assessment is carried out it must be detailed and person-centred so that the solution will suit the individual and their situation. It is also important to emphasise that AT can be effective only when combined with good care.

Many devices can be bought independently, but before doing so it is advisable to contact the person's occupational therapist or GP, or the local authority social services department. Even if they can't offer the products, the person with dementia may be eligible for a proper assessment, help in finding the best product or financial assistance ('**At a glance 60**'; SCIE, 2012).

At a glance 60: Preventing loneliness and social isolation among older people
- Older people are particularly vulnerable to social isolation and loneliness owing to loss of friends and family, mobility or income.
- Social isolation and loneliness have a detrimental effect on health and wellbeing. Studies show that being lonely or isolated can impact on blood pressure, and is closely linked to depression.
- The impact of loneliness and social isolation on an individual's health and wellbeing has cost implications for health and social care services. Investment is needed to ensure that voluntary organisations can continue to help alleviate loneliness and improve the quality of life of older people, reducing dependence on more costly services.

The range of interventions for alleviating loneliness and social isolation can be grouped into one-to-one interventions, group services and wider community engagement. Those that look most effective include befriending, social group schemes and Community Navigators.
- Aim to find solutions that can be integrated into the person's normal routine with minimum disruption.
- Involve the person in decisions about which product or solution to use, and take his or her opinions on board.
- There is a higher chance of success if you can introduce AT when the dementia is still at an early stage, so that the person can gradually get used to the new way of doing things.
- Simple ideas such as a diary or noticeboard can provide a reminder of appointments, important phone numbers and things to do.
- Deciding on a permanent place to keep important items such as keys and labelling; cupboards or rooms may help the person with dementia to remember where things are.

GENERAL ETHICAL PRINCIPLES GOVERNING TELECARE

Researchers at the **Welsh Centre for Learning Disabilities** identified the ethical issues in the use of telecare mainly through the 'Delphi' method. The '**Delphi**' method is a structured process for collecting data and distilling knowledge from a group of experts (Adler and Ziglio, 1996).

The experts in this study included local authority/Northern Ireland health and social care trust telecare leads, occupational therapists, commissioners, providers and third sector representatives. People with learning difficulties and people with dementia were also involved through informing the content of the Delphi questionnaires and in discussions about the findings before they were written up. The Welsh Centre's work also benefited from input by the project advisory group.

The Welsh Centre researchers adopted an '**ethical framework**' to illustrate the potential problems associated with the use of telecare. This framework comprises four important principles. The Social Care Institute for Excellence's report refers to the ways in which the commissioning and provision of telecare can compromise these principles ('**At a glance 24**'; SCIE, 2010).

The four ethical principles are shown in Box 14.1.

BOX 14.1 Four ethical principles

- *Autonomy* – the ability of an individual to make choices. Autonomy is related to the independence and choice in everyday life that is often taken for granted. When people rely on professionals or family carers for their care or for safety monitoring, the introduction of a telecare service can drastically promote or restrict autonomy.
- *Beneficience* – the principle of working for the benefit of the individual. Telecare has the potential to benefit people. It can provide assurance and confidence and can reduce unwanted dependence on professional staff or family carers. It can also increase comfort through environmental sensors and controls.
- *Non-maleficence* – the principle of doing no harm. While telecare can benefit an individual, it also has the potential to expose people to risk. A balance must be achieved between ensuring safety and invading privacy. The potentially stigmatising effect of telecare should be recognised and minimised.
- *Justice* – the moral obligation to act on a fair adjudication between conflicting claims. In the interests of justice, resources for telecare services should be allocated so as to balance the needs of the individual with those of the wider community.

The Nuffield Council on Bioethics (2009) flag up general ethical issues in dementia in their report:

Technologies such as 'smart' home adaptations, telecare, memory aids and monitoring or tracking devices may play an important role in enhancing the lives of people with dementia and their close family and friends. They may promote a person's autonomy and wellbeing by enabling them to live more freely and more independently for longer. Concerns, however, have been raised about possible detrimental effects, such as intrusion on privacy, stigma (particularly with reference to tracking devices) and the risk of reduced human contact. All these issues have the potential to affect both a person's autonomy, for example through feeling controlled or devalued, and their wellbeing, for example through impoverished human relationships.

ETHICAL CONSIDERATIONS OF TELECARE

Telecare offers potential benefits for individual users including safety and independence. It also has the potential to reduce social care costs, allowing the more efficient deployment of direct care staff.

Telecare has the potential to threaten individual users' privacy, autonomy and control. Social care and health professionals need to consider a range of ethical issues when supporting an individual in deciding whether to use telecare. These issues need to be considered before, during and after the installation of a telecare service. Commissioners must ensure that people who are self-funders or personal budget holders have access to relevant information so they can decide what type of telecare service would best suit their needs. Local priorities and commissioning strategies may affect telecare services, including what kind is provided and who receives and pays for it. Service providers must have robust systems and agreements for collection, storage and sharing of data. Proper support for telecare users will have training implications for practitioners. Equipment manufacturers are urged to improve the sophistication of technology to reduce the potentially stigmatising effect of certain types of telecare. They are also urged to improve flexibility in the means of communication between monitoring centres and telecare users.

WELLBEING CONSIDERATIONS ABOUT SOCIAL ISOLATION

Telecare has a potentially isolating effect.

Many advise specifically that telecare should not be considered as an alternative to direct medical, social care or informal support, unless that is the expressed wish of the person using the service with full mental capacity exercising autonomy and knowing all the risks and benefits.

Local commissioning strategies could recognise the potential of telecare for meeting low-level needs. It is important to recognise that a telecare service cannot monitor changes in a person's wellbeing as sensitively as human beings can, and this should be reflected in care planning. Telecare should be combined with direct social care and informal support to maximise people's motivation and to facilitate carers' support of social engagement.

SMART HOMES

About $14 billion was spent on home networking in 2005, and analysts predict that figure will climb to more than $85 billion by 2011 (Regan, 2010).

The design and structure of houses and their facilities are critical to older people's ability to manage independently. This research has focused on the social rented sector in which there are disproportionate numbers of disabled older people, with 6% greater probability of being disabled at all ages, than those in their own home (Grundy *et al.*, 1999). 'Smart homes' might not be appropriate for individuals with marked cognitive problems, and indeed some individuals might end up becoming quite anxious and upset by the introduction of sophisticated technology into their homes (Orpwood *et al.*, 2005).

Smart home technology was first developed in 1975 in the UK jurisdiction, when a company in Scotland developed X10. X10 allows compatible products to talk to each other over the already existing electrical wires of a home. All the appliances and devices are receivers, and the means of controlling the system, such as remote controls or keypads, are transmitters.

Manufacturers have made alliances with these systems to create the products that use the technology. Examples include the following.

- Cameras will track your home's exterior even if it's pitch-black outside.
- Plug your tabletop lamp into a dimmer instead of the wall socket, and you can brighten and dim at the push of a button.
- A video door phone provides more than a doorbell – you get a picture of who's at the door.

Smart homes also provide some energy efficiency savings. Some systems can go to 'sleep' and wake up when commands are given. Electric bills go down when lights are automatically turned off when a person leaves the room, and rooms can be heated or cooled based on who's there at any given moment. One smart homeowner boasted her heating bill was about one-third less than a same-sized normal home. Some devices can track how much energy each appliance is using and command it to use less.

WEBSITES

- AT dementia: www.atdementia.org.uk
- The ROSETTA project: www.fp7rosetta.org

REFERENCES

Adler, M., and Ziglio, E. (1996) *Gazing into the Oracle.* Bristol: Jessica Kingsley Publishers.

Alm, N., Dye, R., Astell, A., *et al.* (2005) *Making Software Accessible to People with Severe Memory Deficits. Proceedings of Accessible Design in the Digital World, Dundee, 23–25 August,* available at: www.computing.dundee.ac.uk/projects/circa/ADDWcirca.pdf

Crick, F., and Koch, C. (2003) A framework for consciousness, *Nat Neurosci,* **6**(2), pp. 119–26.

Department of Health (2009) *Living Well with Dementia: A National Dementia Strategy; Putting people first (Accessible summary.)* London: The Stationery Office, available at: www.gov.uk/government/uploads/system/uploads/attachment_data/file/168221/dh_094052.pdf

Department of Health (2005) *Building Telecare in England.* London: The Stationery Office.

Design Council (date uncertain) *Five Innovative Solutions to Help Individuals with Dementia Live Well,* available at: www.designcouncil.org.uk/our-work/challenges/Health/Living-well-with-Dementia1/Solutions1/

ENABLE. *Enabling Technologies for Persons with Dementia: Experience from the ENABLE Project,* available at: ftp://ftp.cordis.europa.eu/pub/life/docs/topo.pdf

Gaikwad, R., and Warren, J. (2009) The role of home-based information and communications technology interventions in chronic disease management: a systematic literature review, *Health Informatics J,* **15**(2), pp. 122–46.

Gems, D. (2011) Tragedy and delight: the ethics of decelerated ageing, *Philos Trans R Soc Lond B Biol Sci,* **366**(1561), pp. 108–12.

Greenfield, S. (2002) Mind, brain and consciousness, *Br J Psychiatry,* **181**, pp. 91–3.

Grundy, E., Ahlburg, D., Ali, M., *et al.* (1999) *Disability Follow-up to the 1996/97 Family Resources Survey,* available at: www.herc.ox.ac.uk/icohde/datasets/65

Izard, C. (2009) Emotion theory and research: highlights, unanswered questions and emerging issues, *Annu Rev Psychol,* **60**, pp. 1–25.

Löfqvist, C., Nygren, C., Széman, Z., *et al.* (2005) Assistive devices among very old people in five European countries, *Scand J Occup Ther,* **12**(4), pp. 181–92.

McKinney, K.M., Kart, C.S., Murdoch, L.D., *et al.* (2004) Striving to provide safety assistance to families of elders: the SAFE house project, *Dementia,* **3**, pp. 351–70.

National Institute for Health and Care Excellence (NICE) (2013) *Supporting people to live well with dementia (Quality Standard 30),* statement 7, available at: http://publications.nice.org.uk/quality-standard-for-supporting-people-to-live-well-with-dementia-qs30/quality-statement-7-design-and-adaptation-of-housing

Nuffield Council on Bioethics (2009) *Dementia: Ethical Issues.* London: Nuffield Council on Bioethics, available at: www.nuffieldbioethics.org/sites/default/files/Nuffield%20Dementia%20report%20Oct%2009.pdf

Orpwood, R. (2007) Short communication: neurobiological mechanisms underlying qualia, *J Integr Neurosci,* **6**(4), pp. 523–40.

Orpwood, R. (2009) Involving people with dementia in the design process: examples of the iterative process. In: Topo, P., and Östlund, B. (eds) *Dementia, Design and Technology,* London: IOS Press. pp. 75–95.

Orpwood, R., Chadd, J., Howcroft, D., *et al.* (2008) User-led design of technology to improve quality of life for people with dementia. In: *Designing Inclusive Futures,* London: Springer Verlag. pp. 185–95.

Orpwood, R., Gibbs, C., Adlam, T., *et al.* (2005) The design of smart homes for people with dementia: user-interface aspects, *Univ Access Inf Soc*, **4**, pp. 154–64.

Orpwood, R., Sixsmith, A., Torrington, J., *et al.* (2007) Designing technology to support quality of life in dementia, *Technol Disabil*, **19**(2–3), pp. 103–22.

Regan, K. (2007) *Ten Scary Things About Home Networks: Part 1.* TechNewsWorld, 22 February, available at: www.technewsworld.com/story/55882.html

Royal Commission on Long Term Care (1999) *With Respect to Old Age: Long Term Care – Rights and Responsibilities; Alternative models of care for older people.* Research volume 2. London: Stationery Office.

Sixsmith, A., Orpwood, R., and Torrington, J. (2007) Quality of life technologies for people with dementia, *Top Geriatr Rehabil*, **23**(1), pp. 85–93.

Sixsmith, A. J., Gibson, G., Orpwood, R. D., *et al.* (2007) Developing a technology 'wish-list' to enhance the quality of life of people with dementia. *Gerontechnology*, **6**(1), pp. 2–19.

Sixsmith, A., Woolrych, R., Bierhoff, I., *et al.* (2012). Ambient assisted living: From concept to implementation. In A. Glascock & D. Kutzik (Eds.), *Essential Lessons for the Success of Telehomecare*, Amsterdam: IOS Press. pp. 259–86.

Social Care Institute for Excellence (SCIE) (2010) *At a Glance 24: Ethical Issues of Telecare*, available at www.scie.org.uk/publications/ataglance/ataglance24.asp

Social Care Institute for Excellence (SCIE) (2012) *At a Glance 60: Preventing Loneliness and Social Isolation among Older People.* London: Social Care Institute for Excellence, available at: www.scie.org.uk/publications/ataglance/ataglance60.asp

Tinker, A. (2003) Assistive technology and its role in housing policies for older people, *Qual Ageing*, **4**(2), 4–12.

Topo, R., Maki, K., Saarikalle, K., *et al.* (2004) Assessment of music-based multimedia program for people with dementia, *Dementia*, **3**(3), pp. 331–50.

CHAPTER 15

Ambient assisted living and the innovation culture

Clearly, an ageing population presents many challenges, but above all they should be valued by society at large not least because of their social capital.

More than nine million people in England and Wales are now aged over 65. This is a figure that is likely to increase by more than two million in the next few years as the post-war *'baby boomer'* generation retires. This by anyone's standards is a significant number of people, and includes older people in good health and poor health; those who are physically or socially isolated as well as those living with or supported by families; those who are digitally connected; and those who are digitally excluded (Ayres, 2013). The report by the Nominet Trust entitled *Can Online Innovations Enhance Social Care?* argued that technology provides many different ways of connecting people and resources, and that this should enable the design and delivery of appropriate care services to celebrate and value the life experience and wisdom offered by the older people they are supporting.

An **'ambient assisted living'** (AAL) system is seen to have potential benefits for monitoring a range of alert situations – for example, critical events requiring immediate intervention (e.g. heart attack) to non-critical situations requiring longer-term preventive interventions (e.g. exacerbations of a chronic illness). How can one best respond to an individual's desire to *'age-in-place'*? How can one improve services and enhance people's independence and quality of life? How can one best respond to these challenges in the context of limited resources? It is in this context that advances in the area of AAL may play a crucial rôle.

However, the **barriers to the development of AAL markets remain considerable**, reflecting factors such as funding and reimbursement systems, organisation of care services, cultural differences and ethical or legal concerns. Despite these barriers, the case for incorporating information and communications technology (ICT) within the spectrum of care appears increasingly compelling (Sixsmith, 2012).

DEMOGRAPHICS

In recent years in the Western world, improvements in quality of life have led to much greater life expectancies among the general population (Arbeev *et al.*, 2004). With this increase in life expectancy, a shift has occurred in the demographic of Britain, leading to a phenomenon referred to as the ageing population. With this shift comes a dramatic increase in the diseases and syndromes associated with old age such as dementia (Ferri *et al.*, 2005).

AALIANCE (2010) set the following as the backdrop to the use of AAL:

> Not only will the income side of social schemes be affected but expenditures will be too: healthcare systems will be affected as an ageing population will lead to an increase in the proportion of people with disabilities or chronic illnesses. Thus, healthcare systems and social care in general – which is typically organised on a national level and characterised by national differences as regards institutional design – will have to cope with increasing requirements both in quality and quantity and so lead to increasing expenses.

AMBIENT ASSISTED LIVING

AAL services and technologies are designed to help extend the time that older people can live at home by 'increasing their autonomy and assisting them in carrying out activities of daily life' (Wojciechowski and Xiong, 2008). The services offered may include support for functional, activity, cognitive, intellectual and sensory-related activities; for example, providing alarms to detect dangerous situations that are a threat to the user's health and safety, continuously monitoring the health and wellbeing of the user, and the use of interactive and virtual services to help support the user.

These technology-enriched services have evolved from relatively simple telecare services such as emergency fall alarm provision into more sophisticated telehealth services supporting people with long-term chronic health conditions such as dementia of the Alzheimer type. Along with this evolution in the provision of services, there has been a parallel development in the sophistication of the technology that underpins the AAL services and in the complexity and volume of the data from the sensors that monitor the activity of the user in his or her home setting. Such data can include movement information, device usage information, medication compliance data and other rich data that can inform decisions for AAL services.

A major component of AAL systems is '**activity monitoring**', which uses data collected from environmental sensors installed in the home and wearable biomedical sensors to build a profile of the dweller's typical pattern of living and health status, such as when the person gets up and goes to bed, and level and location of movement. Any variation from the typical pattern of activity may be a source of concern – for example, a reduced level of activity during the day may be indicative of a decline in health status. Activity monitoring may be useful in generating health or emergency alerts in the short term, possibly requiring immediate intervention and also for monitoring changes in the health and independence of people in the longer term.

Technology that monitors people's health, keeps their homes secure and helps them stay fit and connected with family and friends will benefit older people more than perhaps any other group – but only if they are able and willing to use it. European Union (EU)–funded researchers are trying to overcome barriers to the acceptance and usability of AAL systems through innovative user-centred designs. Intelligent ambient technology that uses sensors and actuators to control dynamically lighting or heating, warn if a window has been left open or automatically alert emergency services in the event of an accident has come a long way in recent years. For tech-savvy younger generations, smart homes that can be controlled remotely or intelligently are becoming popular.

It is interesting to note that some of the key ideas within AAL have been around for many years. For example, push-button alarms to send an emergency alert to a call centre or carer has been around since at least the 1960s. The idea of smart housing, where the home environment adapts to the needs and preferences of the dweller, has also been around for many decades, while the idea of activity monitoring has been around since the 1980s. However, many of these ideas have failed to get beyond the prototype stage. Care and support for older people living at home remains overwhelmingly based on direct 'face-to-face' contact and markets for commercially available products and services remain patchy.

Meanwhile, intelligent systems are also being put to use in care homes and assisted living environments to help carers keep older people comfortable, safe and secure. However, in between these two models are a large number of older people who could benefit from ambient technology but find it either too difficult to use or potentially too intrusive. AAL refers to intelligent systems of assistance for a better, healthier and safer life in the preferred living environment and covers concepts, products and services that interlink and improve new technologies and the social environment. It aims at enhancing the quality of life (the physical, mental and social wellbeing) for everyone (with a focus on elder persons) in all stages of life. AAL can help elder individuals to improve their quality of life, to stay healthier and to live longer, thus extending one's active and creative participation in the community. Currently there is a vast number of (more or less linked) European and national research activities in the field of AAL involving various technology areas and innovative technology approaches.

THE EUROPEAN UNION PERSPECTIVE ON AMBIENT ASSISTED LIVING

The emergence of AAL technologies can be tracked back over three generations (Sixsmith *et al.*, 2007).

A '**first generation**' of technology refers to personal alarms that are widely available for older persons to raise an alert should they need assistance – for example, if they experience an episode of illness or have had a fall.

A '**second generation**' of technologies has now emerged into the market-place and has included sensors that observe health status and activity levels and passively monitor the safety and security of the person. A third generation involves 'pervasive' technologies that imbed intelligence and communications within the everyday living environment, making digital technology an integral and intuitive part of daily life.

As well as enhancing safety and security, this '**third generation**' of AAL technology could potentially contribute to supporting independent living and enhancing the quality of life for elderly people by facilitating whole range of health and social care interventions.

The EU has a long history of cross-national initiatives in research and development in the area of technologies for older and disabled people. The European Commission has a mandate to co-fund activities to stimulate EU industry, at the same time as enhancing the social participation of marginalised groups through an inclusive 'information society'.

CHALLENGES IN AAL (THE EUROPEAN AMBIENT ASSISTED LIVING INNOVATION ALLIANCE)

Challenged in AAL are summarised in **Table 15.1**.

TABLE 15.1 The 'drivers' behind ambient assisted living

To live independently need:	Electronic support can help a lot in the form of:	But there are challenges:
A secure environment, peace of mind	Proactive environmental sensors and assistive technology	Currently too expensive, reimbursement issues
Food and drink I like	User-friendly communications	Need for standards for smart labelling and packaging
Contacts with friends and family, including giving reassurance	Local media, local activities, employment/occupation, voluntary work	
Physical, social and mental stimulation	Telehealth, sensors, medication reminders, medication management	Little local and personalised content available
Healthcare in my home, comfort, peace of mind	Appropriate response team, proactive calling	Presently telecare and health systems incompatible

To live independently need:	Electronic support can help a lot in the form of:	But there are challenges:
Certainty that my carers will come		
Apppropriate response when things go wrong, peace of mind		How? Can one team deliver? Cross-organisational issues with respect to business models and responsibilities.

Source: AALIANCE (2010). This table of ambient assisted living needs, supports and challenges was deduced to 'present a more detailed and holistic view'. The authors describe that the essence of this holistic approach is presented in this table, which describes the top-level needs, the electronic support that can accommodate these needs and the challenges that need to be tackled.

INFORMATION AND COMMUNICATIONS TECHNOLOGIES ON OLDER PEOPLE

Services based on ICT are already part of everyday life in Europe. However, the complexity and novelty of many new devices and services run the risk of rendering the majority of older people unable to use them. At the same time, research has shown that a large segment of older people in Europe can be offered AAL services that radically improve their quality of life. This has been made possible by recent developments in ambient intelligence and new abilities of software systems to communicate with users in a similar way to 'person-to-person' interaction.

The **social care approach** can be challenged, frustratingly, by a lack of acceptance on the part of potential 'service users'. Despite their promise of increased safety and comfort, service providers find it difficult to persuade clients to accept technology-based monitoring systems. As a result, appropriate systems are introduced too late or not at all. Older people, despite being in need of some help, are wary of giving outsiders intimate insight into and access to their homes. It is evident that many would accept technology-based help more readily if they had more say in what information is disclosed, to whom and under what circumstances. They are willing to accept assistance but not lose independence to outsiders.

AN INNOVATION CULTURE AND THE DIFFUSION OF INNOVATIONS

Ambient assisted living innovations are a major contribution arising from the overall '**innovation culture**' cultivated by the EU. The innovation culture of any organisation can be witnessed through how that organisation manages 'risk'; how it experiments, and how it seeks out with others new ways of doing things.

Innovation is notoriously difficult to define, though surprisingly perhaps various definitions converge on a similar notion. Tidd and Bessant (2009), for instance, comment, 'Innovation is driven by the ability to see connections, to spot opportunities and to take advantage of them.'

Helen Bevan, the Chief Transformation Officer for the 'NHS Horizons' team, argues that healthcare leaders should adopt **three** main types of innovation to give the NHS the best chance of delivering its transformational goals. These are: process, service and strategy innovations (see the article by Bevan (2013) for a clear description of this). It is likely that Bevan's framework will provide a helpful construct for understanding the initiatives in innovation for living well in dementia which are currently being developed in the NHS.

'**Diffusion of innovations**' is a theory that seeks to explain how, why, and at what rate new ideas and technology spread through cultures (discussed in Greenhalgh and colleagues (Greenhalgh *et al.*, 2004)).

Everett Rogers, a professor of rural sociology, popularised the theory in his 1962 book *Diffusion of Innovations*. Rogers described '**diffusion**' as the process by which an innovation is communicated through certain channels over time among the members of a social system. The origins of the diffusion of innovations theory are varied and span multiple disciplines. Rogers (1962) espoused the original theory that there are four main elements that influence the spread of a new idea: (1) the innovation, (2) communication channels, (3) time and (4) a social system. This process relies heavily on human capital. The innovation must be widely adopted in order to self-sustain. Within the rate of adoption, there is a point at which an innovation reaches critical mass. The main categories of adopters are innovators, early adopters, early majority, late majority, and laggards (Rogers, 1962). Diffusion of innovations manifests itself in different ways in various cultures and fields, and is highly subjective to the type of adopters and innovation-decision process.

The **rate of adoption** depends on many factors, including:
- perceived benefits over alternative products
- communicability of the product benefits
- price and ongoing costs
- ease of use
- promotional efficacy
- efficiency of supply and distribution channels
- perceived risks of adoption
- compatibility with existing standards and values
- divisibility (the extent to which a new product can be tested on a limited basis).

Generally, the constitution of the population of people using the innovation is shown graphically in **Figure 15.1**.

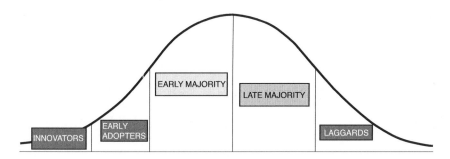

FIGURE 15.1 Adoption of innovations (this curve demonstrates schematically the various different populations of adopters of an innovation, including 'innovators', 'early adopters', 'early majority', 'late majority' and 'laggards')

The population is made up as follows.

- *Innovators*: well-informed risk-takers who are willing to try an unproven product. Innovators represent the first 2.5% to adopt the product.
- *Early adopters*: based on the positive response of innovators, early adopters then begin to purchase the product. Early adopters tend to be educated opinion leaders and represent about 13.5% of consumers.
- *Early majority*: careful consumers who tend to avoid risk, the early majority adopts the product once the early adopters have proven it. They rely on recommendations from others who have experience with the product. The early majority represents 34% of consumers.
- *Late majority*: somewhat sceptical consumers who acquire a product only after it has become commonplace. The late majority represents about 34% of consumers.
- *Laggards*: those who avoid change and may not adopt a new product until traditional alternatives no longer are available. Laggards represent about 16% of consumers.

This is discussed in great detail in Rogers (2003).

The Department of Health in recent years has made accelerating the diffusion and adoption of innovations a clear policy priority.

The Case Study outlined here provides an extract from the Department of Health's long document *Innovation: Health and Wealth; Accelerating diffusion and adoption in the NHS* (2011).

Case Study: *Innovation: Health and Wealth; Accelerating diffusion and adoption in the NHS*

DEPARTMENT OF HEALTH, 2011

There are estimated to be 600,000 people in the UK acting as the primary carers for people with dementia. Caring can be an overwhelming experience, bringing irreversible changes to lives and relationships. Carers can benefit significantly with comprehensive support, including emotional support, assistance with day-to-day caring and access to respite and short breaks.

The costs of caring are significant. Carers save the UK public purse £6 billion every year. Without provision of better support for carers, such as the provision of carer breaks and access to a range of psychological therapies, an increasing number will be unable to continue caring and pressure on the health and care system will continue to grow.

The NHS must ensure that a range of these psychological therapies are being commissioned and are available with the National Institute for Health and Clinical Excellence and Social Care Institute for Excellence guidelines. As set out in the NHS Operating framework 2012/13, the NHS should also ensure that there is better provision of carers' breaks.

We will require the NHS to commission services in line with National Institute for Health and Clinical Excellence and Social Care Institute for Excellence guidance on supporting people with dementia.

Source: Department of Health, 2011.
This extract is reproduced under the UK Department of Health's Open Government Licence: www.nationalarchives.gov.uk/doc/open-government-licence/version/2/. This extract is reproduced under the guidance published in: http://webarchive.nationalarchives.gov.uk/20130107105354/http:/www.dh.gov.uk/prod_consum_dh/groups/dh_digitalassets/documents/digitalasset/dh_134597.pdf. The extract does not imply endorsement of the thesis of this book by the Department of Health. Likewise, the author of this book takes no responsibility of the accuracy of the information contained in this extract.

Increasingly, online innovations are going to play an important rôle in the adoption of innovations. Shirley Ayres in a provocation paper for the Nominet Trust (2013) argues that a major concern about the widespread adoption of technology is fear that it makes everyone, particularly older people, more isolated because they will have less face-to-face contact. However, Ayres also notes that such networks provide some of the most powerful tools available today for building a sense of belonging, support and sharing among groups of people who share similar interests and concerns. Interestingly, a different view of levels of use of an innovation has begun to emerge. This '**concerns based adoption model**' approach is shown in **Table 15.2**.

TABLE 15.2 Levels of use of an innovation: typical behaviours

Levels of use	Behavioural indicators of level
VI. Renewal	The user is seeking more effective alternatives to the established use of the innovation
V. Integration	The user is making deliberate efforts to coordinate with others in using the innovation
IVB. Refinement	The user is making changes to increase outcomes
IVA. Routine	The user is making few or no changes and has an established pattern of use
III. Mechanical	The user is making changes to organise better the use of the innovation
II. Preparation	The user has definite plans to begin using the innovation
OI. Orientation	The user is making the initative to learn more about the innovation
0. Non-use	The user has no interest, and is taking no action

Source: adapted from Hord *et al.* (1987).

SOPRANO

ICT make up an important innovation development. The **SOPRANO** ('Service Oriented Programmable Smart Environments for Older People') project was funded through the European Commission's Sixth Framework and predates the Ambient Assisted Living Joint Programme, through the objectives approaches and methods are consistent with the programme.

SOPRANO is representative of a project that has gone through the full cycle of the research and development process, having started in 2006 and completed in 2011. SOPRANO addressed the broader objective of designing supportive environments through AAL interventions to enable older people to live independently within their own homes. This was achieved by improving safety and security of individuals within the home, helping support everyday tasks of living, facilitating social and community participation and improving information about access to services.

The societal trends SOPRANO is responding to are reported as follows:
- the increase in the proportion of older citizens in the population due to demographic change
- the scale and type of needs of older citizens which society must plan to meet, the rejection of current ICT-based services by many older citizens, and the steady deterioration of non-ICT-based service provision in the Information Society
- the poverty of offer of ICT-based services usable by older citizens
- the difficulty of designing ICT-based services to be usable by older citizens.

According to Professor Andrew Sixsmith and colleagues (Sixsmith *et al.*, 2012), the aim of the SOPRANO analysis was to establish a set of generic situations that threaten the independent living of elderly people, or perceptibly limit their ability to live well. Establishing these requirements for SOPRANO techno-logy commenced with an extensive literature review of human ageing, focused on issues that affect older people as they 'age-in-place' and the limitations of focused interventions in the home environment.

This literature review identified the need to support older people to retain a sense of autonomy and freedom in the process. Overall this sample of literat-ure also identified gaps within existing care support mechanisms that assistive technology could potentially address. This led to the development of a repos-itory of generic situations that threaten older people's sense of independence and wellbeing within the home environment. These situations were then fil-tered by the project partners according to how feasible they were to support within existing technical capabilities and resource constraints of the SOPRANO project. A further process of filtering was undertaken to refine those user situ-ations and ensure that they were applicable across the domains of quality of life affecting older people.

Situations were categorised according to the following domains.

- *Psychosocial domain*: interaction, communication, recreation, exercising, creative activities, communication device use, asking for help.
- *Instrumental activities of daily living*: independence, reassurance of perform-ing, eating and drinking, meal preparation and clean-up, mobility, sphincter control management, personal cleansing and grooming, shopping, control-ling body temperature, care of pets, financial management.
- *Medical treatment*: healthcare, prevention, monitoring, reactive, breathing, sleeping, personal device care (such as hearing aids, glasses, prostheses and adaptive equipment).

Avatangelou and other researchers working in the Soprano project, supported by €7 million in funding from the European Commission, addressed the issue by developing an AAL system designed not only by experts but also by older people themselves. This is described on the CORDIS website (http://cordis. europa.eu/).

Their research, involving 25 academic and industrial partners and telecare service providers in seven countries, focused on developing smart information technology-based assisted living services aimed at promoting independence for older people and improving quality of life in the context of Europe's age-ing population. By following an 'Experience and Application Research' design methodology and holding regular focus group meetings with end users, the researchers ensured that even the smallest details of the SOPRANO sys-tem were fine-tuned to meet the usability and acceptance requirements of users. The emergent themes from the focus groups and interviews are shown in **Table 15.3**.

TABLE 15.3 Barriers to achieving independence and quality of life

Theme	Description	Health and wellbeing impacts
Safety and security	Feelings of having safety and security compromised when in and around the home, for example through leaving doors/windows open and operating home appliances.	Heightened levels of anxiety when in and around the home. Disrupted sleep patterns and increased agitation.
Social isolation	Inability to engage in community activities and sustain important support networks. Restricted opportunities to develop/sustain social networks.	Negative outcomes associated with sense of exclusion, boredom and loneliness. Lack of emotional support and network of informal care.
Keeping healthy and active	Physical restrictions in mobility prevent older people from remaining active and curtail ability to undertake activities of daily living.	Decline in physical health status/ increase in cardiovascular related illness. Impact on body strength, balance and gait which can increase fall risk.
Adherence to medication	Forgetfulness contributes to missed medication and failure to keep appointment times with healthcare professionals.	Side effects of not taking medication/ double-dose medication. Disrupted routines/increased sense of frustration.
Quality of care provision	Quality of the home care received by users inconsistent with the needs of the older person, who require choice and flexibility in care provision.	Compromised independence and ability to self-manage. Impacts on sense of autonomy and freedom.
Access to information services	Not knowing where to get hold of information about local services that might support them.	Barriers to accessing mainstream services. Feelings of dependency when relying on others to access services.

Source: Sixsmith *et al.* (2012); according to Sixsmith and colleagues, the focus groups and interviews were essential for 'capturing user requirements'. The authors write: 'Consulting with older people was necessary to establish an understanding of their experiences in relation to the care they receive, gaps in service provision and other issues that impact on their perceived independence and quality of live while living at home.'

Based on an open architecture that allows different modular applications to be installed and configured depending on individual user needs, the system can intelligently monitor a user's home, tell the user if someone is at the front door, remind the user to turn off the oven or take his or her medication, and even monitor the user's health and alert carers in the event of a fall, among many other potential applications.

THE AALIANCE PROJECT

There is missing however a common vision of AAL that provides and defines the necessary future research and development steps and projects on the way to AAL.

In order to close this gap, the **AALIANCE** project, or the European Ambient Assisted Living Innovation Alliance, was funded within the specific programme 'Cooperation' and the research theme 'ICT' of the Seventh European Framework Programme. It aims at developing such a roadmap and strategic guidance for short-, mid- and long-term research and development approaches in the context of AAL. The strategic research agenda for AAL and its main concepts will be presented in this document.

The AALIANCE project seeks to do the following.

1. **Transform** the existing AALIANCE Community into a long-term sustainable network:
   - create the central entity for all AAL-related issues and stakeholders in Europe
   - to form a European Technology Platform focusing not solely on technology but on integrated solutions for a societal challenge
   - to provide a central node for global interaction.
2. Find solutions for major challenges in AAL that consist of:
   - coordinating the various activities of European industry and research institutions in the field of AAL by building consensus upon research priorities in an AAL Roadmap and Strategic Research Agenda for the upcoming decades
   - standardisation requirements in the field of ICT and wellbeing (including care and healthcare standards)
   - providing recommendations for overcoming market barriers and effective regulations in AAL markets
   - investigating the current state-of-the-art and market developments in AAL in North America and Asia.
3. Support the implementation of coherent strategies of the public and private sectors.

THE NOCTURNAL PROJECT

In the **NOCTURNAL** project, data representing activities of people with dementia are gathered and analysed in order to create behavioural profiles for them. The goal of this project is to develop a solution that supports older people with mild dementia in their homes, specifically during the hours of darkness.

This is a relatively new area of research, and one that was identified as a key area of need for care recipients with dementia according to Carswell and colleagues (Carswell *et al.*, 2009) in their literature review of papers reporting on the quality night-time care of people with dementia. They found that only 7%

of papers addressed night-time-specific issues. It is also of interest because of the negative impact that lack of sleep and consequent anxiety causes for the informal carer in the home of the person with dementia.

The support provided is also relatively unusual in that the AAL services are focused on identifying negative behaviours at night-time such as restlessness and wakefulness (Wang *et al.*, 2010), and then responding to these behaviours with interventions that are designed to have a therapeutic impact. The focus on night-time AAL services centres on lighting and guidance, motion monitoring and intervention decision support. The design is intended for the AAL services to provide reassurance, and to guide the general behaviour of the care recipient to support a healthy circadian rhythm. The types of therapeutic interventions include musical-, visual- and lighting-based interventions.

COACH

Handwashing, a very important 'activity of daily living', can be conceptualised as shown in Figure 15.2. Older adults with dementia require constant assistance from a caregiver when completing activities of daily living. This study examined the efficacy of a computerised device intended to assist people with dementia through activities of daily living, while reducing caregiver burden. The device, called **COACH**, uses artificial intelligence to autonomously guide an older adult with dementia through the activities of daily living using audio and/or audio-video prompts.

Mihailidis and colleagues (Mihailidis *et al.*, 2008) conducted a study with six older adults with moderate to severe dementia. Handwashing was chosen as their target activity of daily living. A single subject research design was used with two alternating baseline (COACH not used) and intervention (COACH used) phases. This is shown schematically in Figure 15.3. Signals from the camera are translated into hand and towel positions by the tracking system. These are passed to the belief monitor, which calculates the probability distribution over the possible states. This belief state is passed to the policy, which selects an action for COACH to take (i.e. prompt, observe user, or call caregiver).

Data were analysed to investigate the impact of COACH on the participants' independence and on caregiver burden, as well as COACH's overall performance for the activity of handwashing. Participants with moderate-level dementia were able to complete an average of 11% more handwashing steps independently and required 60% fewer interactions with a human caregiver when COACH was in use. Four of the participants achieved complete or very close to complete independence. Interestingly, participants' Mini-Mental State Examination scores did not appear robustly to coincide with handwashing performance and/or responsiveness to COACH. While the majority (78%) of COACH's actions were considered clinically correct, areas for improvement were identified.

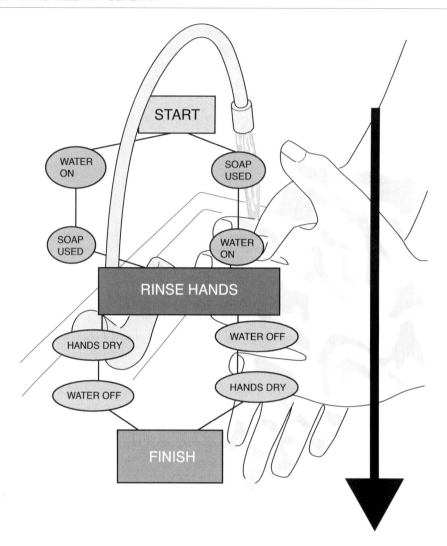

FIGURE 15.2 COACH: the five essential steps of handwashing – successful activity completion was considered to be any sequence of steps that took the participant from start to finish; as the long-term care facility's guidelines required the use of liquid soap, wetting one's hands before getting the soap was not considered an essential step in the activity, therefore the 'water on' and 'soap used' steps are interchangeable (adapted from Mihailidis *et al.*, 2008)

It seems that the COACH system shows promise as a tool to help support older adults with moderate levels of dementia and their caregivers. These findings reinforce the need for flexibility and dynamic personalisation in devices designed to assist older adults with dementia. After addressing identified improvements, the authors plan to run clinical trials with a sample of community-dwelling older adults and caregivers.

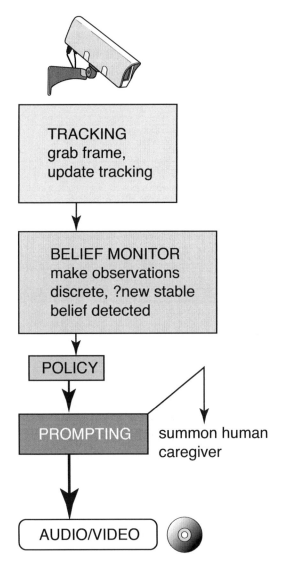

FIGURE 15.3 COACH: motion tracker – a flow diagram of COACH components – images from the camera are translated into hand and towel positions by the tracking system; these are passed to the belief monitor, which calculates the probability distribution over the possible states; this belief state is passed to the policy, which selects an action for COACH to take (i.e. prompt, observe user, or call caregiver) (adapted from Mihailidis *et al.*, 2008)

REFERENCES

AALIANCE (2010) *The European Ambient Assisted Living Alliance: Strategic Research Agenda*, available at: www.aaliance.eu/public/Documents/SRA2010
Arbeev, K.G., Butov, A.A., Manton, K.G., *et al.* (2004). Disability trends in gender and race groups of early retirement ages in the USA, *Soc Prev Med*, **49**(2), pp. 142–51.

Ayres, S. (2013) *Can Online Innovations Enhance Social Care?: Exploring the Challenges of Using Digital Technology to Develop New Models of Support for Older People.* Oxford: Nominet Trust, available at: www.nominettrust.org.uk/sites/default/files/Enhancing%20 social%20care_PP_0113.pdf

Bevan, H. (2013) Helen Bevan: three steps to a new innovation strategy, *Health Services Journal* (4 November 2013), available at: www.hsj.co.uk/home/innovation-and-efficiency/helen-bevan-three-steps-to-a-new-innovation-strategy/5064849.article

Carswell, W., McCullagh, P.J., Augusto, J.C., *et al.* (2009) A review of the role of assistive technology for people with dementia in the hours of darkness. *Technol Health Care*, **17**(4), pp. 281–304.

Department of Health (2011) *Innovation: Health and Wealth; Accelerating diffusion and adoption in the NHS*, available at: http://webarchive.nationalarchives.gov.uk/201301071 05354/http://www.dh.gov.uk/prod_consum_dh/groups/dh_digitalassets/documents/ digitalasset/dh_134597.pdf

Ferri, C.P., Prince, M., Brayne, C., *et al.* (2005) Global prevalence of dementia: a Delphi consensus study, *Lancet*, **366**(9503), pp. 2112–17.

Greenhalgh, T., Robert, G., Macfarlane, F., *et al.* (2004) Diffusion of innovations in service organizations: systematic review and recommendations, *Milbank Q*, **82**(4), pp. 581–629.

Hord, S.M., Rutherford, W.L., Huling-Austin, L., *et al.* (1987) *Taking Charge of Change*. London: Association for Supervision and Curriculum Development.

Mihailidis, A., Boger, J.N., Craig, T., *et al.* (2008) The COACH prompting system to assist older adults with dementia through handwashing: an efficacy study, *BMC Geriatr*, **8**, p. 28.

Rogers, E.M. (1962) *Diffusion of Innovations*. Glencoe: Free Press.

Rogers, E.M. (2003) *Diffusion of Innovations*. Fifth edition. New York, NY: The Free Press.

Sixsmith, A. (2012). Gerontological perspectives on ambient assistive living. In J.C. Augusto, *et al.* (eds.), *Handbook of Ambient Assisted Living: Technology for Healthcare, Rehabilitation and Well-being*. Ambient intelligence and smart environments, volume 11 (pp. 253–7). Amsterdam, NL: IOS Press.

Sixsmith, A., Hine, N., Clarke, N., *et al.* (2007) Monitoring the well-being of older people, *Top Geriatr Rehabil*, **23**(1), pp. 9–23.

Sixsmith, A., Woolrych, R., Bierhoff, I., *et al.* (2012). Ambient assisted living: From concept to implementation. In A. Glascock & D. Kutzik (Eds.), *Essential Lessons for the Success of Telehomecare*, Amsterdam: IOS Press. pp. 259–86

Tidd, J., and Bessant, J. (2009) *Managing Innovation: Integrating Technological, Market and Organizational Change*. Fourth edition. Chichester, UK: John Wiley & Sons Ltd.

Wang, H., Zheng, H., Augusto, J.C., *et al.* (2010) Monitoring and analysis of sleep pattern for people with early dementia. In: *Proceedings of the First Workshop on Knowledge Engineering, Discovery and Dissemination in Health, 2010*, available at: www.infj.ulst. ac.uk/~jcaug/pubytype.htm

Wojciechowski, M., and Xiong, J. (2008) A user interface level context model for ambient assisted living, Smart Homes and Health Telematics, (Online). In: Helal, S.: *Smart Homes and Health Telematics, 6th International Conference, ICOST 2008: Ames, IA, USA, June 28–July 2, 2008; Proceedings.* Berlin: Springer. (Lecture Notes in Computer Science 5120), pp. 105–12.

The importance of built environments for living well with dementia

The previous chapters have considered the design of wards and homes, and also considered a possible rôle for assistive technologies and ambient assisted living as important innovations for wellbeing in dementia. That is clearly not the 'end of the story' for an individual 'living well with dementia'. There are two further important components to consider: first, the outside **'built' environment** (the focus of **Chapter 16**), and second, (the focus of **Chapter 17**), the wider **'dementia-friendly community'**.

According to Liu and colleagues (Liu *et al.*, 2009), recent research suggests that wellbeing in later life is closely related to the physical environment, which is an important mediator of ageing experiences and opportunities. The physical character of the built environments or neighbourhood in particular seems to have a significant impact on the mobility, independence and quality of life of older people living in the local community (Gilroy, 2008). The ultimate goal is a 'built environment for all ages', perhaps (EQUAL, 2010a).

NATURE

According to a Greenspace Scotland report from 2008, 'Trust for Nature' (TfN) is a community-based conservation organisation that focuses on the protection of private land of high conservation value in the state of Victoria, Australia.

Fifty-one TfN group members were questioned about their health, wellbeing and social capital, and the data obtained were compared with data collected from 51 local community members (matched for age, gender and locality) who were not involved in any conservation groups. General health scores were better in TfN members compared to controls, and the number of annual doctor visits was also lower.

The eponymous *'Feel blue? Touch green!'* was undertaken to explore the specific potential of nature-based activities for promoting health among people suffering from depression, anxiety and related social isolation. Self-selected participants undertook at least 10 hours of supported hands-on nature-based activities, with the impacts of the experience on the health and wellbeing of participants being evaluated. The findings of this ongoing study so far indicate that the improved mental health outcomes also relate to increased physical activity associated with project involvement. It appears that civic environmentalism has the potential to promote health, wellbeing and social connectedness for individuals and the wider population, as well as for groups with identified health vulnerabilities.

In recent research by **Inclusive Design for Getting Outdoors (I'DGO)** (Newton *et al.*, 2010), 15% of questionnaire respondents (a large sample, nearing 1000 in sample size) had stumbled or fallen outside within the last 12 months. The real figure is likely to be higher, since past-year falls are often under-reported (Hauer *et al.*, 2006). Research has shown thus far that many of the environmental risk factors associated with outdoor falls appear to be preventable through better design and maintenance; factors including pavement quality, dilapidation and kerb height (Li *et al.*, 2006).

THE CHALLENGES OF AGEING

According to the Academy of Social Sciences and many other stakeholders, ageing is one of the big societal issues of today, if not indeed *the* biggest. As a result of improved diet, healthier living, better healthcare, less hazardous work, safer conditions and medical advances, most of us can now expect to live well into old age and longer. No longer is retirement a short period of deteriorating health prior to death. Today over 14 million people are over the age of 60 and 1.3 million of them are 85 or older and the number is increasing.

There is growing evidence that well-designed outdoor spaces can enhance the long-term health and wellbeing of those who use them regularly. According to **EQUAL's 'competitive advantage of ageing cities'**, ageing populations are often seen as 'a socio-economic challenge', placing a particular burden on social and healthcare systems. The World Health Organization argues that this need not necessarily be the case, stating that *'countries CAN afford to get old if governments, international organizations* [sic] *and civil society enact "active ageing" policies and programmes that enhance the health, participation and security of older citizens.'* (EQUAL, 2010b)

Indeed, it may be possible to improve the competitive advantage of a city–region through supporting the needs of its older citizens and capitalising on their knowledge and skills. This is increasingly recognised by leading thinkers in politics, academia and business, who are pointing to 'a new dynamic in the relationship between ageing and regional competitiveness'. *Urban Green Nation*

(CABE Space, 2010) also revealed that in areas where more than 40% of residents are black or minority ethnic, there is 11 times less green space than in areas where residents are largely white. Furthermore, the spaces they do have are likely to be of a poorer quality.

Interestingly, according to Commission for Architecture in the Built Environment (CABE), people living on a low income in deprived urban areas are more likely to experience worse health and be less physically active. Although where you live is ultimately likely to be quite intimately related to your personal income, as well as the services in the locality, their research found a difference, by ethnicity, over and above what would have been expected for level of income alone. Bangladeshi and Pakistani people and African-Caribbean women, for instance, are more likely to report bad or very bad health, compared with the general population. 'Green space' has a proven track record in reducing the impact of deprivation, delivering better health and wellbeing and creating a strong community. The simple presence of green space is related to a reduced risk of serious problems like depression and lung disease. Living close to green space reduces mortality, which can help reduce the significant gap in life expectancy between rich and poor.

There is furthermore growing evidence, to which OPENspace has contributed, to suggest that a certain level of access to green space and 'nature' of some sort is a key contributor to quality of life and patterns of healthy living (Bell *et al.*, 2004; Ward Thompson *et al.*, 2005; Sugiyama and Ward Thompson, 2007b). Catharine Ward Thompson, Research Professor of Landscape Architecture at Edinburgh College of Art and the University of Edinburgh, has been a major driving force in the field. Various forms of contact with nature, for instance, are known to produce restorative benefits (Hartig, 2007) and OPENspace have found evidence of social and emotional benefits associated with different experiences of the landscape. The early OPENspace research had elucidated that an attraction of natural open spaces and the perceived benefits from them are factors to do with mental wellbeing, stress relief, and psychological restoration, rather than exercise for its own sake.

Abstract experiential qualities such as perceptions of 'safety' and 'attractiveness' have been identified as important factors in stated preferences for parks and green spaces (Bedimo-Rung, Mohen and Cohen, 2005) and there has been much written over many years on landscape aesthetics (e.g. Bourassa, 1991) and how this might influence preference and use (e.g. Kaplan and Kaplan, 1989).

By contrast with research on environment and health, arguably this is a domain rich in theoretical concepts for the mechanisms behind engagement with the environment but poor in terms of tools to measure the detailed spatial and structural qualities of different landscapes in relation to how people actually use and experience them. For landscape designers, this is of crucial interest. There have been, historically, attempts to develop guidance based on general principles, but few tools actually to measure the dynamic spatial experience in practice. A built environment for all ages is conceptualised as one that has been designed so that people can access and enjoy it over the course of their lifetime, regardless of ability or circumstance. Such environments are said to be designed '**inclusively**'.

I'DGO

I'DGO is built around a core group of international academics in three lead-ing research centres: (1) the Edinburgh-based **OPENspace**, (2) **SURFACE** at Salford and (3) the **WISE** (Wellbeing in Sustainable Environments) research unit at the University of Warwick. From 1999, Professor Marcus Ormerod and the SURFACE team have pioneered the development of the discipline of **inclus-ive design** within the UK. They are funded by the Engineering and Physical Sciences Research Council and play an active rôle in its flagship knowledge transfer consortium, KT-EQUAL.

The I'DGO consortium was launched in 2004 to investigate how outdoor environments affect older people's wellbeing and to identify what aspects of design help or hinder older people in using the outdoors. Their focus is on identifying the most effective ways of **shaping outdoor environments inclu-sively**. They support the needs and preferences of older people and disabled people, always seeking to improve their independence and overall quality of life.

I'DGO was set up to explore the ways in which being able to get out into one's local neighbourhood affects older people's wellbeing and what barriers there are to achieving this, day to day. The project asked the crucial question: *Why do we need a built environment for all ages?* The first phase of research, which finished in 2006, involved over 770 people aged 65 or above. Participants were asked about their wellbeing and quality of life, how often and why they went outdoors and what features of their local neighbourhood helped or hindered their activity. Researchers also physically audited 200 residential neighbour-hoods to look for barriers and benefits to getting around as a pedestrian.

The I'DGO research found quickly that older people went outdoors very frequently to socialise, exercise, get fresh air and experience nature. If they lived in a supportive environment – one that made it easy and enjoyable for them to get outdoors – they were more likely to be physically active, healthy and satisfied with life. Walking was by far the most common way that people spent their time outdoors, whether for recreation or transport (*'getting from A to B'*). Participants in the I'DGO study who lived within 10 minutes' walk of an open space were twice as likely to achieve the recommended levels of healthy walking (2.5 hours a week) as those whose nearest open space was not local.

When it came to the problems people faced in getting outdoors, the I'DGO research found that shortfalls in the built environment were often compounded by personal limitations and social circumstances. Sometimes, it was a lack of amenities that provided the disincentive, but sometimes it was the poor condition that neighbourhoods were kept in, fuelling negative perceptions about nuisance and traffic (often disproportionately so). Innovative '**conjoint analysis**' of the findings meant that researchers could look in great detail at the comparative importance of different outdoor attributes, finding that one of the top priorities for most older people was plentiful trees and shrubs. Distance was a major factor for people living alone, and frequent benches crucial to those with impaired mobility have been considered desirable.

As with the first phase of I'DGO, the consortium's current research projects focus on the individual circumstances and priorities of the participants – what the team calls '**personal projects**'. This is crucial as national policy heads towards more person-centred care strategies and plans to enable as many older people as possible to remain in their own homes. The three areas of research place a critical focus on the way in which 'everyday' outdoor environments for older people are influenced by current best practice in regeneration, such as an emphasis on high-density housing and the redevelopment of brownfield land. This is an area in which evidence is still lacking, 10 years since the publication of Lord Rogers' *Towards an Urban Renaissance* (Rogers, 1999).

The I'DGO projects address outdoor environments on a range of scales, starting with gardens and other forms of residential outdoor space (the study being undertaken by the WISE unit in the University of Warwick). After reviewing standardised measures of wellbeing, they identified ways in which being in – or being able to see – a favourite residential outdoor setting could affect an older person positively, again producing a useful point-by-point summary:

- **satisfaction** from being able to use the space for practical activities, such as hanging out washing, growing food, storing property, maintaining vehicles and parking
- **enjoyment** from being able to use the space for leisure activities, such as entertaining visitors, sitting outside, gardening, keeping pets or feeding wildlife
- **pleasure** from the appearance of the space and the way it enhances the dwelling
- **relaxation and comfort**
- **enjoyment** from social interaction with neighbours and passers-by and feeling part of the community
- **wellbeing** from gaining exercise and having access to fresh air.

TACTILE PAVING

A major research goal has been to examine the specific attribute of neighbourhood streets – **tactile paving at steps and crossings** – and asks how this affects the biomechanics of walking and risk of falling in older people (the project run by the SURFACE Inclusive Design Research Centre and their colleagues in

Health, Sport and Rehabilitation Sciences at the University of Salford). The benefits of tactile paving for blind and visually impaired people have been well established yet the system is not without its issues.

Tactile paving is not a policy area without its concerns, and a few in particular emerge from a report by the UK Health and Safety Executive (Loo-Morrey, 2005). This report suggested that there is a need better to understand the extent and implications of incorrectly designed and laid tactile paving, and the toe clearance of an individual in negotiating paving 'blisters' and potential slip hazards. These factors appear to be crucial to older people, since many of the first-phase I'DGO interviewees expressed concerns about falling or feeling unstable on tactile surfaces and fall-related injuries were associated with loss of independence, morbidity and death in older people.

SHARED SPACES

Research is examining the emergence of pedestrian-friendly neighbourhoods, such as Home Zones and other '**shared space**' developments, asking if they are supportive environments for people of all ages and abilities (a longitudinal study being run by the Edinburgh-based OPENspace Research Centre).

'Shared spaces' are created through the physical alteration of the public realm to enhance the pedestrian experience – such as through planting and street furniture – and to calm vehicular traffic at the same time. The OPENspace element of I'DGO TOO is looking specifically at how such interventions influence older people's activity patterns and the knock-on effect this has on wellbeing. An objective is to assess whether living in a 'shared space' residential environment enables older people to go outside more often, spend more time outside, have better social networks and enjoy an enhanced quality of life.

Recently, according to Ward Thompson and Aspinall (2011), it appears that, in practice, much of the use that is made of such natural environments involves physical activity. This suggests that attempts by policymakers and those interested in public health to encourage greater use of natural open space in order to increase physical activity levels may be more effective if promoted as benefiting mental wellbeing rather than physical health. The analysis of the relationship between childhood experience and adult behaviour in these studies suggests that ready access to natural environments in early life is important if such environments are to be perceived as offering opportunities for physical activity in adulthood. This, again, has potentially significant implications for policy and practice in landscape and urban planning.

Methodologies tailored to the preferences and lifestyles of older participants include activity diaries, questionnaires and interviews, the wearing of accelerometers, street audits and measuring, behavioural observations, focus groups, and laboratory testing.

'ENVIRONMENTAL SUPPORTIVENESS'

If we are to understand what qualities of the environment are important to an ability of individuals to '*live well*', we need perhaps to acknowledge the diversity that exists in people's capabilities, experience, desires and needs. This overall is a huge challenge for designers; the response conventionally has been to look for factors in the environment that matter to most people, or to a defined group of people, and to address those factors as if they were equally important. Yet for any individual, different qualities and elements in the environment may be a matter of indifference (e.g. certain colours if you are visually impaired) or vitally important (e.g. proximity of an accessible toilet if you have a weak bladder).

To address this, these research groups explored the notion of '**environmental supportiveness**' as a way of conceptualising the relationship between the outdoor environment and activities undertaken at a personal level (Sugiyama and Ward Thompson, 2007c). They developed two instruments to measure the quality of the environment relevant to older people's level of activity, on the premise that environments that make chosen outdoor activities easy and enjoyable are contributing to a better quality of life.

Such an approach, for example in Ward Thompson and Aspinall (2011) draws on the ecological psychology of Gibson (1979) and Heft (2010), with its emphasis on '**affordance**' and the reciprocal relationship between perceiver and environment. The concept of affordance links environment and human behaviour, or opportunities for action, and is therefore of particular interest in understanding how the environment might encourage or support people to be more active – a primary goal of public health policy. This is an insight of key relevance to investigating human behaviour in the landscape. As Appleton (1975) has put it, more succinctly, for any individual considering their landscape context, it helps us understand '*what's in it for me?*'

UNIQUE ENVIRONMENT–PERSON INTERACTIONS

Of particular relevance here is the use of personal projects (Little, 1983) as a methodological approach, founded on Kelly's (1955) '**personal construct theory**'. In contrast with normative ways of measuring the quality of the environment, where criteria are fixed and are assumed to be equally salient to all, this idiographic method makes it possible to assess environmental supportiveness based on a person's unique needs, wants and a relevant setting within which chosen activities are undertaken.

This research offers a unique way of investigating how well individuals' needs, desires and aspirations are supported or frustrated by their environment and how well people cope with the environment in which they find themselves (Sugiyama and Ward Thompson, 2007a). **One can see therefore emerging in the literature a concept that a person's unique interaction with his or her** environment will have a massive bearing on his or her personal wellbeing, and this has been a pivotal finding to come out from a synthesis of all recent research.

A particular aspect of environment–person interaction highly pertinent to this conference is the notion that there may be salutogenic environments – that is, environments that support healthy behaviours and responses, by contrast with, for example, obesogenic environments that support lifestyles which are conducive to people becoming overweight and obese. Public health concerns over sedentary lifestyles and lack of cardiovascular fitness in the populations of the developed world have led to a particular focus on environments that encourage people to walk more, since walking has been called '*the nearest activity to perfect exercise*' (Morris and Hardman, 1997). This approach requires no specialist skills or equipment. The question for researchers is: what qualities in the outdoor environment (where most walking is likely to happen) make a difference to how much people walk (Sugiyama and Ward Thompson, 2007b)?

ENVIRONMENTAL INFLUENCES AND ACTIVITY

Research in physical activity has become aware of the significance of the environmental influence on activity (Trost *et al.*, 2003). One theory underpinning this research approach is '**social cognitive theory**', originally developed by Bandura (1986). The central idea here is '*self-efficacy*', a belief that one can exercise control over one's activities. However, it also encompasses environmental factors as facilitators or impediments of activities.

Booth and colleagues (Booth *et al.*, 2000) reported that perceived environmental variables (e.g. safe footpaths and access to local recreational facilities) are positively correlated with frequent participation in outdoor activities. Takano, Nakamura and Watanabe (2002) considered that the existence of nearby 'walkable' green spaces is conductive to a more active lifestyle. They found that the 5-year percentage of older people who have easier access to such green spaces is significantly higher than those without access to such places.

Most helpfully, Sugiyama (2004) describes an '**activity model**' that employs physical activity as a proximal predictor of quality of life (*see* **Figure 16.1**). The model postulates that older adults' functional ability and environmental factors interact to shape their activity pattern, which in turn affects their wellbeing.

INCLUSIVE DESIGN

An **inclusive environment** is created by surveyors, architects, planners, building control surveyors, engineers, access consultants and facilities managers. Ultimately, though, creating an inclusive place is in the hands of developers, landlords and service providers. It is their responsibility to ensure that their property is designed, built and operated in line with inclusive principles. It

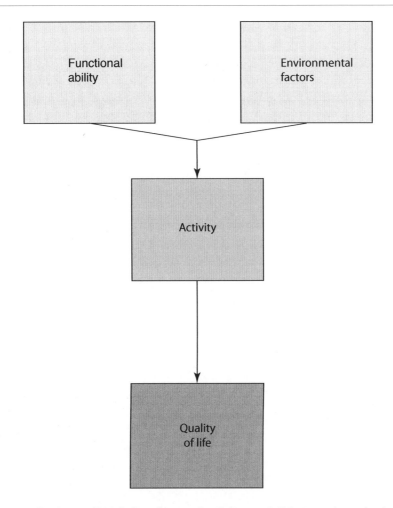

FIGURE 16.1 Sugiyama (2004) describes an '**activity model**' that employs physical activity as a proximal predictor of quality of life

remains an incredibly important policy plank in design for dementia (Imrie and Hall, 2001).

According to truly seminal work by Professor Marcus Ormerod and Dr Rita Newton (Ormerod and Newton, 2005), it has been accepted for some time, not only in England and Wales but also in other countries, that accessibility of the built environment is critical in order to create a **socially inclusive society**. Buildings and the environment facilitate social inclusion for everyone, including disabled people and older people.

If people are excluded from facilities that provide homes, education, employment, leisure, entertainment, services and amenities, then not only does discrimination occur but also opportunities for integration are lost. Integration is also lost if facilities and services are segregated, separate or stigmatising such that disabled people become unnecessarily dependent on others for support in using the built environment. An inclusively designed environment considers people's diversity and removes unnecessary barriers and exclusions in a way that benefits us all.

There are differing terms given to what appears to be *the same underlying goal* – to create a world that everyone can participate in to the fullest extent possible. It is, however, important to challenge the myth that within the context of our participatory world we all come from the same level of understanding. **Accessible design** is design to accommodate specific individuals or groups of disabled individuals, and is usually applied erroneously at the end of the design process as an afterthought, or retrofit to a completed design. However, because in certain situations it may be the only solution for some problems and some users, accessible design will always be necessary. Specialised accessible design is usually more expensive than inclusive or universal design and may segregate and stigmatise the users it is designed to accommodate, highlighting their disability (Story, 2002).

Through the integrative approach of universal design there is improved acceptability of the design and less stigmatising, or exclusion, of individuals. Imrie (2001), however, suggests that while universal design addresses the technical and procedural issues, it fails to address the social and attitudinal barriers. He argues that, by contrast, inclusive design achieves this through working '*with*' rather than '*for*' people as building users and this is an important distinction between the two terms. From these differing views, an appropriate definition of inclusive design would seem to be:

> Inclusive design is a way of designing products and environments so they are usable and appealing to everyone regardless of age, ability or circumstance by working with users to remove barriers in the social, technical, political and economic processes underpinning building and design.

Other definitions of inclusive design have been provided, such as that by the UK Commission for Architecture in the Built Environment (CABE, 2006). CABE have added a further design principle to those suggested by Imrie and Hall (2001), that is **the principle of user engagement in the design process**. This additional principle is further justified during the development of an inclusive design toolkit (Keates and Clarkson, 2004).

The main features of inclusive design are summarised in a very useful booklet by CABE, the Commission for Architecture and the Built Environment. Inclusive design aims to remove the barriers that create undue effort and separation. It enables everyone to participate equally, confidently and independently in everyday activities.

They outline the following essential design principles.

1. *Inclusive design puts people at the heart of the design process.* Design and development should create spaces and buildings that people can use to form strong, vibrant and sustainable communities. To achieve this, you should ensure that you involve as many people as possible on the design. This will help to promote personal wellbeing, social cohesion and enjoyment for all. Latham (1994) and subsequently Egan (1998) have continued to emphasise the need for increased client satisfaction.

2. *Inclusive design acknowledges diversity and difference.* Good design can be achieved only if the environment created meets as many people's needs as possible. Everyone at some point will probably experience limited mobility – as a tourist with excessive bulky luggage, a parent with young children, or an individual with a badly sprained ankle. It is important to identify barriers to inclusion as early as possible within the design process so that good design can overcome them.

3. *Inclusive design promotes choice.* An inclusive environment does not attempt to meet every need. By considering people's diversity, however, it can break down barriers and exclusion and will often achieve superior solutions that benefit everyone. Disabled people are not homogenous, of course, but considering their needs within the design process will secure benefits for everyone.

4. *Inclusive design promotes flexibility.* Meeting the principles of inclusive design requires an understanding of how the building or space will be used and who will use it. Places need to be designed so that they can adapt to changing uses and demands.

5. *Inclusive design provides for buildings that are convenient and convenient to use.* Making environments easy to use for everyone means considering signage, lighting, visual contrast and materials. Access to buildings is not simply a question of their physical layout. It also requires people having sufficient information, often before they leave their house, that makes them feel confident enough to access a building or space. Ensuring this 'intellectual' and 'emotional' access means considering signage, lighting, visual contrast and materials.

The **Equality Act** 2010 brings together nine different strands of discrimination legislation into one unified act, including the **Disability Discrimination Act** 1995. The case law on this, therefore, is not expected to be settled yet. As dementia is covered by the **Equality Act** 2010, there are some legal imperatives too for places, organisations and groups to take the needs of people with dementia into account.

This is important also for '**dementia-friendly communities**', discussed in **Chapter 17**. The **Equality Act** 2010 makes it unlawful for prohibited activities under any protected characteristics to act to the detriment of individuals, so clearly this Act is very relevant to the protection of fundamental rights of citizens under English law.

HOW CAN ENVIRONMENTS BE USED SUPPORTIVELY TO IMPROVE WELLBEING IN DEMENTIA?

The first phase of I'DGO demonstrated that enabling people to remain physically and socially active in and around their own homes is good for their general health and wellbeing; potentially significantly alleviating care costs and Health Service demands.

However, I'DGO research has also found that there is currently little provision for getting outdoors in residential care homes and sheltered accommodation for older people. The tendency is to focus on what individuals cannot do, treating them as totally debilitated, thus leading to defeatism and apathy. The clinical symptom of apathy may be linked to a pathological disease process in particular brain regions such as the anterior and posterior cingulate and dorsolateral or inferior frontal gyrus (Benoit and Robert, 2011).

Supportive built environments are considered, tentatively, to be one of the most effective effective practical interventions for apathy. This may be related to recent research findings linking older people's physical activity levels with better cognitive function in ageing. An important point is that our brains somehow appears to use our surroundings to 'tag' our experiences, making a vital connection between the environment and our memories through complex associative learning neural network mechanisms.

MOVING FORWARD

While consortia like I'DGO have succeeded in making their findings both 'useful and useable' (e.g. Hobcraft (2013)), many other researchers have not seen their work acknowledged by policymakers and practitioners in this way, leading to apparent gaps in evidence. Policymakers have seemed not to grasp the full significance of these important findings yet. Hopefully, this will change in due course.

WEBSITES

- I'DGO (Inclusive Design for Getting Outdoors): www.idgo.ac.uk
- CABE (Commission for Architecture and the Built Environment): http://webarchive.nationalarchives.gov.uk/20110118095356/http:/www.cabe.org.uk/

REFERENCES

Appleton, J. (1975) *The Experience of Landscape*. New York, NY: John Wiley.

Bandura, A. (1986) *The Social Foundations of Thought and Action: A Social Cognitive Theory*. Englewood Cliffs, NJ: Prentice-Hall.

Bedimo-Rung, A.L., Mowen, A.J., and Cohen, D.A. (2005) The significance of parks to physical activity and public health: a conceptual model, *Am J Prev Med*, **28**(2 Suppl. 2), pp. 159–68.

Bell, S., Morris, N., Findlay, C., *et al.* (2004) *Nature for People: The Importance of Green Spaces to East Midlands Communities (Research Report 567)*. Peterborough, UK: English Nature, available at: http://publications.naturalengland.org.uk/publication/50068

Benoit, M., and Robert, P.H. (2011) Imaging correlates of apathy and depression in Parkinson's disease. *J Neurol Sci*, **310**(1–2), pp. 58–60.

Booth, M.L., Owen, N., Bauman, A., *et al.* (2000) 'Social-cognitive and perceived environment influences associated with physical activity in older Australians', in *Preventive Medicine*, **31**(1), 15–22.

Bourassa, S.C. (1991) *The Aesthetics of Landscape*. New York, NY: Belhaven.

CABE (2006) *The Principles of Inclusive Design. (They Include You.)*, available at: http://webarchive.nationalarchives.gov.uk/20110118095356/http:/www.cabe.org.uk/files/the-principles-of-inclusive-design.pdf.

CABE Space (2010) *Urban Green Nation: Building the Evidence Base*. London: Commission for Architecture in the Built Environment.

Egan, J. (1998) *Rethinking Construction*. London: Department of the Environment Transport and the Regions.

EQUAL (2010a) *A Built Environment for All Ages*, available at: http://kt-equal.org.uk/uploads/monographs/built_environment_monograph.pdf

EQUAL (2010b) *The Competitive Advantage of Age Friendly Cities*, available at: www.idgo.ac.uk/useful_resources/Presentations/Age_Friendly_Cities_monograph_FINAL_with_logos_110816[1].pdf

Gibson, J. (1979) *The Ecological Approach to Visual Perception*. Boston, MA: Houghton-Mifflin.

Gilroy, R. (2008) Places that support human flourishing: lessons from later life, *Planning Theory Pract*, **9**, pp. 145–63.

Greenspace Scotland (2008) *Research Report: Greenspace and Quality of Life; A critical research review*, available at: www.openspace.eca.ac.uk/pdf/appendixf/OPENspacewebsite_APPENDIX_F_resource_9.pdf

Hartig, T. (2007) Three steps to understanding restorative environments as health resources. In: Ward Thompson, C., and Travlou, P. (eds) *Open Space: People Space*, Abingdon, UK: Routledge, pp. 163–79.

Hauer, K., Lamb, S.E., Jorstad, E.C., *et al.* (2006) Systematic review of definitions and methods of measuring falls in randomised controlled fall prevention trials, *Age Ageing*, **35**, pp. 5–10.

Heft, H. (2010) Affordances and the perception of landscape: an inquiry into environmental perception and aesthetics. In: Ward Thompson, C., Aspinall, P., and Bell, S. (eds) *Innovative Approaches to Researching Landscape and Health*, Open Space: People Space 2, Abingdon: Routledge, pp. 9–32.

Hobcraft, P. (2013) Thinking about scalable environment, blogpost available at: www.innovationexcellence.com/blog/2013/07/28/thinking-about-scalable-engagement/

Imrie, R., and Hall, P. (2001) *Inclusive Design: Design and Developing Accessible Environments.* London: Spon Press.

Inclusive Design for Getting Outdoors (Date uncertain.) *Do Gardens Matter? The Role of Residential Outdoor Space,* available at: www.idgo.ac.uk/useful_resources/Publications/WISE_MTP_brochure_FINAL.pdf

Inclusive Design for Getting Outdoors (Date uncertain) *Pedestrian-friendly environments.* available at: www.openspace.eca.ac.uk/pdf/appendixf/OPENspacewebsite_APPENDIX_F_resource_5.pdf

Inclusive Design for Getting Outdoors (Date uncertain) *Tactile Pacing: Design, Sitting and Laying,* available at: www.idgo.ac.uk/useful_resources/Publications/Salford_MTP_brochure_FINAL.pdf

Kaplan, R., and Kaplan, S. (1989) *The Experience of Nature: A Psychological Perspective.* New York, NY: Cambridge.

Keates, S., and Clarkson, J. (2004) *Countering Design Exclusion: An introduction to Inclusive Design.* London: Springer-Verlag.

Kelly, G. (1955) *The Psychology of Personal Constructs.* New York, NY: Norton.

Latham, M. (1994) *Constructing the Team.* London: The Stationery Office.

Little, B.R. (1983) Personal projects: a rationale and method for investigation, *Environ Behav,* **15**(3), 273–309.

Li, W., Keegan, T.H.M., Sternfeld, B. *et al.* (2006) Outdoor falls among middle-aged and older adults: a neglected public health problem, *Am J Public Health,* **96**(7), pp. 1192–200.

Liu, C.-W., Everingham, J.-A., Warburton, J., *et al.* (2009) What makes a community age-friendly: a review of international literature, *Australas J Ageing,* **28**(3), pp. 116–21.

Loo-Morrey, M. (2005) *Tactile Paving Survey. Report Number HSL2005/07.* Buxton: Health and Safety Laboratory.

Morris, J.N., and Hardman, A. (1997) Walking to health, *Sports Med,* **23**, 306–32.

Newton, R., Ormerod, M., Burton, E., *et al.* (2010). Increasing independence for older people through good street design, *Journal of Integrated Care,* **18**, Issue 3, pp 24–9.

Ormerod, M.G., and Newton, R.A. (2005) Briefing for accessibility in design, *Facilities,* **23**(7/8), pp. 285–94.

Rogers, Richard (1999) *Towards an Urban Renaissance: Final Report of the Urban Task Force.* London: Department of the Environment, Transport and Regions.

Story, M.F. (2002) Distance education in universal design. In: Christophersen, J. (ed.) *Universal Design 17 Ways of Thinking and Teaching,* Oslo: Norwegian State Housing Bank Husbanken.

Sugiyama, T. (2004). Conceptual frameworks examining the relationship between older people's quality of life and the environment. In: *Open Space People Space Conference,* Edinburgh, Scotland, 27–29 October, 2004.

Sugiyama, T., and Ward Thompson, C. (2007a) Measuring the quality of the outdoor environment relevant to older people's lives. In: Ward Thompson, C., and Travlou, P. (eds) *Open Space: People Space,* Abingdon, UK: Routledge, pp. 153–62.

Sugiyama, T., and Ward Thompson, C. (2007b) Older people's health, outdoor activity and supportiveness of neighbourhood environments, *Landscape and Urban Planning,* **83**, pp. 168–75.

Sugiyama, T., and Ward Thompson, C. (2007c) Outdoor environments, activity and the wellbeing of older people: conceptualising environmental support, *Environ Planning A*, **39**, pp. 1943–60.

Takano, T., Nakamura, K., and Watanabe, M. (2002) Urban residential environments and senior citizens' longevity in mega city areas: the importance of walkable green spaces, *J Epidemiol Community Health*, **56**(12), 913–18.

Trost, S.G., Owen, N., Bauman, A.E., *et al.* (2003) Correlates of adults' participation in physical activity: review and update, *Med Sci Sports Exerc*, **34**(12), 1996–2001.

UK Government (1995) *Disability Discrimination Act*, available at: www.legislation.gov.uk/ukpga/1995/50/contents

UK Government (2010) *Equality Act*, available at www.legislation.gov.uk/ukpga/2010/15/contents

Ward Thompson, C., Aspinall, P.A., Bell, S., *et al.* (2005) 'It gets you away from everyday life': local woodlands and community use; what makes a difference? *Landsc Res*, **30**(1), pp. 109–46.

Ward Thompson, C., and Aspinall, P. (2011) Natural environments and their impact on activity, health and quality of life, *Appl Psychol Health Well-Being*, **3**(3), pp. 230–60.

CHAPTER 17

Dementia-friendly communities and living well with dementia

Statement 10. People with dementia are enabled, with the involvement of their carers, to maintain and develop their involvement in and contribution to their community.

In this penultimate chapter, I make a final change of direction from the person and physical environment, towards the vital importance of human communities. This sense of solidarity, that the whole is greater than the sum of its individual parts, is fundamental to creating a sense of shared value in the living well with dementia architecture. There is a strong message from the National Dementia Strategy (Department of Health, 2009) of the need for individuals living well with dementia to be part of a wider network that creates higher shared value.

> The establishment and maintenance of such networks will provide direct local peer support for people with dementia and their carers. It will also enable people with dementia and their carers to take an active role in the development and prioritisation of local services.

There is, however, a growing realisation that many settings are not in fact particularly 'dementia friendly', which strongly opposes an international drive for improved wellbeing. In the Department of Health's *Improving Care for People with Dementia* (2013), it is described that people with dementia occupy a quarter of hospital beds. To improve health and care services for people with dementia, the current English policy is committed to asking every hospital in England to become 'dementia friendly'. Indeed, the UK government reported in *Improving Care for People with Dementia*, on the UK government website, 25 March 2013, that 'dementia-friendly communities' are a top priority.

> While it's very common, dementia is not very well understood. People often don't ask for help because there's still a stigma attached. Or they think – wrongly – that the symptoms are a normal part of ageing, and that nothing can be done.

It is argued that it will take time for communities to become truly 'dementia friendly'. Groups in over 20 areas have now committed to working towards becoming dementia friendly villages, towns and cities. As a process is developed systematically to encourage dementia friendly communities, this number is expected to grow. For example, at the time of writing, 30 new members had signed up to the Dementia Action Alliance (DAA), taking the number of bodies and organisations to over 100. Each organisation has produced an action plan on what they will do to become more dementia friendly. The DAA is a membership body committed to transforming the quality of life of people living with dementia in the UK and the millions of people who care for them.

CONTEXT

People with dementia and carers have described seven outcomes that must be met to ensure that they live well with the condition (Dementia Action Alliance, 2010).

The history of this 'declaration' is summarised thus:

> Working in partnership with the initial signatories, people with dementia and their family carers described seven outcomes they would like to see in their lives. They provide an ambitious and achievable vision of how people with dementia and their families are supported by society. All individuals and organisations, large and small, can play a role in making it a reality.

The elements are:
- 'I have personal choice and control or influence over decisions about me'
- 'I know that services are designed around me and my needs'
- 'I have support that helps me live my life'
- 'I have the knowledge and know-how to get what I need'
- 'I live in an enabling and supportive environment where I feel valued and understood'
- 'I have a sense of belonging and of being a valued part of family, community, and civic life'

- *'I know there is research going on which delivers better life for me now and hope for the future'*

This work, alongside other research on quality of life for people affected by dementia, shows that many issues influence how well people live, from health and social care, to social relationships, engagement in activities, a sense of belonging and of being a valued part of family, community and civic life.

Other work also highlights the importance of society and developing age-friendly environments.

DOMESTIC AND INTERNATIONAL CONTEXT

The RSA's **'Connected Communities'** project describes itself as, *'multi-faceted comprising several interrelated research projects, through which we aim to gain a better understanding of the conditions under which a new civic collectivism, or social productivity, may emerge – one that is organic, spontaneous, and bottom-up.'*

The World Health Organization's (WHO) **'age-friendly communities'** or **'age-friendly cities'** initiative is also very significant. In 2008, for the first time in history, the majority of the world's population lived in cities. Urban populations will continue to grow in the future. It is estimated that around three out of every five people will live in an urban area by 2030. At the same time, as cities around the world are growing, their residents are growing older. The proportion of the global population aged 60 will double from 11% in 2006 to 22% by 2050.

According to the WHO, making cities and communities 'age friendly', let alone 'dementia friendly', is one of the most effective local policy approaches for responding to demographic ageing. There are parallel movements for communities currently to become consciously more *'child friendly'* and *'wheelchair friendly'*. As mentioned in **Chapter 16**, dementia comes within scope of the **Equality Act** 2010, and this therefore is an important legal consideration now.

According to the WHO:

> The physical and social environments are key determinants of whether people can remain healthy, independent and autonomous long into their old age.
>
> Older persons play a crucial role in their communities – they engage in paid or volunteering work, transmit experience and knowledge, and help their families with caring responsibilities. These contributions can only be ensured if they enjoy good health and if societies address their needs.
>
> The WHO Age-Friendly Environments Programme is an international effort to address the environmental and social factors that contribute to active and healthy ageing.
>
> The Programme helps cities and communities become more supportive of older people

by addressing their needs across eight dimensions: the built environment, transport, housing, social participation, respect and social inclusion, civic participation and employment, communication, and community support and health services.

This WHO initiative provides an international network of good practice in these areas and opportunities to connect the growing number of places interested in dementia-friendly communities to this work. This is obviously useful for domestic policy developments in our jurisdiction. For example, it is argued that in Manchester, England (UK), long-term involvement of older people in planning the development of the city at urban and neighbourhood levels has improved the physical and environmental access for older people, raising their confidence and empowering them to become involved in decision-making.

Social inclusion is becoming, of course, increasingly achievable through online social networks. Shirley Ayres (2013) powerfully argues in a provocation paper for Nominet that social exclusion, loneliness, managing health and disabilities, and unemployment are big issues for society generally. The problems for older people can be exacerbated by ill health, significant life changes such as retirement and transitions – which may require moving to supported living – and the death of partners and close friends. Retaining a sense of worth and value, keeping connected to family and friends, and continuing to contribute to society are important considerations in addressing social inclusion.

WHAT IS A 'DEMENTIA-FRIENDLY COMMUNITY'?

Improving wellbeing and resilience is of course an **international** aspiration (Friedli, 2009).

The definition of the word '**community**' itself is problematic, and in this chapter we have used it both thematically (e.g. ethnic or spiritual group, specific interest group, club or society) and geographically to reflect the various domains of people's lives. Nonetheless, it is relatively **local**.

The AESOP Consortium is an organisation that advises local health and social care systems on reform. They have been worked closely with persons with dementia to produce a working definition of a '**dementia-friendly community**' as one which enables them to:

- find their way around and feel safe in their locality/community/city
- access the local facilities that they are used to (such as banks, shops, cafés, cinemas and post offices, as well as health and social care services)
- maintain their social networks so they feel they still belong in the community.

(Local Government Association and Innovations
in Dementia, 2012)

Furthermore, a society or community that acts consciously to ensure that people with dementia (along with all its citizens) are respected, empowered, engaged and embraced into the whole is one that can claim to be, or is becoming, a dementia-friendly community.

Communities that aspire to become dementia friendly are likely also to be those that constantly strive to build social capital and community capacity for all their local populations of residents, workers and visitors and, in doing so, value the contribution that each makes. This may be summarised by the phrase **'an assets-based approach'**, that is, one that builds on what people can still do, as opposed to a *'deficit-model'* that focuses on what people can no longer do and somehow *'reduces'* them because they cannot contribute to society more fully.

Appreciating the whole person – consistent with Kitwood's (1997) development of the notion of personhood – or the person's valuable individual contribution to the 'citizenry' of a place, community or society is undeniably an important societal aspiration. Community development progresses this aim; civic engagement and increased social capital are its outputs. Mutual gain for everyone is the outcome.

In Scotland, there is growing sense of community activism among people with dementia to redefine the *kind of community* in which they want to live. The University of Stirling Dementia Centre is a leading authority on design for dementia living and has done much research on ways in which the lives of people with dementia, and those who care for them, can be improved in communities.

Elsewhere in Europe, Bruges is leading the way in an expanding movement of towns and cities that are championing the dementia-friendly approach, which include Nantes in France and Ansbach in Germany. Other countries are taking up Bruges' knotted red handkerchief logo, signifying *dementievriendelijk Brugge* ('dementia-friendly Bruges'). Bruges welcome others using the logo too, to increase its chances of becoming a universally recognisable emblem.

WHERE EXACTLY DID THE CONCEPT OF 'DEMENTIA-FRIENDLY COMMUNITIES' COME FROM?

Growing awareness of the demographic changes in the population as the proportion of older people and the prevalence of dementia increase has prompted research and policy development in both age- and dementia-friendly communities.

In 2011, the Department of Health convened a 'think tank' of experts, including people with dementia and family carers, to explore the concept of **'dementia-capable communities'.** In preparation it commissioned Innovations in Dementia to work with people with dementia to find out what makes a good community for people with dementia to live in and what can be done to make this happen (the 'Innovations in Dementia' initiative).

They found that the things that make the most difference are:
- the physical environment
- local facilities
- support services
- social networks
- local groups.

People with dementia suggested that things could be made better by:
- increasing people's awareness of dementia
- having more local groups for people with dementia and their carers
- providing more information, and more accessible information, about local services and facilities
- and making local facilities more accessible for people with dementia.

WHY ENCOURAGE 'DEMENTIA-FRIENDLY COMMUNITIES'?

The growing numbers of people with dementia

All statutory agencies should be familiar with the public health and demographic changes occurring over the next generation, including a doubling of the numbers of people with dementia over the next 30 years and a shrinking of the working population to support those in later life.

By 2019, it is predicted that 38% of the population will be aged over 50, and by 2029 this will have risen to 40% (Audit Commission, 2008).

The economic arguments

In the UK, the economic climate has driven significant cuts in public sector spending that have affected commissioners' abilities to fund services or to invest in future service provision. There has been a wider drive to make 'efficiency savings' in the UK, but these in theory are not supposed to affect front-line clinical care.

This economic programme has also unfortunately coincided with the formation of different health commissioning arrangements. The clinical commissioning groups and the health and wellbeing boards, both still in their transitional infancy, are too new to have had much demonstrable impact yet. While clinical commissioning groups appear to be firmly footed in the new English NHS policy literature, their exact functions are yet to develop.

Arguably, the growing elderly population is a source of spending power that has been overlooked in the past in favour of younger people with apparently more cash to spend.

The value of independence and interdependence

Individuals with dementia often report how distressing it is to feel as if they have become dependent on others.

Even when they recognise that they need help, such individuals remain sensitive to the complexity of nuance and understanding that can be felt on both sides.

The wish to remain connected to communities

Highest on the list of difficulties for people with dementia are the everyday community activities that everyone else takes for granted, such as withdrawing money at the bank, paying bills, shopping and using public transport.

Trying to carry on daily life as before becomes more difficult and problematic for some people. As a result they start to feel disconnected from their old groups, friends, activities and places, getting trapped in a vicious cycle of social isolation.

The interconnectedness of community life

Research and anecdotal reports of people's personal accounts converge on the notion that receiving a diagnosis of dementia is a major life event.

Fear and ignorance of dementia among family and friends, as well as the general population, may mean that others respond negatively.

Many report, in addition, a necessity to make new friends, commonly from the dementia community, as they begin to lose friends and connections in their previous walks of life.

The need to create inclusive local communities

Older people are fellow citizens who should be able to participate in local communities and benefit from universal services to the same extent as other age groups.

Scrutinising local mainstream and universal services in a way non-prejudicial to a particular section of the population may be a beneficial approach generally – as for younger people, families with children, wheelchair users and other disabled groups (Audit Commission, 2008).

Older people should be valued members of society, and thus should have a stake in how universal services, such as transport, parks and gardens, refuse collection and leisure services, are planned and organised.

Finally, through better use of space and the increased use of technology, more older people are able to participate more fully in society. The *Guardian* featured in its reporting the impact of ageing on city life in the future, signalling the growth of environmental gerontology (Mitchell, 2012).

WHY INVOLVE INDIVIDUALS WITH DEMENTIA IN THE DESIGN OF 'DEMENTIA-FRIENDLY COMMUNITIES'?

The Local Government Association and Innovations in Dementia have explained why it is so essential to listen to the views of those individuals with dementia.

The idea of making our communities better places to live for people with dementia is something which engages the enthusiasm and interest of all sorts of people. Traders, leisure companies, transport providers, planners, service providers, health and social care organisations, charities are all potentially affected; all have a role to play in forming a vision about what a dementia-friendly community should look like.

The most important stakeholders in this process of course are people with dementia, and those who care for and support them.

'Nothing about us without us' is a slogan which carries great resonance for disability rights campaigners – and is one which is increasingly being articulated by people with dementia as well. The voices of people with dementia and their carers should be at the start and the heart of the process of creating dementia-friendly communities.

WHAT DO INDIVIDUALS WITH DEMENTIA APPEAR TO WANT FROM 'DEMENTIA-FRIENDLY COMMUNITIES'?

The Local Government Association and Innovations in Dementia have explained that it is important to listen to the expectations of individuals with dementia in formulating a policy on dementia-friendly communities.

Their findings are shown here (Local Government Association, and Innovations in Dementia, 2012).

People told us about the things which make a difference in a dementia-capable community:
- the physical environment;
- local facilities;
- support services;
- social networks;
- local groups.

People told us that they kept in touch with their local communities:
- through local groups;
- through the use of local facilities;
- through walking;
- through the use of support services.

People told us they had stopped doing some things in their community because:
- their dementia had progressed and they were worried about their ability to cope
- they were concerned that people didn't understand or know about dementia.

People told us that they would like to be able to:
- pursue hobbies and interests;

- simply go out more;
- make more use of local facilities;
- help others in their community by volunteering.

People told us that one-to-one informal support was the key to helping them do these things. People told us that a community could become more 'dementia-capable' by:
- increasing its awareness of dementia;
- supporting local groups for people with dementia and carers;
- providing more information, and more accessible information about local services and facilities;
- thinking about how local mainstream services and facilities can be made more accessible for people with dementia.

It is indeed very inspiring that individuals with dementia are beginning to emerge in being local 'dementia champions'.

THE FOUR CORNERSTONES MODEL

Crampton, Dean, and Eley (and the Joseph Rowntree Foundation) (2012) in a report on building a dementia-friendly community in York present an elegant 'four cornerstones' model (*see* **Figure 17.1**). This seminal paper summarised a year-long project in York investigating what it would take to make the City of York a good place to live for people with dementia and their carers. The authors concluded that the city is responding positively in many ways to the needs of people with dementia, but there is still much to do to make sure that people can live well with dementia.

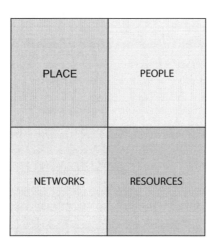

FIGURE 17.1 The 'Four Cornerstones' model (source: Crampton, Dean and Eley, 2012)

Their analysis of previous and parallel work, supported by our findings in York, led us to propose a model for realising a dementia-friendly community. With the voices of people at the heart of the process, it is argued that communities need to consider four 'cornerstones' to test the extent of their dementia friendliness. These are:

1. *Place* – how do the physical environment, housing, neighbourhood and transport support people with dementia?
2. *People* – how do carers, families, friends, neighbours, health and social care professionals (especially GPs) and the wider community respond to and support people with dementia?
3. *Resources* – are there sufficient services and facilities for people with dementia and are these appropriate to their needs and supportive of their capabilities? How well can people use the ordinary resources of the community?
4. *Networks* – do those who support people with dementia communicate, collaborate and plan together sufficiently well to provide the best support and to use people's own 'assets' well?

THE 'SOCIO-ECONOMIC POSITION'

The **'socio-economic position'** (SEP) refers to the position of individuals in the hierarchy and is inherently unequal, shaping access to resources and every aspect of experience in the home, neighbourhood and workplace (Krieger, 2001a, 2001b; Graham, 2004; Regidor, 2006).

Different dimensions of SEP (education, income, occupation, prestige) may influence health through different pathways and so may be more or less relevant to different health outcomes. It is the extent to which SEP involves exposure to psychological (in addition to material) risks and buffers that is of special interest from a mental health perspective.

SEP structures individual and collective experiences of dominance, hierarchy, isolation, support and inclusion. Social position also influences constructs such as identity and social status, which have an impact on wellbeing, for example, through the effects of low self esteem, shame, disrespect and 'invidious com parison' (Rogers and Pilgrim, 2002; de Botton, 2004).

The work of Prof Amartya Sen, a previous Nobel Laureate and Master of Trinity College in Cambridge, and Chairperson of the Commonwealth Commission on Respect and Understanding has previously argued that shame and humiliation are key social dimensions of absolute poverty, and that the 'ability to go about without shame' is a basic capability or freedom (Sen, *cited in* Zavaleta Reyles, 2007).

The use of the term **'psychosocial'** is important because it highlights the psychological/emotional/ cognitive impact of social factors, the effects of which need to be distinguished from material factors. For example, unemployment that leads to loss of income is not psychosocial, whereas the loss of self-esteem that accompanies unemployment is (Martikainen, Bartley and Lahelma, 2002).

Individual psychological resources, for example, confidence, self-efficacy, optimism and connectedness, all appear embedded within social structures: our position in relation to others at work, at home, and in public spaces. Because social position influences emotion, cognition and behaviour, it is an ongoing challenge to separate out contextual effects (Singh-Manoux and Marmot, 2005). Context was first introduced in **Chapter 9**.

AN EXAMPLE OF MAKING A COMMUNITY 'DEMENTIA FRIENDLY'

Hampshire County Council, Innovations in Dementia and the Local Government Association (2012) provide a very good example of steps through which a community can be made more 'dementia friendly'. They cite that memory problems make life difficult, and suggest the following:

- people who understand about memory problems – this can be people in shops, bus drivers, friends and family or anyone you come into contact with
- clear signposting, so people know where they are going and where things are
- clearly-written information on things like bus timetables or leaflets about services
- being able to spend time with other people in a similar situation
- having someone to go with.

THE BENEFITS OF 'RESILIENT COMMUNITIES'

A wide range of research demonstrates the health significance of social relationships and both formal and informal social systems as mediators of psychosocial stress resulting, for example, from inequality or economic transition. The relationship is not always clear-cut (De Silva *et al.*, 2005, 2007). There are different forms of community cohesion with different effects, in low-income countries, for example, or for particular groups where strongly bonded communities may exclude minorities.

Nevertheless, **'resilient communities'** with high levels of social capital, indicated by norms of trust, reciprocity and participation, have advantages for the mental health of individuals, and these characteristics have also been seen as indicators of the mental health or wellbeing of a community (Morgan and Swann, 2004; Lehtinen *et al.*, 2005; McKenzie and Harpham 2006).

The mental health of communities can be both a risk factor (e.g. the concept of social recession) and a protective factor (e.g. the application of herd immunity to mental health) (Stewart-Brown, 1998). A feeling of **'hopelessness'**, which is considered to be a possible risk factor for parasuicidal or suicidal behaviour, is influenced by the neighbourhood culture.

For individuals, social participation and social support in particular, are associated with reduced risk of common mental health problems and better self-reported health. Social isolation is an important risk factor for both deteriorating mental health and suicide (Pevalin and Rose, 2003; Social Exclusion Unit, 2004). A key question is, perhaps, the extent to which social capital mediates the effects of material deprivation. Many studies have found that social support and social participation do not mediate these effects (Mohan *et al.*, 2004; Morgan and Swann, 2004). A recent ecological study of 23 high- and low-income countries found no significant association between trust and adult mortality, life expectancy and infant mortality. Rather, the results supported the importance of both absolute and relative income distribution (Lindstrom and Lindstrom, 2006).

This does not mean, however, that '**neighbourhood effects**' are insignificant. It is hypothesised that indicators of social fragmentation and conflict in communities, as well as high levels of neighbourhood problems, influence outcomes independently of socio-economic status (Agyemang *et al.*, 2007; Steptoe and Feldman, 2001). Mistrust and powerlessness amplify the effect of neighbourhood disorder, making where you live as important for health and wellbeing as personal circumstances (Krueger *et al.*, 2004).

Socially disorganised areas provide a dangerous mix: large numbers of potential offenders who have few opportunities other than crime, many potential victims, and few social organisations or individuals who are capable of protecting others from violence (Krueger *et al.*, 2004). '**Area level effects**' may be particularly significant for some causes of mortality: in Scotland, for example, increases in inequalities in mortality are driven by increases in death rates at a young age in areas of high deprivation (e.g. for liver disease, suicide and assault and mental and behavioural disorders due to drugs) (Leyland, 2007).

It may be that negative symptoms of low morale and psychosocial vulnerability in communities, including anxiety, paranoia, aggression, hostility, withdrawal and retreat, have a greater power than protective factors, or, as we saw in relation to resilient places, that material resources outweigh other factors.

SOME EXAMPLES OF DEMENTIA-FRIENDLY COMMUNITIES
Financial institutions
Financial institutions are working together to create a 'dementia-friendly protocol'. This is something that any financial institution can implement so it can provide better support to customers with dementia and make it easier for them and their carers to be in control of their finances.

Schools
Twenty-one schools (at the time of writing) have formed a 'Pioneer Group' to develop dementia awareness sessions for children and young people across

England. The aim is that the sessions will educate children and young people about dementia, remove stigma and provide the opportunity for interaction with people with dementia. There has been talk of a new '**dementia-friendly generation**' emerging.

A very useful guide to current initiatives in English policy is to be found on the Department of Health's 'Dementia Challenge' page entitled 'Dementia friendly communities: what has been achieved so far' (dated 8 November 2012).

Emergency services

The Fire and Rescue Service have indicated that half of people who die in accidental house fires are over 65 years old. Two-thirds of people who have dementia live in the community. Recognising this, the Fire and Rescue Service have made a 'Pledge on dementia'. The pledge commits Fire and Rescue services to take action to increase the safety of people with dementia, and increase awareness among their staff.

Energy providers

People with dementia can have problems keeping their houses energy efficient and warm, as well as remembering to submit meter readings for utility usage and contacting their utility suppliers if they have a problem.

Leisure

It is hoped that various museums and galleries will commit to becoming age friendly or dementia friendly, if they have not already done so.

The importance of leisure activities was first introduced in **Chapter 7**.

Transport

A travel support card has been launched in a city, aimed to make travel easier for people with hidden disabilities. This is intended to be particularly useful for those with communication, learning or cognitive disabilities, who may find it difficult speaking with staff or asking for assistance.

Retail

When shopping in unfamiliar areas or larger supermarkets, some individuals with dementia said they sometimes lacked confidence or felt pressurised. This is because staff are unlikely to be aware that such individuals have dementia, and that they may need more time or help with certain cognitive functions.

WEBSITES

- Dementia Action Alliance, National Dementia Declaration: www.dementiaaction. uk/nationaldementiadeclaration

- Dementia Friendly Communities: http://dementiachallenge.dh.gov.uk/category/areas-for-action/communities/
- Dementia Services Development Centre, University of Stirling: www.dementia.stir.ac.uk
- Department of Health: The Dementia Challenge: dementiachallenge.dh.gov.uk
- **Disability Discrimination Act** 2005: www.legislation.gov.uk/ukpga/1995/50/contents
- **Equality Act** 2010: www.legislation.gov.uk/ukpga/2010/15/contents
- Joseph Rowntree Foundation, Dementia Without Walls: www.jrf.org.uk/work/workarea/dementia-without-walls
- RSA – Connected Communities: www.thersa.org/action-research-centre/public-services-arts-social-change/connected-communities
- WHO Global Network of Age-Friendly Cities and Communities: www.who.int/ageing/age_friendly_cities_network/en/

REFERENCES

Agyemang, C., van Hooijdonk, C., Wendel-Vos, W., *et al.* (2007) The association of neighbourhood psychosocial stressors and self-rated health in Amsterdam, the Netherlands, *J Epidemiol Community Health*, **61**(12), pp. 1042–9.

Audit Commission (2008) *Don't Stop Me Now: Preparing for an Ageing Population.* London: Audit Commission, available at: www.cpa.org.uk/cpa/Dont_Stop_Me_Now.pdf

Ayres, S. (2013) *Can Online Innovations Enhance Social Care?* Oxford: Nominet Trust, available at: www.nominettrust.org.uk/sites/default/files/Enhancing%20social%20care_PP_0113.pdf

Ayres, S. (2013) *Click Guide to Digital Technology in Adult Social Care [Epub]*, available at: www.lulu.com/shop/shirley-ayres/click-guide-to-digital-technology-in-adult-social-care/ebook/product-20730904.html;jsessionid=F772B09C305EF528BE72FFA61ED53371

Crampton, J., Dean, J., and Eley, R. (2012) *Creating a Dementia-Friendly York.* York: Joseph Rowntree Foundation, available at: www.jrf.org.uk/sites/files/jrf/dementia-communities-york-full.pdf

De Botton, A. (2004) *Status Anxiety.* London: Hamilton.

De Silva, M.J., Huttly, S.R., Harpham, T., *et al.* (2007) Social capital and mental health: a comparative analysis of four low income countries, *Soc Sci Med*, **64**(1), pp. 5–20.

De Silva, M.J., McKenzie, K., Harpham, T., *et al.* (2005) Social capital and mental illness: a systematic review, *J Epidemiol Community Health*, **59**(8), pp. 619–27.

Dementia Action Alliance (2013) *National Dementia Declaration.* London: DAA, available at: www.dementiaaction.org.uk/nationaldementiadeclaration

Department of Health (2009) *Living Well with Dementia: A National Dementia Strategy; Putting people first (Accessible summary).* London: The Stationery Office, available at: www.gov.uk/government/uploads/system/uploads/attachment_data/file/168221/dh_094052.pdf

Department of Health (2012) *Dementia Friendly Communities: What Has Been Achieved so Far*, available at: http://dementiachallenge.dh.gov.uk/2012/11/08/dfcachievements/

Department of Health (2013) *Improving Care for People with Dementia.* London: The

Stationery Office, available at: www.gov.uk/government/policies/improving-care-for-people-with-dementia

Friedli, L.; National Institute for Mental Health in England, Child Poverty Action Group, Faculty of Public Health and Mental Health Foundation (2009) *Mental Health, Resilience and Inequalities*. Cophenhagen: World Health Organization Regional Office for Europe, available at: www.euro.who.int/__data/assets/pdf_file/0012/100821/E92227.pdf

Graham, H. (2004) Social determinants and their unequal distribution: clarifying policy understandings, *Millbank Q*, **82**(1), pp. 101–24.

Hampshire County Council, Innovations in Dementia, and Local Government Association (2012) *Making Hampshire a Dementia-Friendly County: Finding Out What a Dementia Friendly Community Means to People with Dementia and Carers*, available at: www.innovationsindementia.org.uk/DementiaFriendlyCommunities/Dementia FriendlyCommunities_engagement.pdf

Kitwood, T. (1997) *Dementia Reconsidered: The Person Comes First*. Maidenhead: McGraw-Hill (Open University Press).

Krieger, N. (2001a) A glossary for social epidemiology, *J Epidemiol Community Health*, **55**(10), pp. 693–700.

Krieger, N. (2001b) Theories for social epidemiology in the 21st century: an ecosocial perspective, *Int J Epidemiol*, **30**(4), pp. 668–77.

Krueger, P.M., Bond Huie, S.A., Rogers, R.G., *et al.* (2004) Neighbourhoods and homicide mortality: an analysis of race/ethnic differences, *J Epidemiol Community Health*, **58**(3), pp. 223–30.

Lehtinen, V., Sohlman, B., and Kovess-Masfety, V. (2005) Level of positive mental health in the European Union: results from the Eurobarometer 2002 survey, *Clin Pract Epidemiol Ment Health*, **1**, p. 9.

Leyland A.H., Dundas R., McLoone P. *et al.* (2007) Cause-specific inequalities in mortality in Scotland: two decades of change. A population-based study, *BMC Public Health*, **7**, p. 172.

Lindstrom, C., and Lindstrom, M. (2006) Social capital, GNP per capita, relative income and health: an ecological study of 23 countries, *Int J Health Serv*, **36**(4), pp. 679–96.

Local Government Association, and Innovations in Dementia (2012) *Developing Dementia-Friendly Communities: Learning and Guidance for Local Authorities*. London: Local Government Association, available at: www.local.gov.uk/c/document_library/ get_file?uuid=b6401bb0-31a8-4d57-823b-1fde6a09290e&groupId=10180?

Martikainen, P., Bartley, M., and Lahelma, E. (2002) Psychosocial determinants of health in social epidemiology, *Int J Epidemiol*, **31**(6), pp. 1091–3.

McKenzie, K., and Harpham, T. (2006) *Social Capital and Mental Health*. London: Jessica Kingsley.

Mitchell, L. (2012) *Outdoor Design has an Impact on the Quality of Life of Older People*, the *Guardian*, available at: www.theguardian.com/sustainable-business/older-people-ageing-population-supportive-neighbourhood-planning

Mohan, J., Barnard, S., Jones, K., *et al.* (2004) Social capital, geography and health: developing and applying small-area indicators of social capital in the geography of health inequalities. In: Morgan, A., and Swann, C. (eds) *Social Capital for Health: Issues of Definition, Measurement and Links to Health*. London: Health Development Agency, pp. 83–109, available at: www.nice.org.uk/niceMedia/documents/socialcapital_issues.pdf

Morgan, A., and Swann, C. (eds) (2004) *Social Capital for Health: Issues of Definition, Measurement and Links to Health*. London: Health Development Agency.

Pevalin, D.J., and Rose, D. (2003) *Social Capital for Health: Investigating the Links between Social Capital and Health using the British Household Panel Survey*. Wivenhoe: Institute for Social and Economic Research, University of Essex, available at: www.nice.org.uk/nicemedia/documents/socialcapital_BHP_survey.pdf

Regidor, E. (2006) Social determinants of health: a veil that hides socioeconomic position and its relation with health, *J Epidemiol Health*, **60**(10), pp. 896–901.

Rogers, A., and Pilgrim, D. (2002) *Inequalities and Mental Health*. London: Palgrave Macmillan.

Singh-Manoux, A., and Marmot, M. (2005) Role of socialization in explaining social inequalities in health, *Soc Sci Med*, **60**(9), pp. 2129–33.

Social Exclusion Unit (2004) *Mental Health and Social Exclusion: Social Exclusion Unit Report*. London: Office of the Deputy Prime Minister, available at: www.nmhdu.org.uk/silo/files/social-exclusion-unit-odpm-2004-social-exclusion-and-mental-health.pdf

Steptoe, A., and Feldman, P.J. (2001) Neighborhood problems as sources of chronic stress: development of a measure of neighborhood problems, and associations with socioeconomic status and health, *Ann Behav Med*, **23**(3), pp. 177–85.

Stewart-Brown, S. (1998) Public health implications of childhood behaviour problems and parenting programmes. In: Buchanan A, Hudson BL (eds) *Parenting, Schooling and Children's Behaviour: Interdisciplinary Approaches*. Aldershot, Ashgate Publishing.

UK Government (2010) *Equality Act*, available at www.legislation.gov.uk/ukpga/2010/15/contents

Zaveleta Reyles, D. (2007) *The Ability to Go About Without Shame: A Proposal for Internationally Comparable Indicators of Shame and Humiliation*. OPHI Working Paper No. 03. Oxford: Oxford Poverty and Human Development Initiative, University of Oxford, available at: www.ophi.org.uk/wp-content/uploads/OPHI-wp03.pdf

CHAPTER 18

Conclusion

This is the final chapter of my journey into living well with dementia, but for English health policy this really is only the beginning. Modern management of the patient in the UK has a tendency to see the person experiencing medical care in the NHS as a series of *'problems'*. However, modern English policy has made a real effort to see the person in a positive light, and as an individual. This, however, presents a formidable obligation for all those who meet an individual with dementia to get to know him or her properly, and to make an effort to understand that individual even in the absence of obvious physical illness. Whether it is by chance or by design, in recent years, the Social Care Institute for Excellence has advocated an approach based on personalisation, and, for people who come into contact with social care services, aspires for people with dementia to be empowered with real choice and control wherever possible. This could become significant as all political parties consider the value of integrated services in healthcare in the English jurisdiction.

A pervasive theme in this book has been to address all issues with an open mind. Like any faith, it is impossible perhaps to have evidence in enormous detail for you to make personal decisions appropriate for you. Had the decision of 'hip replacement' *versus* 'no hip replacement' been subject to double-blind, randomised control trial, the benefits and outcomes of such a surgical intervention might not have been realised so fast. To be honest, the amount of peer-reviewed trials, pertaining to design of the home or assistive technologies, may be criticised for still being relatively small in number. However, it has become clear that there have been some blatant untruths in the narrative now emerging – for example, newspaper headlines touting a 'cure for dementia', with potential conflicts of interest in the business plans of biotech companies not clearly stated, or a minority of non-clinical policy leaders exaggerating the efficacy of current medications for dementia.

Phrases such as 'there now exist treatments that slow down the rate of progression in dementia in many patients' have been used with little attention to the precise clinical evidence base. What type of dementia? What treatment?

How many individuals with dementia need to be treated to observe any effect? Such questions and answers need to be asked properly by experts in the field, while simultaneously listening intently to the beliefs, concerns and expectations of patients. An inadvertent lack of attention to clinical evidence has led to a number of 'opinions' unfortunately creating considerable noise to the serious academic and professional debate. Many subtle influences seem to be at play, and so it can be difficult sometimes to work out where the English dementia policy has come from.

In the recent report *The Prime Minister's Challenge on Dementia: Delivering Major Improvements in Dementia Care and Research by 2015: A report on progress* (Dementia Challenge Champion Groups, 2013), the following is noted. People who donate to 'research', an aspiration of the Prime Minister's Challenge on Dementia, should have a realistic opinion of what is feasible in such research:

> Significant research continues across all stages of the disease, but this year has brought forward some potentially interesting developments in treating early stage dementia in Alzheimer's disease in particular.
>
> Global trials of the Solanezumab drug by Lilly failed to show benefit for all dementia suffers, but appeared to show some improvements in those with mild dementia, suggesting treatments could be developed to help slow or prevent the disorder if caught early enough.
>
> Whilst the Janssen studies of the Bapineuzumab drug did not show any clear clinical benefits for patients, the drugs did appear to affect the underlying biology of the disease by halting growth in harmful amyloid protein deposits, providing insights to support development of future treatments. Further phase III trials will report in April 2013.

With a finite 'pot' of resources, it is therefore vital that allocation of resources is put into ethical research. I have indeed described a huge range of valid approaches for improving living well with dementia, which do *not* involve any neuropharmacological intervention. Indeed, it is worth noting that Emanuel, Wendler and Crady (2011) begin their consideration of 'What makes clinical research ethical?' with a description that, 'To be ethical, clinical research must be valuable, meaning that it evaluates a diagnostic or therapeutic intervention that could lead to improvements in health or well-being.' Indeed, that would be entirely in keeping with the approach taken in all responsible decision-making in the current policies for dementia in England. The issue of responsible use of information for use by patients, carers and immediates has become massively important, given the deluge of information that is currently available.

More information does not necessarily mean better information, as any Google search will reveal at an instant. Likewise, an earlier diagnosis is not necessarily a better diagnosis, and here the nature of language is vital. To be responsible, it is vital that all policymakers, including politicians, use language with precision. As I mentioned in the introduction to this book, a timely diagnosis is only useful if there can be a useful intervention. It is also abundantly clear that this diagnosis should be correct, as far as possible, and training for all healthcare professionals is vital in this regard.

Critically, it would be extremely unhelpful to say that dementia is the diagnosis in all individuals with memory problems. The diagnosis of the behavioural variant frontotemporal dementia (bvFTD) syndrome remains challenging; while some patients are dismissed as 'normal', others may be misdiagnosed as suffering from psychiatric disorders, because of the presence of complex symptoms such as disinhibition, apathy, impulsivity or overeating. For example, Rascovsky and colleagues (Rascovsky *et al.*, 2011) described the complexity of making the clinical diagnosis of bvFTD, a common diagnosis in the presenium. In fact, the authors of this highly influential paper, arguing for revised diagnostic criteria for bvFTD, argue that, 'Preservation of episodic memory relative to executive dysfunction, can be valuable in differential diagnosis, particularly when the distinction involves bvFTD and Alzheimer's disease'.

One of the worst things that could happen in the drive of English health policy to look for an *'early diagnosis'* is that patients make plans on the basis of an incorrect diagnosis of dementia ('non-maleficence', *see* **Chapter 14** for a discussion of 'ethical principles'). There is a policy drive to look for 'innovative ways of diagnosing dementia early', but even medical students are warned about other conditions that may mimick dementia, particularly in elderly populations. If you were to ask a group of clinical medical students how many of them are worried about their memory just before their finals, you can expect a high proportion of them to be concerned. There are important medical conditions to be considered here. For example, Cordes, Cano and Haupt (2000), in German, report that hypothyroidism remains one of the most important causes of potentially reversible dementia. Their reported case demonstrates a relatively rapid remission of cognitive and noncognitive symptoms within a period of a few months. The authors provide that, for separating dementia in hypothyroidism from dementia with hypothyroidism, cross-sectional and longitudinal assessment of the clinical features is crucial. Furthermore, at around 50 years since Leslie Kiloh's paper titled *Pseudo-dementia* was published (and this term is still debated fiercely), it is still recognised that depression in the elderly can present in a way that can resemble dementia (Snowdon, 2011).

It can be all too easy to get carried away with an innovation 'bandwagon', but it is easy to forget that originally parchment was a disruptive innovation, and that pen-and-paper tests could yet hold the key to a successful timely diagnosis of certain forms of dementia including the dementia of Alzheimer type.

Even if you appreciate that not all dementia is Alzheimer's disease, tests for an early diagnosis inevitably have to be used responsibly and with caution. As described in **Chapter 5** of this book, which included a discussion on the pitfalls of introducing 'screening' into this debate concerning dementia in English policy, the sensitivity and specificity of any test used to try to uncover potential cases of dementia is pivotal. Deficits in a presentation of the **paired associates learning** task have been discovered in other groups (e.g. female inpatients with anorexia nervosa (Fowler *et al.*, 2006) , first episode psychosis, major depressive order (Barnett *et al.*, 2005) and geriatric depression (Beats, Sahakian and Levy, 1996)). Indeed, it is widely recognised that the initial locus of neuropathology in Alzheimer's disease is thought to be the hippocampus (and this is a very consistent finding in the literature) (review, Braak, Braak and Bohl, 1983). Neuroimaging of this task has provided an important rôle of frontoparietal networks in successful performance of this task (Gould *et al.*, 2005). However, that the task may be one probing attentional and spatial cognition, as much as memory is an interesting observation potentially in itself, and consistent with the literature concerning what frontoparietal networks might do in cognition (see, for example, a recent article by Jerde and Curtis, 2013). It is crucial that, amidst the policy momentum of 'QOF' in NHS England for dementia, that the precise evidence base is correctly analysed by people with skills in this niche area.

Attentional deficits may have been thus far relatively underestimated in the presenting features of Alzheimer's disease, but they may actually be entirely consistent with the 'cholinergic hypothesis of geriatric cognitive dysfunction' (reviewed by Robbins *et al.*, 1997). Notwithstanding that complicated cognitive neurology discussion, 'losing your memory' may not be the only presenting feature of dementia. Certainly, there is growing appreciation that not only is a diagnosis of dementia useful, when correct, but also it is very helpful to have the correct diagnosis of dementia (given also that some types of dementia are genuinely reversible) (Gershon and Herman, 1982). For example, in a helpful review by Mosimann and McKeith (2003), the authors review that neuroleptic medication can be relatively contraindicated in patients with dementia with Lewy bodies; this is because these individuals can show severe neuroleptic sensitivity, which is associated with increased morbidity and mortality.

So, one potent message already emerges from the briefest discussion of how English dementia policy has evolved. This is very much one of *primum non nocere* – first, do no harm. You can easily anticipate the 'knock-on effects' of dementia policy that is poorly formulated. A simple observation that many cases of mild cognitive impairment do not in fact progress to dementia within 10 years might lead to individuals incorrectly labelled as having 'preclinical dementia' (Mitchell and Shiri-Feshki, 2009). There is a 'growth industry' from rent-seeking businesses wishing to profit out of the initial dementia diagnosis. Non-maleficence is, however, of course one of the central pillars of medical ethics (Page, 2012; Beauchamp and Childress, 2001). The problem of the 'timely diagnosis' is slowly being considered in different jurisdictions, each with their own legal rules. For example, any national policy to consider whether a person with dementia is allowed to drive will consider the importance of the independence of the individual compared with the personal safety of that individual with dementia. All too often governments might be concerned about other factors, such as lost revenue from tax, petrol sales or insurance from banning people with dementia from driving. Further, GPs have warned about patients not wishing to approach their physicians about receiving a possible diagnosis of dementia, in case this diagnosis has an adverse effect on personal insurance premium(s). A 'timely' diagnosis of dementia could one day lead to a 'timely' loss of a driving licence for that individual, and we are all aware how catastrophic chain reactions can occur.

RESILIENCE

In Professor Felicia Huppert's latest chapter, entitled, 'The state of well-being science: concepts, measures, interventions and policies', to appear in *Interventions and Policies to Enhance Well-being* (Huppert, F.A., and Cooper, C.L., eds, 2014), Professor Huppert re-establishes the perspective that it is possible to demonstrate wellbeing *even* in the presence of a label of a clinical diagnosis. This aligns itself nicely with the thesis that I have been advanced here, that it is possible to enhance the wellbeing of an individual with dementia through careful consideration of his or her environment. For example, one could attempt to make the home or ward better designed, attempt to involve the individual with leisure activities or general activities (such as reminiscence therapy), seek to encourage adoption of assistive technologies or assisted-living technologies, or try to encourage more social activities including participation in a wider community. However, Huppert and So (2013), to establish what components compose wellbeing, have examined carefully the internationally agreed criteria for the common mental disorders (as defined in the Diagnostic and Statistical Manual of Mental Disorders, Fourth Edition, and the International Statistical Classification of Diseases and Related Health Problems, 10th Revision) and for each symptom, listed the opposite characteristic. This resulted in a list of 10 features that represent positive mental health or '**flourishing**'. These are (1) competence, (2) emotional stability, (3) engagement, (4) meaning, (5) optimism, (6) positive emotion, (7) positive relationships, (8) resilience, (9) self-esteem and (10) vitality.

Just as symptoms of mental illness are combined in specific ways to provide an operational definition of each of the common mental disorders, they proposed that positive features could be combined in a specific way to provide an operational definition of flourishing. The diagnostic criteria for a mental disorder do not require that all the symptoms be present; likewise, the operational definitions of flourishing (as, for example, established in Keyes, 2002) do not require that all the features of positive feeling and functioning need to be present. There is currently a relative paucity of literature on the efficacy of psychological techniques such as 'mindfulness' in enhancing wellbeing in individuals with dementia, but it is possible that novel ways of improving any aspects of the multidimensional construct could be developed through such a technique. The following are among the reported benefits of mindfulness training in other populations, which are related to subjective wellbeing, reductions in stress and anxiety, increased positive mood, improved sleep quality, better emotion regulations, greater bodily awareness and increased vitality, and greater empathy (Huppert, 2014).

Clearly, ignoring the economic climate of an individual with dementia is not going to be possible, although I have thus far successfully managed to avoid such a discussion. The data reported in Huppert and So (2013) are from 2006/07, 2 years before the severe economic recession from which many countries have since suffered. Relatively recent data from the Gallup World Poll show almost no impact of the economics crisis on subjective wellbeing in the UK (Crabtree, 2010). However, one clearly has to acknowledge the 'social determinants of health', famously described by Marmot (2012) thus: *'Mental health and mental illness are profoundly affected by the social determinants of health; psychosocial processes are important pathways by which the social environment … impact[s] on … physical and mental health'.* Indeed, McKee and colleagues (McKee *et al.*, 2012) make a constructive but profoundly depressing link between illbeing and austerity:

> For many months, the political and financial aspects of the crisis have filled the headlines. However, behind those headlines, there are many individual human stories that remain untold. They include people with chronic diseases unable to access lifesustaining medicines, persons with rare diseases who are losing income support and forced to care for themselves, and those whose hopes of a better life in the future have been dashed see no alternative but to commit suicide. So far, the discussion has been limited to finance ministers and their counterparts in the international financial institutions. Health ministers have failed to get a seat at the table. As a consequence, the impact on the health and wellbeing of ordinary people was barely considered until they made their feelings clear at the ballot box.

More optimistically, Huppert and So (2013) argue that this parcellation of the positive wellbeing multidimensional construct may be useful for developing targeted interventions:

Psychosocial resilience is a dimension of wellbeing that perhaps will be worth considering in detail, of how an individual and immediates might be able to cope and adapt to future adversity. Given that there might be aspects of life that encourage illbeing, a reasonable strategy might be to strengthen components that can help to improve specific aspects of wellbeing. This would not have been possible had it not been for the work of Professor Felicia Huppert and colleagues emphasising that wellbeing is a multidimensional construct, in the same way that it is widely acknowledged that it is unhelpful to think of dementia as a unitary diagnosis. Therefore, logically, the entire construct of 'living well in dementia' is entirely multidimensional.

The Department of Health (2012) policy document *No Health without Mental Health: Implementation Framework* very nicely produces the contemporaneous backdrop for emphasising the importance of wellbeing in dementia. Their core principles set out 'a clear and compelling vision, centred around six objectives: more people will have good mental health, more people with mental health problems will recover, more people with mental health problems will have good physical health, more people will have a positive experience of care and support, fewer people will suffer avoidable harm, and fewer people will experience stigma and discrimination'.

Notwithstanding this, it appears that the analysis of 'living well in dementia' is now benefiting from an approach that has led to an appreciation that no dementia is clinically the same; nobody's wellbeing is exactly the same, because of the way in which all the contributing parts have come together. This approach is elegant, and it holds incredible promise for the future.

English health policy, rightly, has started identify those who might be particularly vulnerable in coming into contact with health and social care services, and to consider how they might be best supported in the community rather than in a hospital instead. Similar parallels can be drawn with the notion of 'frailty', which is actually very hard to define. As Strandberg, Pitkälä and Tilvis (2011) helpfully observed, in later and end-stage frailty, prevention gives way to palliation, and treatments follow the principles of adequate geriatric care. As with end-stage dementia, it is generally perceived that burdensome interventions should be avoided, and that a reasonable primary goal is to ensure good quality of life and appropriate multidisciplinary care while meeting complex medical, psychological and social needs (not only those of the patient but also those of caregivers).

THE IMPORTANCE OF OTHER DISCIPLINES

Through my own diverse academic journey, I have latterly been struck by the influence that the English law has in influencing policy, especially the **Equality Act** 2010 and **Mental Capacity Act** 2005, and how that 'dismal science' (economics) has shaped our policy. Different stakeholders can have different interests in the conclusions of this discussion (as discussed by Brunet, 2012), but it has genuinely struck me how some subtle interventions could make a massive intervention in dementia for very little cost. If the diagnosis of dementia is correct, and an individual with dementia and his or her immediates is given full support, there is much value to be shared in communities and living independently, if the appropriate resources are put in place. Of course a massive challenge for that individual is to know what resources are available and where, and I hope that this book has been a useful first step in that direction.

CLOSING REMARKS

In summary, dementia then is not a unitary phenomenon, and nor is well-being. That is why writing a book on wellbeing in dementia is an impossible task. Wellbeing fundamentally depends on the 'make-up' of any individual as a person, and how he or she interacts with the local environment. Because of this remarkable complexity, it is hard to articulate few helpful generalisations. For example, this book has emphasised that 'context' is all-important, whether this is for the social cognition of an individual (**Chapter 9**), or the communication of that individual with other people (**Chapter 12**). 'Independence' has also been a very important pervasive theme, bridging a number of chapters in this book including measurement of wellbeing, adaptations, design of the home and ward, ambient assisted living, and advocacy, for example.

I sincerely hope, however, that you have enjoyed thinking about the numerous issues raised in the book, but also that you have a real feel for the very exciting time we are experiencing in dementia care in English health policy, currently. I hope you enjoy the rest of the policy journey. It is built on solid foundations, but it will be a bit of a 'roller-coaster ride' as well.

Shibley Rahman
London
October 2013

REFERENCES

Barnett, J.H., Sahakian, B.J., Werners, U., *et al.* (2005) Visuospatial learning and executive function are independently impaired in first-episode psychosis, *Psychol Med*, 35(7), pp. 1031–41.

Beats, B.C., Sahakian, B.J., and Levy, R. (1996) Cognitive performance in tests sensitive to frontal lobe dysfunction in the elderly depressed, *Psychol Med*, 26(3), pp. 591–603.

Beauchamp, T.L., and Childress, J.F (2001) *Principles of Medical Ethics*. Fifth edition. New York, NY: Oxford University Press.

Braak, H., Braak, E., and Bohl, J. (1993) Staging of Alzheimer-related cortical destruction, *Eur Neurol*, 33(6), pp. 403–8.

Brunet, M. (2012) *Early Diagnosis of Dementia – Cui Bono?* available at: http://binscombe.net/blog/?p=464

Cambridge Cognition website. *Paired Associates Learning (PAL)*, available at: www.camcog.com/paired-associates-learning.asp

Cordes, J., Cano, J., and Haupt, M. (2000) [Reversible dementia in hypothyroidism] [Article in German], *Nervenarzt*, 71(7), pp. 588–90.

Crabtree, S. (2010) Britons' wellbeing stable through economic crisis, *Gallup*, November 24, available at: www.gallup.com/poll/144938/Britons-W%20ellbeing-Stable-Economic-Crisis.aspx

Dementia Challenge Champion Groups (2013) *The Prime Minister's Challenge on Dementia: Delivering Major Improvements in Dementia Care and Research by 2015: a report on progress*, London: Department of Health, available at: http://media.dh.gov.uk/network/353/files/2012/11/The-Prime-Ministers-Challenge-on-Dementia-Delivering-major-improvements-in-dementia-care-and-research-by-2015-A-report-of-progress.pdf

Department of Health (2009) *Living Well with Dementia: A National Dementia Strategy; Putting people first.* London: The Stationery Office, available at: https://www.gov.uk/government/uploads/system/uploads/attachment_data/file/168221/dh_094052.pdf

Department of Health (2012) *No Health without Mental Health: Implementation Framework*, available at: www.gov.uk/government/uploads/system/uploads/attachment_data/file/156084/No-Health-Without-Mental-Health-Implementation-Framework-Report-accessible-version.pdf.pdf

Department of Health (2013) *The Dementia Challenge*. London: The Stationery Office, available at: http://dementiachallenge.dh.gov.uk

Emanuel, E.J., Wendler, D., and Grady, C. (2011) What makes clinical research ethical? *JAMA*, **283**(20), pp. 2701–11.

Fowler, L., Blackwell, A., Jaffa, A., *et al.* (2006) Profile of neurocognitive impairments associated with female in-patients with anorexia nervosa, *Psychol Med*, **36**(4), pp. 517–27.

Gershon, S., and Herman, S.P. (1982) The differential diagnosis of dementia, *J Am Geriatr Soc*, **30**(11 Suppl.), pp. S58–66.

Gould, R.L., Brown, R.G., Owen, A.M., *et al.* (2005) Functional neuroanatomy of successful paired associate learning in Alzheimer's disease, *Am J Psychiatry*, **162**(11), pp. 2049–60.

Huppert, F. (2014) The state of well-being science: concepts, measures, interventions and policies. In: Huppert, F.A., and Cooper, C.L. (eds) *Interventions and Policies to Enhance Well-being*, vol. 6. Oxford: Wiley-Blackwell. pp. 1–49.

Huppert, F.A., and So, T.T.C. (2013) Flourishing across Europe: application of a new conceptual framework for defining well-being, *Soc Indic Res*, **110**(3), pp. 837–61.

Jerde, T.A., and Curtis, C.E. (2013) Maps of space in human frontoparietal cortex, *J Physiol Paris*, pii: S0928–4257(13)00016–8, Epub Apr 18.

Keyes, C.L.M. (2002) The mental health continuum: from languishing to flourishing in life, *J Health Soc Behav*, **43**(2), 207–22.

Marmot M. (2012) Health inequalities and mental life, *Adv Psychiat Treat*, **18**, pp. 320–22.

McKee, M., Karanikolos, M., Belcher, P., *et al.* (2012) Austerity: a failed experiment on the people of Europe. *Clin Med*, **12**(4), pp. 346–50, available at: www.rcplondon.ac.uk/sites/default/files/documents/clinmed-124-p346-350-mckee.pdf

Mitchell, A.J., Shiri-Feshki, M. (2009) Rate of progression of mild cognitive impairment to dementia-meta-analysis of 41 robust inception cohort studies, *Acta Psychiatr Scand*, **119**(4), pp. 252–65.

Mosimann, U.P., and McKeith, I.G. (2003) Dementia with Lewy bodies: diagnosis and treatment, *Swiss Med Wkly*, **133**(9–10), pp. 131–42.

Page, K. (2012) The four principles: can they be measured and do they predict ethical decision making? *BMC Med Ethics*, **13**, pp. 10.

Rascovsky, K., Hodges, J.R., Knopman, D., *et al.* (2011) Sensitivity of revised diagnostic criteria for the behavioural variant of frontotemporal dementia, *Brain*, **134**(Pt. 9), pp. 2456–77.

Robbins, T.W., McAlonan, G., Muir, J.L., *et al.* (1997) Cognitive enhancers in theory and practice: studies of the cholinergic hypothesis of cognitive deficits in Alzheimer's disease, *Behav Brain Res*, **83**(1–2), pp. 15–23.

Snowdon, J. (2011) Pseudodementia, a term for its time: the impact of Leslie Kiloh's 1961 paper, *Australas Psychiatry*, **19**(5), pp. 391–7.

Strandberg, T.E., Pitkälä, K.H., Tilvis, R.S. (2011) Hot topics in geriatric medicine: frailty in older people, *Eur Geriatr Med*, **2**(6), pp. 344–55.

Index

Page numbers in **bold** refer to figures, tables and boxes.

CPD with Radcliffe

You can now use a selection of our books to achieve CPD (Continuing Professional Development) points through directed reading.

We provide a free online form and downloadable certificate for your appraisal portfolio. Look for the CPD logo and register with us at: www.radcliffehealth.com/cpd

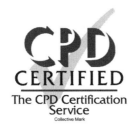

CERTIFIED
The CPD Certification
Service
Collective Mark